HUMAN HORIZONS SERIES

Parkinson's Disease

A Self-help Guide for Patients and Their Carers

Marjan Jahanshahi, BSc, MPhil (Clin Psychol) PhD
C. David Marsden, MRCPsych, DSc, FRS

With contributions from
Richard G. Brown, BA, MPhil (Clin Psychol), PhD
and
Brigid MacCarthy, BA, Dip Clin Psychol (BPS), MSc

A CONDOR BOOK
SOUVENIR PRESS (E&A) LTD

First published 1998 by
Souvenir Press (Educational & Academic) Ltd,
43 Great Russell Street, London WC1B 3PA

ISBN 0 285 63317 1

Typeset by Rowland Phototypesetting Ltd,
Bury St Edmunds, Suffolk

Printed in Great Britain by
The Guernsey Press Company Ltd,
Guernsey, Channel Islands

Contents

Tailpiece

Acknowledgements

We have spent many years treating people with Parkinson's disease and conducting research on the illness. During this period, many of those people have shared their experiences with us, and in so doing have been instrumental in teaching us what we know. Others have been generous with their time, participating in studies evaluating the impact of Parkinson's on daily living, or in more experimental tests. We see this book as a way of repaying our debt of gratitude. We will find it rewarding indeed if it goes some way towards making living and coping with Parkinson's disease easier for those who have the illness, their carers and their families.

We should also like to thank the following for permission to quote from copyright material: Macmillan Publishers Ltd. for *Ivan: Living with Parkinson's Disease* by Ivan Vaughan; Seven Locks Press for *Parkinson's Disease: A Patient's View* by Sidney Dorros; Windrush Press for *A Shadow Over My Brain* by Cecil Todes; Bellew Publishing for *The Spaces in Between* by John Harris; John Wiley & Sons, Inc. for *Living Well with Parkinson's Disease* by Glenna Wotton Atwood (with L. Green Hunnewell), Copyright © 1991 by Glenna Wotton Atwood, adapted by permission; the Parkinson's Disease Society of the United Kingdom for *An Old-age Pensioner at Eighteen* by Helen Rose, *Parkinson's Disease and Employment* ed. John Williams and *Parkinson's Disease: Doctors as Patients* ed. John Williams.

Marjan Jahanshahi
David Marsden
London 1998

Preface

Parkinson's disease is one of the most common neurological disorders. One person in every thousand of the population has it. Although young adults can develop the illness, it is usually a disorder of old age. In Western countries, increased life expectancy means that the proportion of elderly will also increase. Since the risk of developing Parkinson's increases with age, there will be more people with it.

What is Parkinson's disease?
What is the cause?
Is there a cure?
Can it be treated?
What other symptoms will I get?
How quickly will I deteriorate?
Can I carry on working?
Will it affect my mind?
Will I be confined to a wheelchair?
Is there anything I can do to alleviate my symptoms?
Will my children get Parkinson's disease?

These are some of the questions that will be asked by someone who has been diagnosed as having Parkinson's disease. In the limited time available for an initial consultation, most doctors can provide only minimal information about the nature of the disorder and its drug treatment. Some of these questions may not come to mind when the individual is first told that he or she has Parkinson's. It is usually after leaving the consulting room, and during the following days and weeks, that some of the questions will surface. The subsequent medical management of the illness mainly focuses on adjusting the level of medication to control the symptoms. The patient and his or her family are often left unaided, to anticipate and adapt to the long-term social implications.

The aim of our book is to fill this gap in patient–doctor communication, and to provide the individual and his or her family with the essential information about the nature of the illness, its diagnosis and medical treatment, its implication for their daily lives, and about how best to cope with the changes brought about by it.

A number of very informative books about the experience of living with Parkinson's disease have been written by people who have it, and there are some excellent books by health professionals providing information about the illness and its management. Our book differs from these publications in three main ways.

1   We provide much more detailed information about the symptoms of the disease, its possible causes, the process of diagnosis and its medical treatment. We have tried to collate in a single book all the information that people with Parkinson's disease and their carers may want access to. By its nature, much of this information is very technical, but we have assumed that our average intelligent reader will find it enlightening.

2   The symptoms of Parkinson's disease, the associated disability and progression, vary from person to person. We have tried to portray these varied experiences. The lives of the spouse or partner and of the family who live with and care for the person with Parkinson's, the carers as we call them, are also affected by the illness, and so we also consider their experiences and needs, which are often overlooked.

3   In addition to medical treatment, there are many other ways in which the Parkinson's patient and his or her carer can soften the impact of the illness on their lives. We describe a range of self-help strategies that can help people cope better with disability, and reduce its effects on their daily activities, mood and social relationships.

The book is organised into three main parts. The first, 'Parkinson's Disease: The Medical Facts', provides up-to-date medical information about the symptoms, what is known about the possible causes, the aims and procedures of different tests used in diagnosis, and treatment with medication or surgery. In this era of modern health care, the ill person is considered an active participant in his or her health care rather than a passive recipient of treatment. 'Patient education' – or providing the chronically ill person with information about his or her illness and its medical treatment – is considered to be beneficial in two main ways. First, it can alleviate the anxiety and anticipation experienced when an individual faces the unknown. By creating a sense of familiarity, information can generate a sense of choice and control. Second, it provides the individual with the opportunity of actively participating in his or her own health care. The person diagnosed with Parkinson's disease has to travel many novel and personally uncharted waters in the course of the illness. The general medical information provided in

Part I may serve as signposts to guide the patient and his or her family on this journey. Informed decisions are often more rational, and their consequences easier to live with, and we hope that the information provided in Part I will facilitate such informed decisions.

The onset and development of a progressive and disabling illness such as Parkinson's constitute a traumatic life crisis that can have a major impact on the pyschological well-being and social functioning of both the patient and his or her family. The knowledge that one's experiences are not unique, that they are shared by others in the same predicament, can be reassuring and take the edge off the threatening aspects. The experience of Parkinson's disease is shared by 120,000 people in the UK alone. As the great variability of symptoms across individuals would imply, there is no one form of the disorder. This, combined with the very individual way in which each person responds to stress and change, means that no standard experience of the illness exists either. Nevertheless, by portraying some of the common experiences of living with it, we aim to offer some assurance to those who have to experience it. Part II, 'Living with Parkinson's Disease', deals with the impact of chronic illness on the individual. His or her feelings and reactions to the illness are traced from the shock and anger experienced in the early acute phase, through the sense of loss and mourning, to the ensuing acceptance and adjustment that occur in the later, more chronic, stage. The effect of Parkinson's disease is considered in terms of the changes brought about in the various spheres of life, ranging from everyday activities, work and finance, to family, marital, sexual and social relationships. These psychosocial changes are considered from the perspective both of the ill person and of the carer. Although, as we noted, it is in the majority of cases a disorder of old age, it can develop before the age of forty. A minority, about 15–20 per cent of patients, become demented – that is, their memory and intellectual abilities become impaired. The special needs of the person with Parkinson's disease and dementia and of the 'young-onset' patient are considered in Chapters 7 and 8.

Faced with the challenge of a chronic illness such as Parkinson's, the individual has to overcome the effects of the symptoms on his or her mobility and health, and strive to preserve his or her identity, lifestyle and social relationships from the assault of the illness. Part III, 'Coping with Parkinson's Disease', focuses first on the various external sources of help. It describes a multitude of health professionals as well as outside agencies such as the Parkinson's Disease Society, and details precisely the kind of help that they can offer. Strategies that can be used by the patient for controlling the symptoms and reducing the associated disability are proposed in Chapter 10. In human terms, the main impact of the disease may be on the individual's identity. Self-help techniques are suggested to help him or her to come to terms with the reality of the illness, to optimise his or her coping with its effects, to prevent depression and anxiety and to maintain emotional well-being. The ultimate goal, of course, is to ensure that the individual possesses the necessary resources to meet the many challenges and to achieve the best quality of life possible within the confines of the illness. To ensure a good quality of life, the physical and psychological well-being of the carer is as important as that of the patient. Also considered in Part III are methods that can be used by the carer to minimise and cope with the stresses produced by the illness.

In the last part of the book, a history of the illness and of the research that has been carried out on it provides the background for a discussion of future horizons. The outstanding questions yet to be answered, and the directions for future research, are considered. The book ends with an Appendix containing an A–Z of useful organisations and a list of other publications that readers may find of interest.

As neither of us, nor our two co-authors, have Parkinson's disease, our writing about living and coping with the illness is undoubtedly second-hand, gained by treating, working with and talking to many patients and their relatives over many years. But by quoting from people with Parkinson's disease, and their relatives, we have been able to reflect first-hand experiences of what it is like to live with the illness. These quotations come from two sources: from patients we have known, treated or worked with ourselves, and from books by people who have the illness. When reproducing the words of people known to us, we have changed details such as names, professions and so on to protect their identity and to ensure confidentiality. When we have used quotations from books or other texts, we have of course, referred directly to the authors.

We hope that the particular order we have imposed on the information gathered here will be perceived as a logical way of conveying it. However, this does not mean that the book has necessarily to be read from page 1 to the end, chapter by chapter. We hope that most of our readers will have the interest and the time to do so, but for those who haven't, each chapter has been written to stand alone, without the need to read preceding or subsequent ones in order to understand the information. This also provides the reader with the option of referring to specific chapters as the need arises, or of refreshing his or her memory on any particular aspect.

We have deliberated over which terms to use when referring to the person who has Parkinson's disease and the person who is most involved in looking after him or her. We are aware of the inadequacies and the possible derogatory interpretations of the terms 'Parkinsonian', 'patient and 'sufferer'. When a person gets a cold or develops an infection he or she consults a doctor and while ill he or she is a 'patient', but once the illness is cured, the individual is no longer ill *or* a patient. There is a tendency to refer to people with progressive neurological illnesses such as Parkinson's disease who are not 'cured', as 'patients'. This is acceptable in the context of doctors, hospitals, drug regimes and so on, but is less appropriate in relation to the individual's everyday life at home and in society. Therefore, we have used 'patient' as little as possible. This book is addressed to *people who have Parkinson's disease*. To emphasise this focus on 'personhood', we have sometimes used the term 'the person with Parkinson's disease'. Unfortunately, this is too unwieldy to use very often. We hope that simply referring to him or her as 'the individual' or 'the person', which we frequently do, will be acceptable. The term 'sufferer' we have vetoed altogether – it has lost its original meaning and has negative connotations that are objectionable to those who cope well with the demands of illness.

With the term 'carer', there is less of a problem. It usually refers to the person most involved in looking after the 'patient'. The Carers' National Association defines the word to mean 'anyone whose life is in some way restricted because of the need to take responsibility for the care of a person who is mentally ill, mentally handicapped, physically disabled or whose health is impaired by sickness or old age'. Not all people who have Parkinson's have or need a carer – or at least, not in the early, milder, stages of the illness. So they may object to the idea of having a partner, spouse or other relative assigned as their 'carer'. Nevertheless, in our experience most people with Parkinson's disease need, at some stage in the course of their illness, a greater degree of care and looking after than the average person of their age. We therefore find 'carer' a useful summary term to refer to whoever is most involved in looking after the ill person.

It would be difficult indeed to find two people with identical symptoms of Parkinson's and consequently two people with very similar experiences of the illness. One might say that there are as many experiences of living with Parkinson's disease as there are people with the disorder. Although we use case examples to illustrate and clarify certain issues, inevitably much of the book is written in general terms that may not be easily applicable to any individual person. But we hope that everyone with Parkinson's disease and every carer who reads this book will find in it something of value.

*   *   *

We would like to thank all the individuals who have over the years shared with us their experiences of living and coping with Parkinson's disease. Our special thanks go to Paul Rayner and Colin Moat, who have been indispensable volunteers for our research studies, who read through the text and indicated places where we had been overzealous in our use of medical jargon. Last but not least, we would like to thank our two co-authors, Richard Brown and Brigid MacCarthy, for their significant contributions.

Marjan Jahanshahi and David Marsden
London, 1998

Note: All books referred to in the text are listed in the Appendix under 'Further Reading'; all organisations mentioned are listed in the 'A–Z of Useful Organisations'.

Part I

Parkinson's Disease: The Medical Facts

1

What Is Parkinson's Disease?

Parkinson's disease is a neurological illness, meaning a disease caused by a dysfunction of the brain or the spinal cord, the two main parts of the central nervous system, or of the peripheral nervous system and muscles. Tremor, slowness in starting and carrying out movements (bradykinesia), rigidity or muscle stiffness, and problems with balance and walking are the major symptoms. The disorder is named after James Parkinson, the British doctor who first described it in 1817 (the history of the discovery of Parkinson's disease and the research into its causes and treatment are outlined in Chapter 13). In this first chapter, our aim is to provide you with the basic medical information.

HOW COMMON IS IT, AND WHO GETS IT?

One person in every thousand develops Parkinson's disease. As it is commonly a disorder of old age, the risk of contracting it increases with age. Amongst those over 65, the incidence rises to 1 in 100. For those over the age of 80, 1 person in 50 develops Parkinson's. It is estimated that about 120,000 people in the United Kingdom have it. The illness starts between the ages of 50 and 60 in 40 per cent of cases, which makes the sixties the average age of onset. However, about 1 in 7 of those with Parkinson's have developed the symptoms before the age of 40. In so-called young-onset Parkinson's disease, the illness develops between the ages of 21 and 40. The focus of Chapter 8 is on the special needs of those with young-onset Parkinson's. 'Juvenile Parkinsonism', in which the illness starts before the age of 21, is relatively rare.

Men and women are equally likely to develop Parkinson's disease, although some studies have suggested that men are slightly more prone to it. The illness is not selective in terms of either social class or occupation—all classes and occupations are about equally affected. This is reflected in the varied professions of the famous people who have had Parkinson's: Sir John Betjeman (Poet Laureate), Ray Kennedy (Liverpool and England football player), Chairman Mao Tse-tung (Chinese Communist leader), General Douglas Macarthur (American military leader), Kenneth More and Sir Michael Redgrave (actors), A.J.P. Taylor (historian), Terry-Thomas (actor and comedian). The only exceptions to the non-selectivity of the illness is boxers, who, over many years of receiving blows to the head are more likely to get it— witness Muhammad Ali, the great American boxer.

Evidence available since 1855 from the Registrar General of England and Wales, which keeps epidemiological records of all illnesses, suggests that the prevalence of Parkinson's has not substantially changed over the years. And in general, distribution figures in various countries demonstrate that, with a few exceptions, the disorder is not limited to a particular part of the world.

One intriguing finding is that, in studies of large samples of people with Parkinson's disease, there are many who have never smoked and very few current smokers. In other words, people who have never smoked are over-represented and smokers are under-represented. This has led to the proposal that perhaps cigarette-smoking in some ways protects against the disease. The reasons for the association between cigarette-smoking and lower vulnerability to Parkinson's are not known. One possibility is that people with Parkinson's who have smoked die earlier of illnesses associated with smoking. But this can't be the full explanation. The fact that few with Parkinson's disease are smokers, is also true of people who develop it at an early age. Of course, once the illness has started, smoking is unlikely to be of benefit. So no need to go rushing to the tobacconist!

Since the 1970s, when levodopa therapy became the main medical treatment for Parkinson's, the life expectancy of patients has been about the same as for the general population, particularly during the first five years of the illness. After ten to fifteen years, the life expectancy of people with Parkinson's disease drops to about 75–65 per cent of the general population. People with Parkinson's die of the same causes as other people of the same age, except that there is a negative association between Parkinson's and cancer. In other words, people with Parkinson's are less likely to die of cancer, perhaps because they are less likely to smoke.

THE SYMPTOMS

A list of the symptoms of Parkinson's disease is given in Table 1. Each will be described in more detail in the following pages. When looking at the list, it is important to remember a number of things.

● Doctors usually distinguish between major and minor symptoms of a disease, Table 1 observes this distinction. The major symptoms are those present in the majority of people with Parkinson's disease, and one or more have to be present before a person is said to have the illness. The minor symptoms are not encountered in every case. But this distinction overlooks the fact that which symptoms are experienced as major or minor may be different for each individual. For example, for someone who has mild tremor or bradykinesia the symptom of dribbling may be major in the sense of causing most distress and embarrassment. For an actor, the major symptoms may be the dysphonia, or soft and monotonous voice, while for an architect it may be the tremor. Nevertheless, this medical differentiation between major and minor symptoms is useful when talking in general terms, particularly when considering the effectiveness of treatment.

Table 1   The symptoms of Parkinson's disease

Major symptoms
Tremor
Rigidity (muscle stiffness)
Bradykinesia (slowness of movement)
Akinesia (poverty or absence of movement)
Balance and walking problems

Minor symptoms
Dysphonia (low soft voice)
Micrographia (small size of and difficulty with handwriting)
Masked facies (loss of facial expression, 'poker face')
Seborrhoea (excessive greasiness and scaliness of the skin)
Dysphagia (difficulty in swallowing, and dribbling)
Autonomic symptoms (postural hypotension, urinary urgency, sweating)
Pain and other sensory symptoms
Fatigue
Cognitive dysfunction and dementia
Depression
Sleep disturbance
Sexual problems

- Not everyone with Parkinson's disease will necessarily develop all the symptoms.
- No two cases are alike. There are great differences between people with Parkinson's in terms of (1) what the first symptom is, (2) the order in which, and precise time after onset of the first symptom that, other symptoms develop, (3) the severity of the symptoms. The course of the disorder can vary from slowly progressive with relatively little disability, to a more aggressive form with faster progression and faster decline and disability.
- The symptoms may show daily fluctuations in severity. Some people with Parkinson's report a period in the early morning when the symptoms are less evident, or milder. In his book *Ivan: Living with Parkinson's Disease*, Ivan Vaughan describes this morning benefit:

  For a long time I had noticed an extraordinary boost in muscular fluency which flooded my body some time around dawn.

  As the symptoms are not static across time, and fluctuate even in the course of a day, it may be difficult to ask the person with Parkinson's disease to give a clear picture of his or her symptoms.
- It is important not to confuse the symptoms with the side-effects of the medication used to control those symptoms. After a number of years of levodopa therapy, most patients develop dyskinesias, or involuntary movements of the limbs and face. These dyskinesias are side-effects of levodopa therapy and not a symptom of the disease. The distinction between the symptoms and the side-effects of medication may sometimes be difficult to make because some of the symptoms may be made worse by certain types of medication. For example, constipation is a symptom of the disease that can also be a side-effect of anticholinergic medication. The side-effects of medication are listed for each type of drug in Chapter 3.
- In most cases, as already noted, Parkinson's is a disorder of old age. The elderly patient may also have other illnesses such as arthritis, or heart or lung disease, each of which has its associated symptoms. So in some cases, some symptoms may be related to these other disorders and not to Parkinson's.

The history of two people with the illness will illustrate the large individual differences in the type, severity and time of onset of the symptoms, and in the course of the illness and the efficacy of treatment. Susan was fortunate, as her Parkinson's disease remained mild and well controlled for many years. In contrast, Helen's illness had progressed relatively rapidly and after a while medication had failed to produce symptomatic control, bringing on moderate to severe disability within a relatively short time.

Susan is a 70-year-old married woman who at the age of 57 noticed the first symptoms of Parkinson's, which were tiredness and a general feeling of awkwardness, together with a slight tremor of the left hand. She was diagnosed as having the illness two years later. Although her symptoms remained relatively mild and were well controlled with medication, Susan took early retirement from her job as a hospital nurse because of her increased susceptibility to fatigue. Her symptoms remained well controlled on Sinemet and selegiline for eight to ten years, and were associated with mild to moderate disability. During this period she was a very willing and co-operative volunteer, giving generously of her time in order to participate in many experimental studies and research programmes on Parkinson's disease. During the last two to three years, her illness had progressed and the associated disability had increased mainly as a result of 'end-of-dose deterioration' and the development of dyskinesias. She put it this way: 'The period of time when medication controls my symptoms is growing shorter, and the involuntary movements are unpleasant. I still manage to give myself a short "on" period, but I am caught by the unpredictable "running out of steam".'

Helen, married with two young children, had developed Parkinson's disease at the age of 42, a few years after opening her own beauty salon. With a lot of hard work, she had built up a busy and successful business in the span of two years, employing two other stylists. She had been aware of feelings of tiredness and being generally 'run down' for many months before a slight tremor of her right hand appeared. She ignored this for a while, hoping it would go away. When it persisted she consulted her GP, who referred her to a neurologist who diagnosed Parkinson's and started her on medication. For the next three years, the medication controlled her symptoms well. During this period, she carried on with her work at the salon, although she was slower and could see fewer clients. Gradually, the medication stopped controlling her symptoms and the involuntary movements made shampooing, cutting and setting her clients' hair impossible tasks. She was persuaded by her husband to take on a less active role in the salon and to employ a third stylist to stand in for her. This eased the pressure on her and she continued in her managerial role for the next eighteen months. With further progression of the illness and worsening of the symptoms, even dressing and leaving the house in the morning became difficult. Six years after the first appearance of tremor, she was forced to sell the salon. Having spent most of her adult life working outside the home, she welcomed her new role of housewife and focused on busying herself with household chores, with a little help from her mother who visited daily and some input from her teenage daughter after school hours.

The Major Symptoms

Tremor

Tremor is the symptom by which Parkinson's disease is known to most people. In about 50 per cent of cases it is the first symptom. On the other hand, about 15 per cent of people with the illness never develop it. Tremor in Parkinson's disease has a number of typical features that allow a doctor to distinguish it from other forms of tremor present in other movement disorders.

- The tremor in Parkinson's is mainly a *resting tremor*. This means that it is only or mostly present when the individual is at rest, not using or moving the part of the body that has the tremor. For example, the resting tremor of the hands is most noticeable when the hands are resting in the lap. In fact, in some cases the resting tremor of Parkinson's tends to be reduced, or even disappears completely, when the individual moves the hand or uses it to reach towards an object or to grasp something. This is a blessing in a way, since it means that tremor often does not interfere too much with active movements. However, in about 40 to 50 per cent of cases, besides resting tremor there may also be some *action* and *postural tremor*. These are the types of tremor that become evident when, respectively, moving a limb or keeping it in a particular position.
- The second typical feature of the Parkinson's tremor is that it is regular and rhythmic and occurs at a particular rate, about four to six beats per second—in other words, the affected hand or leg shakes or trembles about five times in a second.
- In Parkinson's disease, tremor can affect either a few or many different parts of the body, and can be either mild or severe. For example, at one extreme it may be limited to a single finger of one hand, while at the other extreme it may be present in both hands and legs and even in the muscles of the chest, jaw, tongue and lips. The head

and voice are hardly ever affected by tremor. Usually, the tremor is unilateral – that is, it starts on one side of the body—then the other side is affected later (the tremor becomes bilateral) as the disease progresses. Not only the extent but also the severity of the tremor varies considerably from person to person. It may be so mild that it is only noticeable to the patient. Often, tremor of the chest or abdomen is felt as an internal quivering or shaking that cannot be seen by others. At the other extreme, the tremor can be so severe as to result in violent shaking of the limbs and body. When the tremor of the hands is severe, the thumb may move back and forth in front of the fingers. To the early physicians who used to mix and prepare their own medication by hand, this to-and-fro movement gave the impression of rolling a pill, which gave rise to the label, *pill rolling tremor.*

- The fourth characteristic of tremor in Parkinson's is that it is quite variable and can change considerably with the person's circumstances. It disappears when he or she is sleeping deeply, and is reduced when he or she is very relaxed or sedated. It often becomes worse when the individual is anxious or under stress, or has to concentrate hard. Some people can suppress the tremor for a limited period of time through an effort of will.

Dyskinesias, the involuntary movements associated with medication, can be a cause of embarrassment later on in the illness. In the early stages, tremor is probably the symptom that is most noticeable and that can be embarrassing. As a result the patient may go to great lengths to hide it. Some sit on their affected hand. Others hide it in their trouser or coat pocket, or behind a newspaper. Yet others cover the trembling hand with the unaffected one.

Rigidity, or muscle stiffness

At least in the earlier stages, rigidity, in contrast to tremor, is often something that people with Parkinson's disease are not too aware of. Only relatively later in the course of the illness will rigidity be experienced by the patient as muscle stiffness, and be evident to others as a stooped posture, with the knees and arms bent at the joints. Earlier on, rigidity becomes apparent only during clinical examination by a doctor. It can be brought out by having the patient move one arm while the other arm is moved passively by the doctor. When the doctor passively moves the joints in order to stretch the affected muscles, he or she encounters increased resistance to the movement. This resistance has been compared to bending a lead pipe—hence it is called *lead-pipe rigidity.* Also, during the clinical examination the resistance to passive movements may have a regular jerking characteristic, which has been labelled *cog-wheel rigidity*. The extent and severity of rigidity vary considerably and can affect one arm or one leg or all four limbs. With the progression of the disorder, rigidity can become so severe that the muscles look and feel tense even when they should be relaxed—for example, when the individual is at rest. Rigidity gives rise to aches in the shoulder and neck, back pain resulting from the stooped and forward-leaning posture, muscle cramps in the legs or feet and sometimes even chest pain.

Slowness of Movement—Bradykinesia and akinesia

The word bradykinesia is of Greek origin, *brady* from a word for slowness and *kinesia* from a word meaning movement. It refers to the slowness in initiating as well as in executing movement. In Parkinson's disease, when a movement is repeated several times it becomes gradually slower and 'smaller'. The slowness affects all forms of movement, but slowness in initiating and executing movement is more evident in certain types of movement. Activities involving *repetitive movement* such as brushing the teeth, stirring a saucepan and polishing shoes are particularly affected. So is the performance of *fine movements* such as changing a plug, turning the page of a newspaper or doing up buttons. *Bimanual movements* (movements carried out with both hands) are usually slower than movements with one hand. *Doing two things at once* such as getting up from a chair while talking may become difficult or almost impossible. Activities involving *sequential movements* such as doing up buttons are also slowed down because there is an increased pause between the individual movements in a sequence, which slows down the whole process. Certain movements such as walking, swinging the arms when walking, and blinking and swallowing, are normally done automatically without paying attention to their performance. But in Parkinson's disease such *automatic movements* are more affected than *learned* ones, so that the patient may still be able to perform previously learned dance steps or play the piano.

Rigidity, or muscle stiffness, can add to slowness of movements, but is not the cause of it. Slowness can be present even when there is no rigidity. The severity of bradykinesia may vary from situation to situation. Normally, slowness is evident during movements such as getting out of a chair or walking in and out of a room, and can become worse with increased fatigue. However, under certain circumstances the person with Parkinson's disease can overcome the slowness. The extreme example of this is *paradoxical kinesis*, when an individual who is ordinarily chair- or bed-bound moves at normal speed—for instance, when in danger. Paradoxical kinesis reportedly happened in the case of a usually wheelchair-bound and immobile man with Parkinson's disease who jumped into the water and saved a drowning man! In general, movements that are triggered by external stimuli are less affected than movements initiated by the individual under his or her own steam. For example, despite experiencing problems walking on flat surfaces, the person with Parkinson's can climb stairs remarkably well because each stair acts as a stimulus for taking a step.

A related symptom is *akinesia*, which means absence, or poverty, of movement, and in Parkinson's disease refers to the reduction of spontaneous movements. Akinesia is particularly noticeable in the lack of automatic movements such as blinking and swallowing—in other words, movements than are normally carried out without the individual paying attention to them or expending any effort in doing them. For instance, in Parkinson's disease, during walking the arm swing is lost; when sitting still, the individual does very little fidgeting; while he or she talks, there is little gesturing with the hands or change in facial expression or blinking; the reduced rate of swallowing results in the accumulation and drooling of saliva. The effect of the reduced rate of blinking is that the normal lubrication of the eyes fails to occur, and the eyes become irritated, dry, red, crusted and sore.

The loss of automaticity in performing movements is a particularly disturbing aspect of akinesia and bradykinesia. The person with Parkinson's disease has to consciously think about each phase of the simplest movement.

'Freezing—that is, an inability to move that lasts a few seconds or longer—is another example of akinesia. It occurs during walking, so that the person feels glued to the spot and unable to lift the feet so as to take steps. Freezing often happens when he or she approaches doorways or other confined areas, or when trying to turn. Sudden freezing while walking can lead to falls: the feet stick to the ground, but the momentum of the body continues, so that the person falls forward.

One of the reasons why bradykinesia and akinesia occur may be that in Parkinson's disease the muscles are not sufficiently activated at the appropriate moment. As a result, movements are not only slow but are also often 'smaller' than is needed. For example, when reaching for an object such as a cup, the individual undershoots and the hand falls short of the target, so that the normally smooth and rapid aiming movement is replaced by a slow, stepwise approach to the cup. These problems affect not only the muscles of the hands, arms and legs, but all muscles. For example, the co-ordination of the muscles that move the eyes may be impaired, resulting in difficulty in focusing on nearby objects or slowness in shifting the gaze.

Slowness can be frustrating for the person with Parkinson's. Subjectively, bradykinesia is experienced as a sort of a block between willing a movement and its actual performance. People often feel that they are no longer the masters of their own muscles. Movements previously performed automatically become effortful, and this often calls for a great input of will in order to start them and to overcome what sometimes appears like a counterforce preventing them. This is partly the cause of the excessive fatigue.

As well as producing difficulty with the kind of daily activities described above, bradykinesia and akinesia are also at the root of communication problems arising from the expressionless face (see p. 15), the monotonous voice (see p. 14) and the absence of gesturing.

Balance and walking problems

People with Parkinson's have problems controlling the balance of their bodies. These problems are evident when the individual is sitting or standing, as well as when walking and moving about. When he or she is standing, the balance deficits are seen as a stooped posture, with the body bent slightly forward—as already mentioned, this is a result of rigidity as well as of problems with balance control. In an attempt to compensate for the balance problems, the legs are bent at the knees and the arms at the elbows, and the arms are often held in front of the body. While sitting, the person may tilt to one side, and will be unable to correct this without help. The person with Parkinson's has problems getting out of chairs or bed or in and out of cars because he or she cannot bring about the necessary changes of balance and shifting of body weight to achieve these movements.

The balance problems are particularly evident during walking and turning. In Parkinson's disease, walking (or gait) has a number of characteristic features.

- The individual has difficulty with starting to walk. This is called *start hesitancy*. He or she has problems lifting the foot in order to start walking, and takes a few small uncertain steps before walking at a steady pace.
- The automatic swinging of the arms during walking is lost.
- The individual walks by taking a series of small, short steps, known as a *shuffling gait*. This derives from the reduced length of the stride, in which the feet are not raised high enough while walking.

- The individual walks with the bulk of the body weight on the front part of the feet, so that there is no striking of the heels.
- These last two features result in the so-called *festinant* (or hurried) *gait*, in which walking consists of a series of small, short, shuffling steps which become increasingly rapid.
- Propulsion and retropulsion (literally, forward-pushing and backward-pushing) are the effects of the festinant gait. *Propulsion* occurs when the individual starts walking faster and faster with shorter and shorter steps while leaning forward, until he or she falls forward or is stopped by an obstacle. The tendency to lean backward and take a few hurried backward steps is called *retropulsion*.
- The individual has difficulty with turning while walking. The body turns in one piece without the head twisting first, followed by the trunk and legs. There is also some hesitation when turning is carried out in a number of steps rather than smoothly.
- The loss of righting reflexes—that is, reflexes that compensate for an unexpected loss of balance—causes problems that result in falls. About one-third of people with Parkinson's fall relatively frequently. To prevent themselves from falling forward, they flex their knees.
- When falls occur, Parkinson's patients cannot quickly throw out their arms in order to correct their balance or even to protect themselves. For this reason, falls often cause injuries.
- *Freezing* can occur during walking. As mentioned on p. 11, it mainly happens in doorways. A freezing episode lasting ten minutes is very clearly described by Miss D., a woman with post-encephalitic Parkinsonism (see p. 16) whose case history figures in Oliver Sacks' book *Awakenings*:

> It's like they [her feet] had a will of their own. I was glued there, you know. I felt like a fly caught on a strip of fly-paper . . . I have often read about people being rooted to the spot, but I never knew what it meant—not until today.

The festinant gait, propulsion and retropulsion are partly brought on by the fact that, as a result of the stooped, forward-leaning posture, the centre of gravity is not over the feet, and because the arms are not moved during walking the appropriate stabilisation is not provided.

The Minor Symptoms

Speech problems: dysphonia

Dysphonia in Parkinson's disease is an inability to raise the voice, which results in a very low-volume soft voice that is barely audible to others. It is caused by bradykinesia and rigidity affecting the many muscles of the chest and throat that are involved in the production of speech by regulating air flow through the larynx. The reduction in the volume of the voice is often first noticed by the spouse or by colleagues, who may complain that the individual is mumbling. Dysphonia is sensitive to the individual's emotional and physical state and may become worse when he or she is tired, depressed or anxious. In the early stages of the illness, however, he or she may be able to raise the volume through conscious effort or when feeling emotional. With time, not only is the voice of low volume, but its normal modulation and rising-and-falling intonation, the familiar sing-song of speech, are lost, and it becomes more monotonous.

Besides dysphonia, speech may also show a number of other abnormalities, some of which mirror the problems seen during walking. There may be hesitation in starting to talk or when answering questions, and inappropriate silences in the middle. The person may get stuck on the first word of a sentence and repeat it several times. Also, the 'festination', or hurrying, experienced during walking may also be present when talking, so that the speech may speed up towards the end of a sentence. In addition, there may be some slurring. These changes in speech affect communication with other people—for instance, they can cause problems when the individual is using the phone.

Writing problems: micrographia

Micrographia, a reduction in the size of handwriting, becomes evident when current and previous samples of a patient's handwriting are compared. The letters are well formed but small, and the script gets smaller as writing continues. The alteration in the size may be accompanied by cramps in the muscles of the hand and arm during writing—known as 'writer's cramp'. Writing problems generally improve with treatment.

Skin problems: seborrhoea

This excessive greasiness and scaliness of the skin is especially noticeable around the forehead and nose, which appear shiny, and in the eyebrows, which can be full of dandruff. Another aspect of seborrhoea is excessive sweating: sudden drenching sweats may occur for no apparent reason, requiring frequent changes of clothing.

Loss of facial expression: masked facies

Masked facies (pronounced fayshees), or an immobile and expressionless face, is often combined with a fixed stare. The failure to produce the variations of facial expression that normally accompany speech or emotional change results from the poverty of action and rigidity of the face muscles. Nonverbal cues are thus lost, making communication with the person with Parkinson's disease difficult. On the positive side, the immobility of the face muscles may give him or her a wrinkle-free and youngish-looking skin.

Swallowing problems: dysphagia

Dysphagia, a problem with swallowing, is caused by the reduced ability to transfer food from the mouth to the throat and by a reduced motility of the muscles of the oesophagus, the tube that connects the throat to the stomach. As a result, saliva is not swallowed frequently enough, which causes dribbling. And the disturbance of posture which tilts the head forward so that the chin points down makes the dribbling worse.

Autonomic symptoms

Autonomic symptoms are produced by the dysfunction in the autonomic nervous system, the part of the nervous system that controls the involuntary functions of the body such as blood pressure, heartbeat, breathing rate, movements of the stomach and intestines, the bowel and the bladder, and the sexual organs. The main autonomic symptoms of Parkinson's are postural hypotension, flushing, excessive sweating, urinary frequency and urgency, and constipation.

People with Parkinson's often have low blood pressure, particularly when standing; the pressure tends to fall when they stand up from a sitting position. This drop in blood pressure with change of body posture from sitting to standing is called *postural hypotension*, and may be experienced as feelings of dizziness and light-headedness.

The bladder may not be properly emptied, so that several visits to the toilet may be necessary instead of one. In addition, an urgent need to empty the bladder, even when only small volumes of fluid have accumulated, may result from a tendency for the bladder to be irritable. Such frequency and urgency can disturb night sleep. Constipation, a frequent complaint, arises from the reduced motility of the bowels, and is made worse by the general lack of physical activity and by treatment with anticholinergic drugs.

Pain and other sensory symptoms

Although Parkinson's disease is a motor disorder, about 40 per cent of people also experience sensory symptoms, such as pain, numbness and tingling. However, on clinical examination or investigation these sensory symptoms are not found to be accompanied by any sensory deficits and sight, hearing and touch remain normal, although the sense of smell is affected in about 90 per cent of people.

The pain that is frequently experienced by people with Parkinson's disease is partly a result of rigidity and reduced movement of the joints. Sometimes a dull aching in a limb may be felt many months or even years before the first appearance of tremor or other symptoms. A number of people also report a burning sensation. Pain is experienced mostly in the neck, shoulders and arms and sometimes in the legs. The forward-leaning stooped posture during sitting, standing and walking can also give rise to back pain.

Fatigue

Fatigue, or excessive tiredness resulting from a relatively small amount of physical activity, is common in Parkinson's disease. Everyday tasks calling for physical exertion, such as cleaning or gardening, require more effort to carry out. The person with Parkinson's may need frequent periods of rest to be able to complete such tasks. The fatigue is not purely physical—and some people talk of a sort of mental fatigue, or lethargy. The exaggerated fatigue reaction means that the individual often feels that both physical and mental activity require excessive exertion. Over time this may lead to avoidance of many activities, so that in the later stages of the illness he or she may spend many hours at a stretch simply sitting idle.

Cognitive deficits and dementia

Cognitive functions comprise intellectual abilities and other activities concerned with perceiving, remembering, thinking, reasoning, language and speech. Most people with Parkinson's do not show any intellectual decline or major cognitive deficits. However, more subtle cognitive change may be noticeable over time, such as difficulty in remembering, inability to concentrate or to keep attention focused on a task, sluggishness in thinking and talking. Some of these problems were expressed by Stephen, who had had Parkinson's for seven years:

> I am less alert and more forgetful and unable to express my thoughts. I know what I want to say but the words just don't come out properly.

In general, people with Parkinson's show cognitive deficits when the tasks they have to deal with are difficult and require effort. Such cognitive impairment seems to be magnified when the individual has to plan and do intellectually demanding tasks in his or her own head without any external aids or reminders.

The age of onset of the disease is an important determinant of cognitive decline. Those who develop it after the age of 65 tend to be cognitively more impaired. Those with a mainly tremulous Parkinson's disease tend to be less cognitively impaired than people for whom bradykinesia and rigidity are the core symptoms.

Cognitive deficits are by no means universally present, as is evident in the case of Michael, a 71-year-old man who had had Parkinson's disease since the age of 61. He reported:

> Between the ages of 65 and 70, I undertook two years' A level study at a college and three years at the University of the Third Age, where I have graduated with a BA degree. I found the mental stimulus of studying helped alleviate my symptoms.

A minority of people with Parkinson's develop *dementia*, which is a syndrome of intellectual decline and memory impairment severe enough to interfere with an individual's occupational and social functioning. About 15 to 20 per cent of Parkinson's patients become demented, compared to about 7 to 10 per cent of the elderly population as a whole. This means that the risk of dementia is about 10 to 15 per cent higher than the expected risk in the general population of the same age. Age of onset and rate of progression of the illness predict the likelihood of dementia; it is more likely when the disease first develops at a later age and when it progresses more rapidly. The nature of dementia in Parkinson's disease, and particularly the special needs of the Parkinson's patient who has become demented, are discussed in more detail in Chapter 7.

THE CAUSES

Understanding the cause or causes of the disease may be the first step in designing a cure for it. For this reason, questions about its cause or causes have always been a primary focus of medical research. Unfortunately, the cause of Parkinson's disease is not yet discovered. We know that it develops in the aftermath of a drastic reduction of *dopamine*, one of the chemical messengers in the brain, as a result of the degeneration of the neurones, or nerve cells, that produce it in a little part of the brain called the substantia nigra (see p. 21). What we do not know is what causes the degeneration of the neurones in this area. To explain it, a number of different theories have been suggested. Although none of these has yet proved correct, we will describe some of them in more detail later.

First, in considering the causes of Parkinson's disease, a distinction is usually made between primary and secondary Parkinsonism.

Primary and Secondary Parkinsonism

What has become clear since the 1960s is that the core symptoms of Parkinsonism, rigidity and bradykinesia, can have a multitude of causes and be present in a number of disorders other than Parkinson's. About 76 per cent of those who were diagnosed as having primary or *idiopathic*—that is, without a known cause—Parkinson's disease in life are found in post-mortem examination to have a specific abnormality in the brain. This abnormality is a degeneration of the dopamine-producing neurones in the substantia nigra, accompanied by the presence in the remaining nerve cells of things called Lewy bodies (see p. 23). Idiopathic Parkinson's disease is diagnosed when three of the five main symptoms (resting tremor, rigidity, bradykinesia, postural and walking problems) are present, when there is no history of injury or illness or any other known cause of the symptoms, and when there is a good response to levodopa therapy.

For the remaining 24 per cent, there are other causes, and they are therefore considered to have Parkinsonism secondary to another illness or known cause. These various types of Parkinsonism are listed in Table 2.

We now briefly consider the most common causes of secondary Parkinsonism; besides those listed below, it can, very rarely, be caused by a tumour or head injury.

Post-encephalitic Parkinsonism

Between 1916 and 1926 there was an epidemic of a viral infection, identified first in Vienna and other European cities, which subsequently spread throughout the world and which, among a host of other symptoms, also produced Parkinsonism. The neurologist von Economo called this illness encephalitis lethargica, or sleeping sickness. The name derived from the fact that it involved inflammation of the brain (encephalitis) and one of the first symptoms was sleepiness (lethargica).

Many of the sufferers died in the early phases of the illness. In countries across the world a number survived, but were severely disabled and confined to long-stay hospitals. The traumas of these patients and their short-lived periods of 'awakening' with levodopa were

Table 2   The various types of Parkinsonism

---

1   IDIOPATHIC OR PRIMARY PARKINSON'S DISEASE

2   SECONDARY PARKINSONISM
Post-encephalitic Parkinsonism
Drug-induced Parkinsonism
(a)   Major tranquillisers, e.g. chlorpromazine
(b)   Medication to reduce high blood pressure, e.g. reserpine

Parkinsonism caused by toxins, e.g. MPTP, carbon monoxide, manganese

Parkinsonism as part of other neurodegenerative disorders
(a)   Multiple-system atrophy
           Olivopontocerebellar atrophy
           Striatonigral degeneration
           Shy-Drager syndrome
(b)   Steele-Richardson-Olszewski syndrome
(c)   Corticobasal degeneration
(d)   Wilson's disease
(e)   Guam disease
(f)   Vascular Parkinsonism
(g)   Parkinsonism associated with dementia, e.g. Alzheimer's disease
        and diffuse Lewy body disease

Parkinsonism due to other causes: boxing, other head injury, hydrocephalus

Other causes of juvenile Parkinson's disease

---

movingly portrayed by Oliver Sacks in his book *Awakenings*, mentioned earlier, which was later dramatised into a film. Few survivors of the epidemic are alive today. New cases of post-encephalitic Parkinsonism have rarely been documented, and encephalitis lethargica is no longer a major cause of Parkinsonism.

Drug-induced Parkinsonism
About 7 per cent of people with Parkinsonism have developed the movement disorder following chronic treatment with particular medication. Any drug that blocks the action of dopamine—referred to as a *dopamine antagonist*—is likely to cause Parkinsonism. Major tranquillisers used to treat schizophrenia and other psychotic disorders can cause it, as can drugs such as reserpine and methyldopa (Aldomet) used to treat high blood pressure, and some drugs used to treat indigestion such as metoclopramide, or dizziness, such a prochlorperazine. The major characteristic of drug-induced Parkinsonism is that it will

disappear when the medication is stopped. It may take a month or more after withdrawal of the drugs for the symptoms to disappear.

Parkinsonism caused by toxins

Environmental toxins can also cause Parkinsonism. The condition sometimes develops following carbon monoxide or manganese poisoning, although this is very rare. The most intriguing demonstration of the ability of a toxin to produce Parkinsonism is the 'MPTP story'. In 1982, there were reports from California that a number of young drug addicts had developed Parkinsonism symptoms virtually overnight. Further investigation by the neurologist William Langston and his colleagues revealed that all those affected had taken a 'designer drug', synthesised to produce effects similar to heroin. The development of the classic symptoms of Parkinsonism—tremor, rigidity and bradykinesia—was related to the presence of a substance called MPTP (1-methyl-4-phenyl-1,2,3,6-tetrahydropyridine) in the drug, which in the body was converted to MPP+. MPP+ acted as a specific toxin, causing the death of the dopamine-producing neurones in the substantia nigra, the part of the brain that is affected in idiopathic Parkinson's disease.

Parkinsonism as part of other neurodegenerative disorders

Since the mid-1960s, a number of other, related, disorders have been recognised which have the Parkinsonism features of slowness and rigidity. In addition, these disorders have numerous other symptoms, an underlying disease process and a course that are different from those of idiopathic Parkinson's disease. So a distinction is made between these 'Parkinsonism-plus' syndromes and idiopathic Parkinson's disease. The Parkinsonism-plus disorders include various types of multiple-system atrophy, or MSA (striatonigral degeneration, olivopontocerebellar atrophy, Shy-Drager syndrome), Steele-Richardson-Olszewski (SRO) syndrome, Wilson's disease, other causes of juvenile Parkinsonism, and Guam disease. Post-mortem studies have shown that MSA and SRO account for about 20 per cent of all cases of Parkinsonism encountered. As some of these disorders will be described in the next chapter (see p. 46), only Guam disease needs to be mentioned.

Guam disease was recognised after reports of a higher than usual incidence of a Parkinsonism and dementia together with motor neurone disease amongst the Chamorro natives of Guam. This was subsequently traced to the increased use of cycad seeds as part of their diet. These seeds contain a neurotoxin which causes Parkinsonism.

Finally, there is the question of whether a stroke or a disorder of the blood vessels supplying the brain can cause Parkinsonism. When a blood vessel is blocked by a clot, or bursts, the blood supply to an area of the brain is cut off, brain cells are deprived of oxygen and nutrients, and these brain cells die. The resulting area of dead tissue is known as an infarct. The basal ganglia (see p. 24) have a rich blood supply, and rupture of the blood vessels rarely occurs there. In an elderly population, vascular or arteriosclerotic Parkinsonism may be due to the overlap of cerebrovascular disease and Parkinsonism, in which symptoms appear after a number of small strokes, perhaps as a result of sclerosis, or hardening, of blood vessels. Because of this possible overlap, vascular Parkinsonism, which probably accounts for about 1.5 per cent of all cases of Parkinsonism, is sometimes called pseudo-Parkinsonism.

Dopamine, the Substantia Nigra and the Basal Ganglia

The brain is our most complex organ. It is made up of many hundreds of millions of cells. Neurones, or nerve cells, are designed in such a way as to maximise communication with other neurones. As shown in Figure 1, each neurone has a cell body, a long axon and many shorter dendrites. The dendrites allow cross-talk between adjacent neurones. Dendrites receive messages from neighbouring neurones and pass them on to the cell body, which sends a response down the axon and to the terminal buttons. Here a neurotransmitter (a chemical signal) is released, which transmits the message to another neurone via a synapse (shown in Figure 2), which is a cleft between two neurones that forms a communication bridge between neighbouring neurones.

Idiopathic Parkinson's disease—the type for which no apparent cause is found in the course of taking the history, in clinical examination or from laboratory tests—develops when there is a degeneration of dopamine-producing neurones in that small area at the base of the brain called the *substantia nigra* (meaning, literally, 'a black substance'). It is called this because it contains black-pigmented neurones—neurones that are normally black because they contain a pigment called neuromelanim. These neurones normally produce the chemical dopamine, already mentioned, which is a neurotransmitter—that is, a chemical in the brain that helps convey messages between neurones. When the brains of people with Parkinson's disease have been examined after death, the substantia nigra is not black because it has lost its melanin-containing neurones. As we said earlier, the cause of this degeneration of dopamine-producing neurones is not known.

The substantia nigra is connected to other groups of neurones located at the base of the brain, called the *basal ganglia*. The location of the

Figure 1   A neurone

basal ganglia in relation to other parts of the brain such as the *frontal cortex* (front section of the brain), the *thalamus* (the relay station connecting the basal ganglia to the frontal cortex) and the *cerebellum* (another area of the brain involved in motor function, located at the back of the skull) is shown in Figure 3. The basal ganglia consist of two parts, the striatum and the globus pallidus. The striatum is further subdivided into the caudate nucleus and the putamen. Reduction of dopamine in the substantia nigra results in reduction of dopamine in the striatum, particularly in the putamen. The symptoms of Parkinson's disease become manifest when nearly half of the neurones in the substantia nigra have degenerated and the dopamine in the brain is reduced

Figure 2   Communication between two neurones across a synapse through release of a neurotransmitter

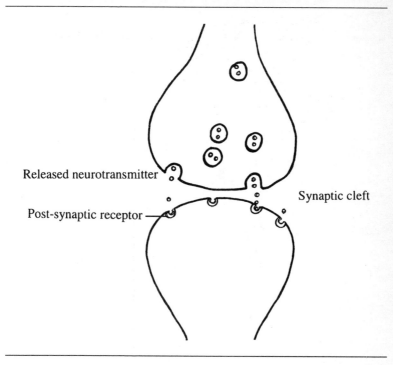

Released neurotransmitter

Post-synaptic receptor

Synaptic cleft

by 80 per cent. For this reason, Parkinson's is considered a dopamine-deficiency syndrome. Another pathological hallmark of the disorder is the presence of smooth spherical 'bodies' with a pale halo called Lewy bodies (named after Frederick Lewy who first described them) in the remaining neurones of the substantia nigra.

Besides the dramatic reduction of dopamine in the striatonigral (from 'striatum' and 'substantia nigra') system, dopamine is also diminished in other areas of the brain. Nor is it the only chemical messenger, or neurotransmitter, that is affected in Parkinson's disease: others include *noradrenaline, acetylcholine* and *serotonin*. Acetylcholine is another important neurotransmitter that is present in the striatum and in all other parts of the brain too. Dopamine and acetylcholine seem to have a see-saw relationship, affecting each other in a reciprocal manner so that a decrease of dopamine is associated with an increase of acetylcholine. This is the case in Parkinson's disease, so that the pharmacological treatment of the illness centres on substances that enhance the action

Figure 3   The location of the basal ganglia in relation to some other parts of the brain (Adapted from J.L. Wilkinson, *Neuroanatomy for Medical Students*. Wright & Sons: Bristol, 1986.)

of dopamine (*dopaminergic medication*) or inhibit the action of acetyl-choline (*anticholinergic medication*).

Possible Causes of Idiopathic Parkinson's Disease

From a scientific perspective, Parkinson's disease is important. It was the first neurological disorder in which a specific chemical dysfunction in the brain was demonstrated. But although we know that the symptoms are due to the degeneration of dopamine-producing neurones, what we don't know is what causes this degeneration and the subsequent dopamine depletion in the basal ganglia. A number of factors have been considered as possible causes.

Inheritance

The question of whether Parkinson's disease is an inherited or a genetic disorder has been addressed in several ways. First, by determining what percentage of identical twins both have Parkinson's disease. Since they are the product of the splitting of a single fertilised egg, identical twins have identical genetic make-up. Similar rates of Parkinson's in twins of this sort would support the notion that genetic factors play a part in the disease. For comparison, also studied are non-identical twins—that is, twins born of two separate eggs fertilised at the same time and so bearing as much genetic similarity as ordinary sisters and brothers. Recent studies have found 17 per cent of identical and 10 per cent of non-identical twins to be concordant—that is, both twins in these instances have Parkinson's disease. These rates are higher than the respective rates of 8 and 5 per cent reported by earlier investigators.

The second line of evidence concerns the percentage of people with Parkinson's disease who have an affected relative, with whom they share some genetic material and would therefore have a greater genetic similarity than with strangers. About 10 to 15 per cent of people with Parkinson's report that they have a relative with similar symptoms. When these relatives have been examined by a neurologist only about half of them are found to have Parkinson's, and the rest have other disorders such as essential tremor. This actual percentage, of about 5 to 7 per cent, is no higher than what we would expect from chance alone. On the other hand, in cases of familial Parkinson's disease— that is, families with many members having the disorder over several generations—also extensively studied, the evidence suggests that her- edity does play a part. However, the weight of the evidence favours the proposition that in the majority of cases the genetic contribution to Parkinson's disease is not of primary importance.

Viral infection

As we noted on p. 18, the post-encephalitic Parkinson's disease of the 1920s epidemic was caused by a viral infection. The existence of this version of the illness has led to the hypothesis that Parkinson's disease may be a result of a slow-acting virus that could have invaded the brain early on in life, many years before the onset of the symptoms. During the intervening years a slow degeneration of the dopamine-producing cells might have occurred, which is compensated until a level is reached beyond which compensation is no longer possible, at which point the symptoms become manifest. So far, the search for a viral agent has proved fruitless, but if the pathologic process giving rise to Parkinson's disease *does* start many years before the appearance of the symptoms, risk factors arising much earlier in life need to be examined.

Environmental toxins and endogenous toxic processes

The current interest in environmental and endogenous (internally gener- ated) toxins as possible causes of Parkinson's disease has been sparked off by two events: first, the report of Parkinsonism in drug addicts induced by MPTP; second, the report of Parkinsonism as an aspect of Guam disease amongst the Chamorro natives (see p. 20). These two phenomena have led to the suggestion that perhaps Parkinson's disease results from a toxin that gradually accumulates in the brain, causing the degeneration of particular neurones in the substantia nigra. This toxin could build up either through exposure to an environmental, or external, toxic source or as a by-product of an endogenous, or internally generated, process in the brain. Alternatively, it is possible that the disorder arises from exposure to a toxin in early life, together with the later natural ageing of the striatonigral system.

With regard to the *environmental toxin* hypothesis, the focus has been on finding a toxin that generates substances known as free radicals—oxygen molecules missing an electron which are attracted to other substances from which they can derive one. Free radicals can kill neurones by interfering with the fundamental metabolic processes that take place in mitochondria, the tiny vesicles contained in all cells. Mitochondria are power-houses of living cells where material is metabolised, or broken down, in order to generate energy. No such environmental toxin has yet been discovered. Again, there may be some difficulty in detecting the possible effects of environmental toxins if they had their causal effect early in an individual's life.

The suggestion that an environmental toxic material such as industrial pollutants, herbicides and pesticides may cause Parkinson's disease has led to a search for variations in prevalence in different parts of the world and between rural and urban areas. No firm evidence has been obtained from these studies. Furthermore, the fact that the prevalence of the disorder has not altered significantly during the last hundred years, and that it is not confined to areas of the world where industrial or agricultural pollutants and toxins may be more prevalent, makes it unlikely that a modern industrial pollutant or agricultural herbicide is the culprit.

As far as the *endogenous toxic mechanisms* hypothesis is concerned, there is evidence that as part of the natural ageing process the number of neurones in the substantia nigra declines. The elderly exhibit in mild form some symptoms that are reminiscent of Parkinson's disease, such as slowness of movement, a stooped posture, shorter strides and a greater number of falls. This raises the question of whether the degeneration of the striatonigral dopamine system in Parkinson's disease represents an accelerated ageing process. More specifically, it has been suggested that in Parkinson's the by-products of dopamine metabolism may act as endogenous toxins in the brain and may be the root of the degenerative process in susceptible neurones. The breakdown of dopamine produces free radicals and hydrogen peroxide, which can have toxic effects by interfering with normal oxidative metabolism in mitochondria and by damaging the membranes of neurones. That 'oxidative stress' might be a possible mechanism of neuronal degeneration in Parkinson's is partly supported by studies that have shown mitochondrial abnormality in the disease. In addition, in the course of post-mortem study, iron which catalyses, or mediates, oxidative reactions has been found in increased concentrations in the brains of people with Parkinson's, even in the early stages of the illness. This also supports the notion of increased oxidative stress being a possible mechanism of neuronal degeneration. However, the nature of the trigger that sets off this chain of oxidative stress in Parkinson's disease is unknown. Also, it is not clear whether these changes are primary and causal or a consequence of the disease, or even a result of medication. Future research needs to throw light on these alternatives.

Other factors

As conscious beings with the ability to reflect on our experiences, we try to make sense of our lives and of what happens to us. So the tendency to seek reasons for or to identify the causes of our ills is quite natural. Since the precise cause of idiopathic Parkinson's disease is unknown, doctors cannot provide any causal explanations. However, this does not stop most people with the disease from searching for causes for their own illness. Helen Rose, the author of *An Old-age Pensioner at Eighteen: or My Life with Parkinson's Disease*, exemplifies such attempts at causal attribution:

> Who can I blame? Can I blame my parents? They both contracted polio when they were young children and were left with severe disability. But polio is an infectious disease—Parkinson's disease is not. So of course it is not their fault. Was it my own fault for banging my head when I fell from a railing that I was sliding down? No. There is no medical evidence to prove that theory. Is it because I was an unmarried mother? What a ridiculous idea. When I pull myself together, I give myself a thorough telling-off. How can anyone be to blame? But as yet, there are no explanations as to why the disease occurs. So, for the time being, I blame the operator on the assembly line for letting me through Quality Control.

Most people with Parkinson's sometimes worry that any one of a number of other factors may have caused their illness, such as stress, diet, their personality, a tumour or head injury. As we mentioned before, tumours or head injury very rarely cause Parkinsonism. With regard to stress, some patients when questioned report experiencing some form of stress or trauma before the start of the illness, such as loss of a loved one, undergoing an unwanted divorce, or redundancy. But such events are also reported by people who suffer from other illnesses, so they cannot be considered as playing a specifically causal role. It *is* possible, though that stress or trauma just before the first symptoms appear in fact precipitate those symptoms in individuals already predisposed to developing the illness.

With the current emphasis on the importance of diet, and the popularity of the idea that 'we are what we eat', it is not surprising that some worry about the role that diet may have played in their illness. But with the exception of the cycad seeds consumed by the Chamorro Indians, evidence shows that diet does not play a part in the development of Parkinson's. People who eat the same food over long periods, such as husbands and wives and people living in institutions such as prisons, show rates of Parkinson's disease no higher than those in the general population.

The notion that this particular disease was in some way brought on by the individual's personality will not bear scrutiny, either. Personality consists of the habitual patterns of thinking, feeling and behaving that make each one of us a unique individual. Our personality is shaped by the temperament we are born with and our subsequent life experiences. There have been some suggestions that certain 'pre-morbid' personality types—those marked by rigidity, inflexibility, punctuality, precision and obsessionality—are predisposed to get Parkinson's disease. But there is little evidence to support this. Retrospective assessment of the pre-morbid personality—that is of the personality before the start of the illness—is virtually impossible. Furthermore, any similarities that are observed in the personalities of people with Parkinson's disease are more likely to be the effect of common experiences of living with a chronic, progressive and disabling illness. This is borne out by the fact that some people with other chronic illnesses such as essential tremor or dystonia (another movement disorder) are also found to have similar personality characteristics—which indicates that such personality traits are in no way specific to any particular disorder.

KEY FACTS 1

What is Parkinson's disease?
Parkinson's is a neurological illness—that is, a disease affecting the functioning of a small part of the brain. Slowness of movement, tremor, rigidity, problems with balance and walking are its main symptoms.

How common is it?
It is a relatively common disorder. About one in a thousand people get it.

Who gets it?
Age is the only known risk factor. Usually, symptoms appear after the age of 50 and the risk of getting the illness increases with age. However, in some cases it starts before the age of 40. Smoking is the only factor that shows a reverse association with Parkinson's disease—people who smoke seem less likely to develop it.

What causes it?
The symptoms of the disorder develop when dopamine-producing neurones in the substantia nigra degenerate and dopamine in the striatonigral pathways are reduced by 80 per cent. In idiopathic Parkinson's disease, the cause of this degeneration and of dopamine deficiency are unknown. But we do know that the illness does not result from something the individual has done, from his or her diet, or from stress. With the exception of people with familial Parkinson's disease, heredity does not play a major causal role. What *is* possible is that some individuals have a genetic susceptibility to develop Parkinson's disease—for example, by being unable to deal with infectious agents or toxic material whether induced by environmental factors or by some endogenous internal mechanism. There are numerous theories about the possible causes of the illness, but none is yet proved. Most investigators believe that the cause is likely to be multifactorial—that is, that many factors may play a role.

Is Parkinson's disease life-threatening?

Parkinson's is not a 'killer disease'. Treated with medication, it is to be feared no more than hypertension or diabetes when they are controlled with the appropriate medication. Parkinson's disease affects the individual's daily activities and 'quality of life'.

Will it affect the intellectual faculties?

Only a minority of cases develop a true dementia—that is, intellectual decline and loss of memory. Many with Parkinson's complain of isolated cognitive problems such as absent-mindedness, slowness of thinking, difficulty with mentally effortful tasks. Others experience no noticeable change in their cognitive abilities.

2

Diagnosis and Prognosis

Diagnosis is the process by which a doctor decides what illness a person is suffering from. Diagnosis is important because it determines what the doctor does next—what advice he or she gives, and the choice of treatment. The term we use is 'the process of diagnosis', and we use it for two reasons. First, because in most cases there is a delay between the first appearance of symptoms and their diagnosis, or labelling, by a doctor as Parkinson's disease. Second, because it is not always possible to establish the diagnosis on the basis of a single consultation or test result. In some cases, the way the disease changes over time may alter the diagnosis.

A doctor diagnoses Parkinson's mainly by taking a history of the development of the symptoms from both the patient and a close relative, then making a clinical examination of the patient. A number of laboratory tests and scanning procedures are also carried out in order to exclude other causes of the symptoms. These tests are mainly for differential diagnosis—that is, to distinguish idiopathic Parkinson's disease from other causes of Parkinsonian symptoms. The *prognosis*, or prediction of the likely course of the illness, in any one individual is difficult. Nevertheless, there have been some attempts to identify factors that may predict the course or that may have prognostic significance.

In this chapter our aim is to provide you with information about the process of diagnosis and the factors that may affect the prognosis.

FIRST SYMPTOMS: THE PRE-DIAGNOSTIC PHASE

Usually the symptoms of Parkinson's disease develop very gradually. The onset can be so gradual that the individual may have difficulty recollecting precisely when the symptoms first appeared. This slow onset means that he or she may be aware of something being wrong for years before the symptoms become manifest to family or friends, or evident enough to warrant a diagnosis of Parkinson's disease by a doctor. This early phase may be marked by periods of worry interspersed with self-reassurance, denial and minimisation of the significance of the perceived change.

The initial symptoms noticed by the individual vary from person to person. As mentioned in Chapter 1, tremor is the most commonly reported one. A number of less well defined symptoms usually precede the first appearance of tremor. A sense of weakness, slowness or clumsiness of one arm or leg is commonly reported. The person may notice loss of manual dexterity or difficulty in using one arm during writing or daily activities such as shaving, doing up buttons and putting on make-up. Getting out of chairs and cars or rolling over in bed may have become difficult. Some complain of a sense of internal trembling before the development of resting tremor. Others remember feeling generally tired, and being unable to perform tasks such as gardening or cleaning the house for long periods without taking a rest. The voice may lose its power and become inaudible to others. Pain, especially in the neck and shoulders, can be a common early complaint and may lead to a misdiagnosis of cervical spondylosis or arthritis.

The symptom or change in function that is perceived first and that brings the individual to medical attention probably also depends on his or her profession. For example, for a draughtsman or architect, slowness of hand movements or muscle rigidity that interferes with the ability to draw may be most noticeable. For a lecturer or a singer a lower voice may be noticed first, although it may not necessarily have been the first symptom to have developed.

Occasionally, early changes in posture and balance, or loss of facial expression, are evident in photographs taken a number of years before the diagnosis of Parkinson's disease. Sometimes it is someone close to the individual who first notices that there is a change or that there is something wrong; slowness of movement or change in posture may be perceived by relatives. Alternatively, it may be someone who has not seen him or her for some time who first comments on changes such as lack of facial expression, sluggishness of action or change in posture. Gradual change can go undetected by those who see us daily.

In the majority of cases, the symptoms of the disorder start on one side of the body and over time progress to the other. In some the asymmetry may persist, and one side may be affected more severely than the other for the duration of the illness. In the early pre-symptomatic phase, the change may be so mild that a doctor may be unable to detect anything amiss in the course of the neurological examination. Or the clinical examination may reveal one noteworthy change, which on its own does not add up to anything and would be insufficient for a diagnosis, but which the doctor may record but not mention to the patient so as not to cause unnecessary alarm. Or again, at this pre-symptomatic phase when the initial symptoms are often only noticeable to the patient, it is possible for doctors to dismiss them and write them off as being neurotic—in the individual's mind rather than real.

Alternatively, the process of diagnosis may take multiple referrals over years, as illustrated by the following comments:

It took a long time for me to be diagnosed, although I think my symptoms were obvious.

My initial symptom was slowness of movement of my fourth finger. I went to see my GP. The first diagnosis was pinched nerve. Later on, the second diagnosis was arthritis. On a subsequent visit I was referred to a rheumatologist, who finally referred me to a neurologist.

FIRST CONTACTS WITH THE MEDICAL PROFESSION

Eventually the disease will progress, and one or more of the symptoms will become noticeably manifest. This brings the individual to medical attention and a doctor diagnoses the illness. When the symptoms appear, most people are likely to go first to see their GP, who either makes the diagnosis or refers the individual to a neurologist or occasionally, if he or she is elderly, to a geriatrician. The majority of those referred to a neurologist are seen in the out-patient clinic of a general or teaching hospital. A minority may initially, or at a later stage, be admitted to hospital for assessment. Others may see a neurologist privately. Here we briefly describe the first contact with the GP and the procedures followed during neurological consultations, focusing on what you can expect during a visit to an out-patient clinic or during hospital admission.

The GP

Apart from his or her role in arranging a referral to a consultant neurologist, contact with the GP is very important in the management of Parkinson's disease in several ways:

- He or she is the doctor with whom you have probably been in contact for a considerable length of time, and who therefore knows the most about you and your general health and is best suited to discuss your specific needs.
- Your GP is the person who will be concerned with the management of any other problems that you may have, whether an ear infection, arthritis or heart trouble.
- Access to most other sources of local help is usually arranged through referral by the GP.
- Repeat prescriptions of medication are usually obtained from the GP.
- Most importantly, as Parkinson's disease is a chronic illness, continuity of care from a single doctor or members of a group practice has many advantages, not the least of which is the possibility of developing a warm and personal patient–doctor relationship that overcomes the need to explain afresh the history of your symptoms and your circumstances at each consultation.

In her book *Living Well with Parkinson's Disease*, Glenna Wotton Atwood lists her expectations of both specialists and GPs:

Will listen to me, will treat me as a whole person, will not rush me, will respect my feelings, will explain his findings and will answer my questions, will educate me about my illness, will respect my intelligence and have me take an active role in decision-making, will be willing to refer to other doctors if their expertise might help me, will write up my visit and send me a copy for my records, will be available or will have an alternate who will be available after office hours in case of emergency, will be a person with whom I can feel comfortable.

These qualities would probably match what most people expect of any good doctor, and two of them are particularly important. First, the person with Parkinson's disease should be actively involved in the management of his or her illness, because he or she is the best person to inform the doctor about the benefits and side-effects of any treatment. Second, doctors should be aware that besides needing medical treatment of the symptoms, the patient and his or her carer also need emotional and practical support. There is much to recommend a holistic approach—that is to say, an approach which, in addition to treating the illness and its symptoms, considers the whole person and his or her circumstances and needs, while also attempting to manage the personal, emotional and practical problems associated with the illness.

However, a good patient–doctor relationship depends on the patient's behaviour as well as the doctor's. If you need more time to discuss your worries, try to do so even if the doctor seems pressed for time. If you don't understand a particular term or piece of information, ask for clarification. Clearly state your preferences about possible medical and complementary treatments. Every GP is likely to have about four or five patients with Parkinson's disease on his or her register, so he or she should know something about it. If, over time, because of your personal interest you find that you have become more knowledgeable about the illness than your GP, don't let it overshadow your relationship. Remember that every GP has to deal with a long list of disorders and that his or her role is to be able to recognise any one of them at its onset so as to make an appropriate referral to a consultant, and to participate in the day-to-day management of all of those disorders. Material is available from the Parkinson's Disease Society, specifically aimed at informing GPs about the finer details of treating and managing the disease. If you feel that you are not getting the best care from your GP or that there is simply a personality clash, it is possible to change doctors. The local health services can tell you how to do this.

The Neurologist

A neurologist is a medically trained doctor who specialises in the diagnosis of neurological illness and its management. One of the rights stated in the Patients' Charter is that of 'being referred to a consultant acceptable to you when your family doctor thinks it necessary, and to be referred for a second opinion if you and your family doctor agree this is desirable'. The type of consultant involved in the diagnosis and care of Parkinson's disease is a neurologist with a special interest in movement disorders. In the UK there is roughly one neurologist for every three hundred thousand of the population, and few specialise in the diagnosis and treatment of Parkinson's disease or movement disorders. For most people with Parkinson's, their illness is initially diagnosed during a consultation with a neurologist. There may then be follow-up contacts with the neurological team for a number of years to tailor medication so as to achieve optimal control of symptoms and minimise disability. When complications arise, or when close monitoring of response to or alteration of medication is required, admission to hospital for brief periods may be arranged by the neurological team.

The Neurological Out-patient Clinic

Out-patient clinics are run by doctors working in a team. The teams in a neurological out-patient clinic are headed by a consultant neurologist who may have a number of other doctors, including a senior registrar, a number of registrars and senior house officers, working with him or her. If the team work in a multidisciplinary fashion, there may also be a psychologist, a physiotherapist, a speech therapist, an occupational therapist and a social worker or a community nurse attached. The consultant has overall clinical responsibility for the patients, and each member of the team plays a particular role in patient care. Where such multidisciplinary teams exist, not all members will necessarily become involved in each individual case—the involvement of particular team members may be dictated by the needs of each individual case.

The way in which out-patient clinics are organised in the UK means that there are many people to be seen, by too few doctors, in too short a time. This means that there is likely to be a delay before you see a doctor, and that you may not necessarily see the consultant neurologist you were referred to. The first visit is likely to take several hours. As with most hospital appointments, prepare yourself for a wait and don't expect to be seen at the time specified on the appointment letter.

On your first visit to a hospital neurological team, you are likely to be first seen by a doctor other than the consultant. This doctor will take down the history of the development of your symptoms and ask some additional questions about your health since childhood and the health of your family; then there will be a neurological examination (described in more detail on p. 43). This procedure can take up to an hour. A waiting period may ensue, during which the doctor you have just seen reports back to the consultant and other members of the team, and provides them with a summary of your history and the results of the clinical examination. While you are waiting, you may be asked to have a number of blood and urine tests or X-rays. Later, you may briefly see the consultant neurologist, who may ask further questions and carry out a short clinical examination. Alternatively, you may see again the doctor you saw before. At this stage you are usually given a diagnosis, either by the consultant or by the doctor. Some general information about the illness and a broad outline of what to expect in the coming years are provided by these doctors, together with suggestions about possible medical treatments.

Hospital Admission

As an alternative to attending an out-patient clinic, you may be admitted to hospital. This will usually be to a neurological ward of a district or teaching hospital. Your stay can last from one to several nights, usually a maximum of a week. During the day you will probably wear your own clothes, so besides your night-clothes and toiletries you may want to take a change of clothes. During the first day of your stay you will be visited by the senior house officer (SHO), a doctor in training. The SHO will take a history of the development of your symptoms and conduct a neurological examination. You will be referred to other departments of the hospital to have a range of tests done (described on p. 45). You may be seen by the consultant neurologist during one of his or her weekly ward rounds (times when the consultant visits the ward with other members of the team). Then the histories, the results of the clinical examinations and other tests are considered in order to arrive at decisions about the diagnosis or treatment of every person on the ward. On most neurological wards visiting hours are not limited, but it is best to tell your family to visit outside working hours, since during the day you will be undergoing a range of tests. When relatives or friends visit you can leave the ward and walk around or go to local cafés and restaurants. You just have to let the ward nurse know where you are going and when you will be back.

If you are seen in a teaching hospital, much of your contact with the consultant neurologist is likely to take place rather publicly. Both in the out-patient clinic and in the ward round, you are likely to see him or her in the presence of a number of other people, usually doctors in various stages of their neurological training. You may find the presence of so many others during your consultations, especially at such a potentially stressful milestone in your life, particularly intrusive. You should be offered the option of not having others present at these times, and your wishes should be respected. But do bear in mind that young doctors have to learn somehow, and that the out-patient clinic and ward round are integral parts of medical training. On occasion, while you are in hospital your case may be presented to a large number of doctors in the course of a 'clinical case presentation'. You may be invited to attend this meeting, to be examined in front of the other doctors. A case presentation has two purposes. First, it allows consultation with a larger number of experts and, second, it is another occasion for teaching the more junior doctors. On the positive side, it is worth bearing in mind that most teaching hospitals are 'centres of excellence' and keep up to date with the latest medical developments.

Receiving the Diagnosis

Early diagnosis is important for several reasons. First, delay in diagnosis delays effective management and treatment of the disorder. Second, a delay in diagnosis may be demoralising both for the patient and for his or her family. Knowing the correct diagnosis brings the reality of the illness home. It allows patient and family to start the process of acceptance and adjustment and to consider the implications for their work, their finances, their daily life and their future prospects; and to start preparing and planning. After being given the diagnosis either by the GP or by a neurologist, some people obtain a second opinion by consulting a neurologist privately or by seeing a neurologist with a specialist interest in Parkinson's disease and other movement disorders. This seeking of a second opinion is further confirmation of the reality of the diagnosis, and it may in fact be this that finally brings the truth home.

For most people, contact with the neurological team at the hospital has a number of shortcomings. As well as the possibility of a long wait before seeing a doctor, and the relatively public nature of most neurological consultations:

- You may see a different doctor each time.
- Medical consultations often involve rather one-sided communication. Most of the conversation centres on answering specific questions asked by the neurologist. For this reason, the patient and the accompanying relative may feel frustrated that they have not had a chance to ask any questions or express their worries.
- The neurologist may know very little about the individual's life circumstances and about him or her as a person. The doctor often relies on what he or she is told by the patient, before arriving at diagnostic or therapeutic decisions. Research studies suggest that about 40 per cent of people who are hospitalised with neurological disorders have psychiatric problems such as depression, most of which (about 70 per cent) remain undetected by neurologists. It appears that most neurologists simply don't ask about, and patients fail to report, any emotional or adjustment problems. So you, your carer and your family should be alert to this fact and bring any feelings of depression or anxiety to the attention of the neurologist.

In addition, many people when asked also recount some displeasure with the manner and circumstances in which they were first given the diagnosis. A rather extreme example of tactless disclosure is given by Helen Rose in *An Old-Age Pensioner at Eighteen*:

> The consultant put his head round the screens and said, 'Mrs Rose, you have Parkinson's disease', then he left. Here I sat in a strange ward with screens closed round me, shut off from the rest of the world, or so it seemed, wondering what Parkinson's disease was.

As the following quotations illustrate, people can be upset by such things as the length of time taken for a final diagnosis to be arrived at, by the lack of privacy, and by the detached and sometimes rather unsympathetic manner in which diagnosis is given.

> I would have preferred to have the news communicated to me in a more private setting, not in front of an entourage of medical students. One of the students recognised my feelings and she stayed behind talking to me, which I found comforting.

> At the time of diagnosis, I did not feel that I was given any support. I was given very little information.

> In retrospect, my initial diagnosis, which lasted five minutes, was pretty brusque. As I was, at that time, only marginally affected it didn't upset me. However, to someone more incapacitated it could have been very traumatic.

> The registrar who gave me the diagnosis did so in a very abrupt manner and responded to my devastation and disbelief with a flippant 'You have at least five good years ahead', and appeared very dismissive of my 'It's a life sentence' response! However, an hour later when I saw him again, he did put a very comforting arm around my shoulder. I think he realised then how shocked I was. I then spent some time having tests and coffee with a nurse— I'll never forget her, she was so caring and kind. I also wrote down many questions, as I was to see the consultant before leaving the hospital. I feel that this second consultation was well timed and conducted, as many decisions about taking medication, work and family had to be made eventually. The information gathered that day set me in motion, and concentrated my thoughts really well on those aspects which were of most importance.

> Supposing Parkinson's disease to be a 'killer', my very first reaction was one of horror, but once the consultant explained some of the basics of the condition and suggested I joined the Parkinson's

Disease Society, I quickly accepted the situation. I find the PDS literature of tremendous help to the 'newcomer', and for consumption by friends and family too.

Most doctors tell the person the diagnosis, unless otherwise requested by a relative. This mirrors the fact that most people would want to know it. Apart from a relative's wish to shield the patient from the reality of his or her illness, failure to convey the diagnosis can occasionally arise from the doctor's discomfort. Despite the potentially negative impact that the diagnosis may have on the individual and the accompanying friend or relative, it is important for doctors to portray a realistic picture. Therefore, the question is not whether to tell the patient or not, but rather *how* to tell him or her, and what and how much information to convey. The manner in which information is conveyed about the illness early on may have paramount and lasting effects. A true expert diagnostician is a doctor who has up-to-date medical knowledge and astute powers of observation that enable him or her to diagnose even rare and unusual cases, combined with an understanding of the needs, hopes and fears of the patient that allow him or her to communicate with that patient with sympathy and tact. That this is possible is reflected by the following experiences:

I found some doctors were very caring and absolutely marvellous, whereas others were hardly interested.

I cannot speak too highly of the way in which both my own GP and the neurologist dealt with me. If anyone could make such an occasion a pleasant experience, this particular neurologist could.

The manner in which the news was first broken to me was very professional and sympathetic.

Telling an individual that he or she has a chronic and progressive neurological illness amounts to conveying unpleasant and sometimes devastating news. Clearly, this is not an easy task, and doctors may have difficulty in communicating the diagnosis in an empathic and caring manner for several reasons. First, like all other professionals, individual doctors differ widely in their personal manners and communication skills. Second, it is only relatively recently that the social nature of medicine has been emphasised in medical schools and the need to specifically train doctors in the art of communication has been recognised. Third, there is the inevitable process of habituation to dealing with trauma that occurs in the course of medical training and practice. Fourth, diagnosis is not always a straightforward exercise. Doctors, especially more junior ones, can get so engulfed in the task of history-taking, clinical examination and recording their observations that they forget the important interpersonal aspect of the consultation.

These reasons may help explain the shortcomings of some doctors in the field of good communication, but they should not serve as excuses. The purpose of medical training at all stages, and the duty of each individual doctor, should be to cultivate such interpersonal and communication skills. Caring communication means being sensitive to the needs of each patient. People differ in the extent to which they want information, and with sensitivity the doctor can pick this up. The information should be tailored to the capacity of the individual. The truth should not be hidden, but neither should it be thrust upon someone who is indicating that he or she is not ready to deal with it. People come to terms with the reality of illness at their own pace. Obviously, communication is a two-way process and the person with Parkinson's and/or the accompanying relative need to be assertive enough to air their concerns if they don't want to leave the consulting-room in a bewildered state and with a bagful of unvoiced questions. In his book *Ivan: Living with Parkinson's Disease* Ivan Vaughan, a psychologist, writes about both his immediate and his delayed reactions to being told by a neurologist that he had the illness:

> I tried to remain casual and got up to leave, remembering the Marx brother's joke: 'I've got Parkinson's disease, and he's got mine.'

But shortly later:

> As I passed through the doorway on my way out at the end of the interview a host of unasked questions began to crowd into my mind.

What is often overlooked by the doctor in the course of a busy outpatient clinic is that it is essential to *make* the time to convey information, to deal with worries, answer questions and reassure the patient and his or her relative.

A more productive approach to the provision of services by a neurological team was developed in the Romford Neurocare Project, the aim of which was to develop standards of good practice in relation to the management of Parkinson's disease. This project devised a multidisciplinary approach in an NHS neurology department, with a focus on three main areas:

1   telling the patient the diagnosis and providing subsequent infor-
    mation and support
2   attending to the social and emotional needs of the patient and
    carer(s)
3   actively involving the patient and carer(s) in decision-making.

The multidisciplinary team consisted of a consultant neurologist, a social worker or counsellor who acted as co-ordinator, a physiothera-pist, a speech therapist and a dietician. For each individual with newly diagnosed Parkinson's disease, one member of the team acted as the 'key worker' (see p. 221). Through home visits and other forms of contact immediately after diagnosis and at least every 12 months there-after, the key-worker assessed early on the needs of each patient and facilitated referral to other members of the team or other services when required.

The objective here is to provide a co-ordinated and flexible service that bridges the hospital–community divide. Emphasis is placed on the provision of adequate information and support at the time of diagnosis.

In the Romford Project, a model for giving the diagnosis was developed, as follows. The first clinic appointment is kept relatively short. After the neurological examination, the neurologist asks the indi-vidual what he or she thinks is wrong with him or her in order to get some idea of any particular worries and fears that can be alleviated in discussion. Then the patient is told that the illness is in fact Parkinson's disease. Before giving further brief details about the illness, its treat-ment and management, the neurologist asks the patient what he or she knows about Parkinson's. This provides an opportunity for the neurologist to correct any misconceptions that the person may have. The period immediately after the diagnosis is likely to be traumatic for the patient and for whoever may be accompanying him or her. At such times it is difficult to take in and make sense of a mass of information, so the patient and his or her family need to be given a chance to assimilate the news before being provided with more detailed infor-mation. To facilitate this, a nurse practitioner (see p. 222) or social worker accompanies the patient and relative from the clinic and spends some time discussing the diagnosis with them and providing them with information sheets about the Parkinson's Disease Society, and other sources of help such as occupational therapy, physiotherapy and speech therapy.

A second appointment is made for a few weeks later. By this time both patient and relative will have had a chance to think about the practical implications of the illness. At this second appointment, their questions are answered and they are given more detailed information about the illness and its management.

The model developed by the Romford Neurocare Project has been adopted in a number of other out-patient clinics in the UK. Such multidisciplinary approaches should improve communication between neurologists and their patients and provide a better quality of care for people with Parkinson's disease. The availability of a key-worker within the multidisciplinary team should ensure that each person's needs are adequately met by appropriate referral. This approach could be important in preventing premature disability and handicap and also avoid duplication of effort through inefficient liaison. Hopefully, before long the model of good practice developed in the Romford Project will be adopted in all neurological clinics.

THE NEUROLOGICAL EXAMINATION AND THE DIFFERENTIAL-DIAGNOSIS TESTS

No single test exists that would reliably lead to the diagnosis of Parkinson's disease. This particular diagnosis is a clinical decision arrived at by a doctor on the basis of his or her observation of the patient's appearance and behaviour, from clinical examination and from consideration of the history of the development of the disease in the case concerned. In addition, the patient may be referred for a number of laboratory tests, which are usually carried out in order to exclude other diseases. We briefly describe here what these various procedures entail.

The Neurological Examination

The neurological consultation has three major components: observation, history-taking and neurological examination. By the time the patient has walked through the door, said hello and sat down, the neurologist will have made a number of important observations about his or her posture and gait, about the presence or absence of arm swing, and the tone of voice. In the course of the consultation, the doctor continues to observe the patient's behaviour—noting, for example, whether spontaneous changes of posture, crossing and uncrossing of the legs, automatic hand gestures during talking, blinking, changes of facial expression are present or absent.

The neurologist combines this observation with taking the history of the illness from the patient and the accompanying relative. This account covers a number of topics, such as the course of the illness from the onset to now—what were the first symptoms noticed? when did they develop? what happened subsequently? any previous medical consultations, tests or treatments?—plus any history of other illnesses or hospitalisations or medication taken, any periods of psychological trauma and stress or physical injury, any family history of similar symptoms or disorders. Questions of a more personal nature may also be asked—about marital status, occupational history, social and leisure activities.

Then comes the neurological examination, which may first concentrate on assessment of the functioning of the sensory organs: the eyes, ears and senses of touch and sometimes smell. The doctor may move on to examine the functioning of the muscles, and of the nerves that connect them to the spinal cord and the brain, by asking you to tense particular muscles or to move parts of your body against resistance. The doctor assesses muscle tone by passively moving each body part while it is relaxed, to determine if rigidity is present. A special hammer is used to test reflexes. To bring out any slowness in initiating and executing movements and any worsening of bradykinesia with certain types of movement, the doctor will ask you to carry out different movements. You are asked to perform these movements with both the right and the left hands, in order to determine whether bradykinesia is bilateral or confined to one side of the body. As mentioned in Chapter 1, tremor is a symptom of other disorders besides Parkinson's: it can be present in essential tremor, cerebellar disease, anxiety states and thyroid disease. The doctor may spend some time doing a differential diagnosis (see below) of tremor in order to distinguish the Parkinson's tremor from the other forms.

Posture while standing, walking, sitting and getting out of a chair is noted. Balance is tested by recording the effects of a gentle push on your stability. Also, you will be asked to write a short sentence, as a sample of your handwriting. To bring out any writing tremor, you will be asked to draw a number of concentric circles. The body temperature may be taken and the pulse and blood pressure assessed while sitting as well as while standing. The neurological examination usually includes a number of quick tests of mental state. General orientation in time and place will be assessed by asking you the date and the name and location of the hospital. Ability to do mental tasks is evaluated with the 'serial sevens' test, which involves asking you to count backwards from 100 in steps of seven. Memory is tested by asking you to retain and then recall after a few minutes a series of words.

The Laboratory Tests Used for Differential Diagnosis

To rule out other illnesses, the neurologist may recommend a number of laboratory tests such as a blood test, urine analysis, and tests of autonomic function; recording the electrical activity of the brain (the electroencephalogram, or EEG) or of the activity of muscles and nerves (the electromyogram or, EMG; and nerve conduction studies, or NCS); and maybe one or more types of brain scan (computed tomography, or CT; magnetic resonance imaging, or MRI). Occasionally, a lumbar puncture to examine the spinal fluid may be required. These tests, which are described in more detail below, allow the doctor to arrive at the diagnosis of idiopathic Parkinson's disease (cause unknown) by a *process of exclusion*.

The first purpose of these tests is to exclude any treatable cause for the observed symptoms. For example, low levels of the hormone thyroxine produced by the thyroid glands located at the front of the neck can result in hypothyroidism, which can also slow down movements. A blood test will reveal such a deficiency, which can then be easily treated. As we said in Chapter 1 and as is evident from Table 1, the symptoms of Parkinson's can be an integral part of a number of disorders other than idiopathic Parkinson's disease. The second purpose of the tests is to allow the doctor to distinguish between the various syndromes that can cause the symptoms of Parkinsonism.

According to the diagnostic criteria set out by the 'brain bank' of the Parkinson's Disease Society, a person is considered to have idiopathic Parkinson's disease when bradykinesia is present together with at least one other symptom, which can be muscular rigidity, or resting tremor or postural instability. Other positive criteria that would support the diagnosis are unilateral onset or persisting asymmetry of symptoms, the progressive nature of the disorder, excellent initial response to levodopa lasting five or more years, severe levodopa-induced abnormal movements, and a clinical course of ten or more years.

As mentioned above, there is no test on the living patient that will result in a definite diagnosis of idiopathic Parkinson's disease; the clinical diagnosis of the disorder can be confirmed only by post-mortem pathological examination. Nevertheless, despite being largely based on clinical judgement, the accuracy of such a diagnosis is relatively high. Studies at the PDS brain bank and elsewhere have shown that in about 80 per cent of those diagnosed during life as having idiopathic Parkinson's the diagnosis is confirmed post-mortem. In such cases, besides degeneration of the substantia nigra, the presence of Lewy bodies (spherical bodies surrounded by a halo), mentioned earlier, is a characteristic pathological finding. The remaining 20 per cent of cases are found to have other causes for their symptoms. Multiple-system atrophy, Steele-Richardson-Olszewski syndrome (progressive supranuclear palsy) and corticobasal degeneration account for the majority of the misdiagnoses. These disorders are called akineto-rigid or Parkinsonian-plus syndromes, because akinesia and rigidity are their symptoms; they also have a number of additional symptoms not seen in idiopathic Parkinson's disease.

Multiple-system atrophy, progressive supranuclear palsy and corticobasal degeneration are distinguished from idiopathic Parkinson's disease in three major ways:

1 Unlike idiopathic Parkinson's, the Parkinsonian-plus syndromes are rarely responsive to levodopa therapy; even if it seems to help a little at first, its long-term efficacy is relatively limited. By contrast, in idiopathic Parkinson's disease, once the symptoms have become disabling, the introduction of levodopa produces a clear beneficial effect which persists for many years before the appearance of complications such as on-off fluctuations and dyskinesias.
2 Parkinsonian-plus syndromes show additional symptoms and signs that are atypical of idiopathic Parkinson's disease. For example, in Steele-Richardson-Olszewski syndrome a downward-gaze palsy (inability to move the eyes down), and a more frequent and certain occurrence of dementia, are additional features. Presence of apraxia (inability to carry out symbolic movements on command such as blowing a kiss or waving goodbye) and alien limb phenomenon (not feeling in control of the activities of an arm or leg) are characteristic of corticobasal degeneration. Early and severe autonomic symptoms (such as fainting and urinary incontinence) and the presence of cerebellar ataxia (unco-ordinated movement) or pyramidal signs (spastic muscles and brisk tendon reflexes) are the distinct features of multiple-system atrophy.
3 Two other features can also help in the differential diagnosis. The absence of resting tremor and frequent falls early in the course of the disorder are usually indicative of a diagnosis other than idiopathic Parkinson's disease.

Distinguishing these Parkinsonian-plus syndromes from idiopathic Parkinson's is not always easy, because some abnormalities of eye movement or mild autonomic dysfunction can occur in idiopathic Parkinson's disease, and dementia, as noted in Chapter 1, is a late feature of the disorder in a small proportion of patients. Furthermore, it is usually only when the patient has been seen on a number of occasions over many years and when changes in symptoms during this follow-up period have been observed that it becomes possible to distinguish these disorders from each other.

We now describe some tests commonly used to distinguish idiopathic Parkinson's disease from the Parkinsonian-plus syndromes and to exclude other causes for the symptoms.

Blood and urine analysis

Examination of the urine and blood can be useful indicators of the normality or abnormality of the levels of various chemicals secreted by the body's glands or organs and of the presence of infections. These analyses usually focus on tests of thyroid and liver function. There are no changes in blood count or blood chemistry that would help in the diagnosis of Parkinson's disease. The results of the blood and urine analysis are usually normal in Parkinson's, unless the individual is suffering from other disorders such as thyroid disease or diabetes.

X-rays of the chest and neck

The X-ray is a radiological technique that uses small amounts of radio-active material to provide a picture of an internal part of the body. A chest X-ray provides an image of the lungs and the heart, while from an X-ray of the neck, the cervical spine (vertebrae of the neck) can be seen. The results of the chest X-ray are normal in Parkinson's disease, unless the individual has an infection or a cardiac or pulmonary disorder. In some people the neck X-ray is likely to reveal a degree of cervical spondylosis, or deformation of the neck vertebrae, that occurs as a result of age in a proportion of the population.

Electroencephalography

The brain emits electrical activity that can be detected with the right equipment. Electroencephalography, also referred to as EEG, is a method of measuring the electrical activity of the brain using sensors that are temporarily glued to the surface of the scalp. Tumours, strokes and epilepsy can affect the EEG, which will show an abnormal pattern of activity in such cases. The EEG results are normal in Parkinson's disease.

Special kinds of EEG-recording, involving the presentation of certain light flashes or patterned visual stimuli, auditory tones or clicks, or small electrical stimuli applied to the skin, are used to assess the functioning of particular sensory areas in the brain and of the corresponding sensory pathways in the nervous system. These are called visual evoked potentials (VEPs), auditory evoked potentials (AEPs) and somatosensory evoked potentials (SSEPs), and respectively assess the visual, auditory and somatosensory pathways in the nervous system. AEPs and SSEPs are normal in Parkinson's disease, while VEPs are reported as abnormal; this may be related to the reduction of dopamine normally present in the retina.

Electromyography

The electromyogram (EMG) is recorded in order to assess the functioning of the skeletal muscles (the muscles attached to the skeleton, including the spine, that produce movement). The electrical activity generated by the muscles is measured by means of special sensors placed over the muscles of the arms or legs. The EMG may reveal the presence of resting tremor before it becomes noticeable. In Parkinson's disease, the size of the first 'muscle burst' that triggers the muscle into activity is reduced. This may be partly responsible for deficits in force generation and slowness of movement in the disorder.

The measurement of nerve conduction velocity

Here the aim is to measure the speed with which information is conveyed from the motor areas of the brain, via the motor neurones, to the muscles. To do this, a motor neurone is stimulated at two separate points along its course over the skin, and the time of the onset of activity (motor unit potentials) produced in an associated muscle is recorded. From this the delay between the stimulus and the start of the contraction of the muscle is measured, which allows the rate of conduction of the impulse along the motor neurone to be calculated. The stimuli used are usually small electrical shocks that can be perceived but are relatively painless. Nerve conduction velocity is normal in Parkinson's disease.

Computerised tomography

The CT scan is a form of X-ray of the brain that reveals any abnormal changes in its structure. The head is placed in an X-ray tube containing many radiation detectors, which can rotate around the head and take pictures at various angles. A large number of measurements are taken, and from these a computer reconstructs a series of images which can reveal the presence of any tumours or other structural abnormalities such as signs of previous strokes. In Parkinson's disease, the CT scan may show a number of non-specific changes—that is, changes that are also found in other disorders and may be partly associated with the normal process of ageing.

Magnetic resonance imaging

The MRI scan is a more sensitive method of obtaining information about any changes in brain structure. (MRI does not involve radiation or the use of radioactive substances.) The head is placed in a tube that contains a powerful magnet, which aligns all the water molecules in the head with the magnetic force. In the presence of radio waves, the water molecules emit electromagnetic energy which is detected by special sensors; a computer then constructs images from these measurements. The MRI scan does not show any structural changes in the brain specific to Parkinson's disease, although some investigators have reported that the intensity of the signal received from the substantia nigra is reduced.

Positron emission tomography

The PET scan provides functional anatomical information about the brain. This means that with PET scans it is possible to assess the functioning of different parts of the brain while the individual is carrying out a particular movement or engaging in a specific mental activity. With PET it is also possible to examine the state of particular neurotransmitter receptor sites in the brain. PET scans require the use of radioactive material in very small quantities, usually equivalent to the radioactive exposure during a transatlantic flight. The dopamine systems in the brain can be assessed with PET scanning. Fluorodopa scans have shown that the capacity to take up levodopa and convert it into dopamine in the striatum (see p. 22) is decreased in Parkinson's disease. This, in effect, has confirmed the specific dopamine deficiency of Parkinson's in living patients. Single-photon emission tomography (SPECT) is a cheaper but far less sensitive alternative to PET.

The Lumbar Puncture

The cerebrospinal fluid (CSF) is a clear and colourless liquid that fills the ventricles, or cavities, of the brain and the middle of the spinal cord and acts as a protective cushion for brain and spinal cord against external pressure. The exchange of chemical material that occurs between the CSF can be of value in the diagnostic process. A specimen of the CSF and the blood allows the removal of metabolic waste products from the nervous system. Examination of the chemical contents of the CSF is obtained by a doctor carrying out a lumbar puncture. He or she will ask the patient to lie curled up in a foetal position, then insert a needle, under local anaesthetic, into the lumbar region (lower back) below where the spinal cord ends. Microbiological assessment and examination of the chemical contents of the CSF usually reveal no abnormalities in idiopathic Parkinson's disease.

Autonomic-function tests

The aim of these tests is to evaluate the functioning of the autonomic nervous system (see p. 15). Tests of autonomic function include assessment of blood pressure with changes in body position—from lying to tilting, to sitting, to standing. Changes in blood pressure are also assessed in a number of other situations: before, during and after exercise, while doing mental arithmetic; while hyperventilating (taking fast and shallow breaths), or before and after putting one hand in ice-cold water for about two minutes. Autonomic disturbance such as excessive sweating and salivation, urinary urgency, constipation and postural hypotension do occur in idiopathic Parkinson's disease, as we noted earlier, but severe autonomic symptoms, particularly in the early stages of the illness, are usually indicative of multiple-system atrophy, one of the Parkinsonian-plus syndromes discussed on p. 46.

Vestibular-function tests

The aim of these tests is to assess the vestibular system located in the inner ear, which plays a role in the control of body balance. The main components of the vestibular system are three fluid-filled semicircular canals located at right angles to each other, which detect and compensate for changes in body position. Vestibular function is tested by using manoeuvres that stimulate these semicircular canals, such as quick changes of body position from standing to lying, or quick turning of the head to the right and left. Alternatively, caloric stimulation may be employed to assess vestibular function: during the caloric test, the right and left ears are in turn irrigated with cold and then warm water. This stimulation results in slow movements of the eyes that occur like the beating of a metronome, the duration and direction of which are noted. Vestibular function is not impaired in Parkinson's disease.

The neuropsychological assessment

People with Parkinson's disease are often referred to a clinical psychologist or neuropsychologist for a neuropsychological assessment. The main purpose of this is twofold. First, this kind of cognitive assessment may confirm the presence of dementia which, particularly in the early stage of Parkinson's disease, would be considered atypical and would suggest a diagnosis other than idiopathic Parkinson's. Second, mild cognitive dysfunction does occur in Parkinson's disease, and neuropsychological assessment establishes a baseline against which any future change can be assessed. Such an assessment usually takes between one and two hours, during which the patient does a number of tests of cognitive function, including tests of intellectual ability, memory, attention, language, verbal fluency and planning.

While, despite the various clinical and laboratory tests, no diagnostic marker of Parkinson's disease exists, the search for a specific test continues. This is outlined in more detail in Chapter 13.

Research-related tests

In addition to the clinical tests that are carried out to help in the diagnosis of Parkinson's disease, you may be asked to take part in studies for research purposes. This can happen while you are staying in hospital, or when you are being seen as an out-patient. The purpose and procedures of these research studies will be explained, so that you can decide whether or not to participate. Although they may be of no particular value to any one patient, it is important to remember that such research studies are the stepping-stones to our fuller understanding of Parkinson's disease, its causes and its optimal treatment. All the same, you always have the option of declining to take part in them— your decision will in no way affect your medical treatment.

In his book *Parkinson's Disease: A Patient's View*, Sidney Dorros, an American with Parkinson's disease who took part in the initial clinical trials to assess levodopa therapy, talks about the rewards of being a pioneer patient:

> I've often been helped over difficult emotional periods by reflecting on my role as a pioneer experimental patient in the development of a medication that is helping thousands of fellow victims of Parkinsonism. This satisfaction is enhanced by my recent discovery of the significance of some of the incidental basic research studies that were conducted on me while I was hospitalized six different times between 1970 and 1973 . . . During these few years, I estimate that I contributed hundreds of gallons of urine, dozens of quarts of blood, and a few pints of spinal fluid to the NIH [National Institute of Health] laboratories— all taken under special conditions designed to add to the basic information about the mechanisms of Parkinsonism, the drugs used to treat it, and the reactions of the body to both. Some of the information has been of direct help to me; some has led to improved treatment for Parkinsonism over a long time, sometimes indirect, route . . .

PROGRESSION AND PROGNOSIS

What comes after diagnosis? Invariably one of the immediate concerns of the person who has been diagnosed as having Parkinson's disease is to find out what the course of the illness is likely to be.

Parkinson's is a progressive illness, which means that the symptoms gradually get worse over time. How quickly this progression occurs is difficult to determine. The only thing that can be said with any certainty is that it varies from person to person. For this reason, it is difficult to predict the likely course of the illness or to give a definite prognosis for any one individual. The symptoms may remain mild and unchanged for decades. Both before and after the levodopa era, a proportion of cases—about 5 to 10 per cent—have been reported as following a mild course, with little disability during the first ten years. Alternatively, the illness may rapidly progress to severe disability over a few years. About 6 to 15 per cent of cases show such a progression. The majority of cases lie somewhere between these two extremes.

Research studies have tried to determine whether the rate of progression, and the prognosis, are different for particular types of Parkinson's disease. The results of several research studies have suggested that three clinically distinct types of the illness can be distinguished in this respect.

1 *Classical type* Most people with Parkinson's can be considered to have the 'classical' disease, with akinesia, rigidity and tremor. This type starts before or after the age of 60, is initially unilateral, then gradually develops into a bilateral disorder. Patients respond well to levodopa, and fluctuations do not develop until three to five years after starting such therapy.
2 *Akineto-rigid type* This subgroup represents about 6 to 15 per cent of all cases, and tends to have a less favourable prognosis. Initial response to levodopa is not outstanding, and response fluctuations and involuntary movements may develop soon after starting treatment. Dementia and depression are also more common with this type of disease.
3 *Tremulous type* Having tremor as the first presenting symptom and as the predominant symptom subsequently, has been found to be prognostically favourable. This type of Parkinson's disease shows a slow progression and is less likely to be associated with depression and dementia. It probably constitutes about 5 to 10 per cent of all cases.

There is some evidence supporting the distinction between these three subtypes. But there is also evidence that Parkinson's with tremor as the dominant feature and Parkinson's with predominantly akineto-rigid symptoms are not necessarily different in terms of prognosis. Furthermore, it may not be easy, whether immediately after the onset of the illness or in the early stages, to classify individual cases as being of one kind or another. Since the various symptoms develop at different times, classification may be possible only after observation of the clinical course of the disease. In addition, it is not clear whether the three subtypes of Parkinson's—the classical, the tremulous and the akineto-rigid—differ in terms of the underlying disease process. A preliminary post-mortem study of small groups of people with Parkinson's disease did not find any pathological differences between the akineto-rigid and tremulous types.

Progression has been examined in a number of ways. Various schemes for quantifying the severity of the illness over time have been developed. One such procedure involves the use of a stages-of-illness scale, devised by Drs Hoehn and Yahr and their colleagues and subsequently known as the Hoehn and Yahr scale. This classifies Parkinson's disease into stages 1 to 5 (from mild to very severe).

- *Stage 1*   The main symptoms—tremor, rigidity, bradykinesia and postural abnormalities—are unilateral.
- *Stage 2*   The disease has become bilateral, and other minor symptoms such as facial masking, swallowing and speech difficulties may have developed.
- *Stage 3*   The same bilateral symptoms are present, but may be somewhat worse. The important feature is that balance problems have appeared for the first time.
- *Stage 4*   The patient has become increasingly disabled, and needs help with some or all activities of daily living.
- *Stage 5*   The patient is confined to a wheelchair or bed and needs complete assistance.

With the Hoehn and Yahr stages-of-illness scale, an index of progression was obtained by determining the average duration of the illness at each of the five stages, both for patients receiving levodopa therapy and those whose illness was untreated. At stage 2, the average duration of illness for treated cases was 9 years, compared to 6 years for untreated ones; at stage 3, it was 12 and 7 years, respectively, for treated and untreated cases; at stage 4, 12 years as opposed to 9 years; and at stage 5, 18 years compared to 14.

From these figures it is clear that levodopa delays progression through the stages by three to five years. However, levodopa therapy does not appear to alter the *rate* of progression of the illness. Many studies have tried to find out whether there are any associations between levodopa therapy and progression, but the results have been contradictory. Despite the controversy, however, comparison of data from the pre-and post-levodopa era suggests that treatment with levodopa has increased the life expectancy of people with Parkinson's disease. Some investigators argue that the prolonged life expectancy is dependent on starting levodopa therapy early in the course of the illness. Others disagree, reasoning that early levodopa treatment simply means that the drug will lose its efficacy and fluctuations will develop earlier in the course of the illness. The latter group propose that the primary guideline for starting levodopa therapy should be the indication that the symptoms in any given case are associated with moderate to severe disability that is interfering with the occupational and social life of the individual.

As will be discussed in the next chapter, the use of a class of medication called monoamine oxidase inhibitors type B (MAO-B inhibitors) has been shown to 'protect' laboratory animals against MPTP-induced Parkinsonism. MAO-B type medication such as selegiline has therefore been used in the treatment of Parkinson's disease, with the possibility that it may slow down the progression of the illness. The evidence at the moment is contradictory, and further investigations are required. The development of medication that can slow down progression is a focus of current research.

KEY FACTS 2

What will the process of diagnosis involve?

Usually, the symptoms of Parkinson's disease develop very gradually. In the UK the process of diagnosis usually starts when the individual consults his or her GP. The GP may diagnose the disease, or refer him or her to a neurologist or geriatrician. Most people are seen at a neurological out-patient clinic; less frequently, the patient may spend a few days in hospital. Besides taking the history of the development of the symptoms and conducting a neurological examination, the neurologist may recommend that a number of laboratory tests be carried out, the results of which will help in the process of differential diagnosis, to distinguish idiopathic Parkinson's from other conditions that produce Parkinsonism. There is no marker or specific test that helps in the diagnosis of the illness. It is diagnosed on the basis of clinical examination of the patient by a neurologist and by exclusion of other causes for the symptoms.

How will the symptoms evolve over time?

Parkinson's is a progressive disorder, which means that the symptoms become more severe over time. However, the rate of progression varies widely. The time between the onset of the symptoms and severe disability and dependency varies between three and thirty or more years. The course can vary from a very mild disease that remains static for many years to a more aggressive form of the disorder, with rapid progression and severe disability within a few years.

Can the likely course of the illness be predicted?

It is not possible to predict the likely course of the illness in any one case. However, there is some evidence that the predominance of tremor may indicate a good prognosis, whereas the akineto-rigid form of the disorder may be associated with a less favourable one.

Can the progression be stopped or slowed down?

It cannot be stopped completely, but the development of medication that can slow it down is a major focus of research.

Will the medication remain effective in controlling the symptoms?

Over time, most types of medication become less effective in controlling the symptoms of Parkinson's disease. But once again, there are major individual differences. Some patients require only minor changes in medication, or in the timing of taking it, in the course of the illness. For others, frequent and major alterations of medication may become necessary to adequately control the symptoms.

Will I become totally incapacitated?

With progression of the illness and with the loss of efficacy of the medication after prolonged use, a proportion of people with Parkinson's become incapacitated, wheelchair-bound and dependent on others for most daily activities. For most people, this is likely to happen, *if* it does, many years after first developing the illness.

3

The Medical and Surgical Treatment of Parkinson's Disease

Although there is still no cure for Parkinson's disease, its medical treatment has come a long way since the first description of the disorder in 1817 by James Parkinson. In his *Essay on the Shaking Palsy*, Parkinson recommended that 'blood should be first taken from the upper part of the neck, unless contra-indicated by any particular circumstance. After which vesicatories should be applied to the same part, and a purulent discharge obtained.' Although prescribing what was probably relatively standard treatment for most illnesses in the 1800s, Parkinson was acutely aware of the gaps in knowledge about the disorder; he also wrote, 'Until we are better informed respecting the nature of this disease, the employment of internal medicines is scarcely warrantable.' The difficulty in finding an effective treatment was also acknowledged by Jean-Martin Charcot, the famous French neurologist, who in the course of his lectures at the Salpêtrière Hospital noted: 'Everything, or almost everything, has been tried against this disease.'

This state of affairs changed only when a series of discoveries in the 1950s and 1960s revolutionised the medical treatment of Parkinson's disease. It was in 1957 that dopamine was discovered to be one of the neurotransmitters, or chemical messengers, in the brain. This was shortly followed by the demonstration that dopamine deficiency was the hallmark of Parkinson's disease. The new therapeutic era of the disorder dawned in the 1960s, when *levodopa* was administered to patients, and was found to control the symptoms effectively when given in large enough dosages. In the intervening years, experience of long-term therapy with levodopa has highlighted the possible complications that can occur and has led to further refinement of this form of drug treatment. Partly in response to the long-term complications of levodopa therapy, other avenues have been explored and developed, resulting in treatment with *dopamine agonists* (chemical substances having a similar effect to that of dopamine) and neuroprotective therapy, to slow down the progression of the disease. The 1980s and 1990s have been marked by other therapeutic explorations, mainly the development of a number of new surgical procedures for treating Parkinson's disease.

The aim of this chapter is to provide information about the two main forms of treatment currently used in Parkinson's disease: treatment with *medication* and treatment with *surgery*. Other kinds of therapy employed in the management of the illness will be considered in Chapter 9.

MEDICATION

Medications are commonly available as tablets or capsules. Tablets have the advantage that they often have a groove on one side that makes it easy to break them in half for smaller doses; capsules are easier to swallow. More sophisticated methods of drug delivery have recently been developed. For example, controlled-release tablets of Sinemet are manufactured in such a way that they are gradually broken down and absorbed in the stomach, making levodopa available in the brain for a longer period. Small portable pumps (see p. 71) have also been used for the continuous delivery of dopamine agonists such as lisuride and apomorphine. The majority of drugs are available in several different strengths, or dosages. The dosage, 50mg, say, refers to the amount of active ingredient contained in the tablet or capsule. For most medications there are recommended therapeutic dosages, which are achieved by taking one or more tablets of a particular dosage each day. This optimal daily amount may vary somewhat from person to person, depending on body weight and metabolism.

Most drugs have two types of label: a generic and a brand name. The generic name is the scientific name of the medication, sometimes referring to the composition of the drug—that is, the chemicals it contains. For example, trihexyphenidyl, the generic name for Artane, refers to its active contents. The brand name is the trade label given to the medication by the drug company that made it. Different companies give different brand names to the same drug, and the same drug is often produced under different names in different countries. The generic and brand names of the medications most frequently used in the treatment of Parkinson's are given in Table 3.

Table 3   Medication commonly used in the treatment of
Parkinson's disease

Type of medication	Brand name	Tablet dosage (mg)	Daily dose (mg)
LEVODOPA			
levodopa	Levodopa	500	100–1,000
levodopa + carbidopa	Sinemet LS	levodopa 50, carbidopa 12.5	100–1,000
	Sinemet 110	levodopa 100, carbidopa 10	
	Sinemet-Plus	levodopa 100, carbidopa 25	
	Sinemet 275	levodopa 250, carbidopa 25	
	Sinemet CR	levodopa 200, carbidopa 50	
levodopa + benserazide	Madopar 62.5	levodopa 50, benserazide 12.5	100–1,000
	Madopar 125	levodopa 100, benserazide 25	
	Madopar 250	levodopa 200, benserazide 50	
	Madopar CR	levodopa 100, benserazide 25	
	Madopar Dispersible		
DOPAMINE AGONISTS			
bromocriptine	Parlodel	1, 2.5, 5, 10	15–80
lisuride	Revanil	200 micrograms	1–5
pergolide	Celance	50, 250 micrograms	2–5
apomorphine	Britaject	2 or 5ml ampoule	
ANTICHOLINERGICS			
benzhexol/ trihexyphenidyl	Artane	2, 5	4–15
benztropine	Cogentin	2	1–4
orphenadrine	Disipal	50	100–300
procyclidine	Kemadrin	5	7.5–30
MAO-B INHIBITOR			
selegiline	Eldepryl Deprenyl/Jumex	5	5–10
OTHER			
amantadine	Symmetrel	100	200–300

General Principles

Since the cause of Parkinson's disease is unknown, treatment is not aimed at eliminating the cause, but at controlling the symptoms. However, the aim of drug therapy is not to make the individual completely free from symptoms, but rather to prevent those symptoms from causing severe disability and handicap, so that he or she can continue living and working independently. More recently, as we noted in Chapter 2, medical treatment has also been aimed at slowing the progression of the illness—an aspect of therapy that is still in its infancy.

The aim of all medication currently used to treat Parkinson's disease is to normalise neurotransmitter function in the affected areas of the brain, particularly the striatonigral region (see p. 23). As we noted earlier, Parkinson's is characterised by a reduction in dopamine and an increase in another brain chemical, *acetylcholine*. As a result, the medical treatment of Parkinson's centres on substances that enhance the action of dopamine (*dopaminergic medication*) or inhibit the action of acetylcholine (*anticholinergic medication*). As the disorder is primarily a dopamine-deficiency syndrome, dopaminergic medications are much more effective than the anticholinergics, which produce only about 25 per cent symptomatic relief.

So the main focus of treatment is to boost dopaminergic transmission in the brain, which can be achieved by several different strategies:

- by increasing the synthesis of dopamine in the brain, which is achieved by administering levodopa in combination with a peripheral decarboxylase inhibitor such as carbidopa and benserazide, which prevent the conversion of levodopa into dopamine *outside* the brain
- by administering dopamine agonists such as bromocriptine, lisuride, pergolide and apomorphine
- by inhibiting the breakdown of dopamine, which is the mode of action of selegiline
- by enhancing dopamine release, which is the mode of action of amantadine
- by blocking dopamine re-uptake at the synaptic terminals (see p. 73 for an explanation of synapses), which is the effect of other classes of medication such as tricyclics and of benztropine, sometimes used to treat Parkinson's disease.

The major and minor symptoms of the disease are differentially responsive to treatment. The various forms of medication produce their beneficial effects on different symptoms. In general, bradykinesia and akinesia respond well to treatment and are often much alleviated; rigidity is usually alleviated by levodopa therapy. Tremor also responds to medication, but it may not be completely eliminated. Balance and walking problems are usually the least remedied. The more minor symptoms such as oiliness of the skin, sweating, aches and pains may also be relieved with medication.

All medications are chemicals that affect brain function. Ideally, they would only operate on and normalise function in the affected areas of the brain, but there is currently no way of restricting the action of any given medication to the affected areas. So most medications give rise to unwanted side-effects as well as to the desired symptomatic relief. Usually the side-effects are minor, and outweighed by the benefits. But at times they can be so severe or disturbing that the patient cannot cope with them. In such cases the drug is discontinued or altered, whatever its beneficial effects might have been. The severity and the interfering nature of side-effects differ from drug to drug. There are also some differences between people in terms of the severity and tolerance of the side-effects. The aim of drug therapy is to strike a balance between obtaining maximal benefit and incurring the minimum of side-effects.

It will by now be clear that there exists no specific recipe or formula for treating Parkinson's disease with medication. It is always necessary to tailor the precise kind of drug therapy, and the point at which it starts, to the symptoms of the individual patient. Treatment will not necessarily be started, especially in the case of levodopa therapy, immediately after the diagnosis. And decisions about which drug to use and when to start it are ruled by the social and occupational circumstances of the individual, as well as by his or her particular symptoms. This means that comparing notes with other patients about when treatment was first started and specific medication regimens is unhelpful and may be misleading. Clinical decisions about medication are not simply taken on the strength of a single consultation at the outset of the disorder. With the progression of the illness, the drug therapy may be revised, and adjustments may be necessary every six months or so to accommodate any changes in the symptoms and the associated disability. For this reason, continuity of care from either the GP or the hospital neurological team is important.

But although the specific nature and timing of drug therapy are determined in each individual case, there are some general guidelines that doctors follow:

- When symptoms are so mild that there is no resultant disability, there is no need for medication.

- When the symptoms of tremor and akinesia become noticeable, or interfere with daily activities or cause social embarrassment, then anticholinergics or occasionally dopamine agonists may be introduced.
- When excessive stiffness or slowness appear, amantadine may be added to the anticholinergics. Temporary benefit may be produced by amantadine, which has weak dopaminergic effects as well as anticholinergic properties.
- When walking and balance are affected and work and daily activities are disrupted, then dopamine therapy is started. The choice will be between levodopa and a directly acting synthetic dopamine agonist. Levodopa will be effective in most cases; a dopamine agonist such as bromocriptine will be of benefit in only one third of cases. Because of the major long-term drawbacks of levodopa therapy, when first introducing dopaminergic drugs most doctors rely on the strategy of using low dosages of levodopa (Sinemet or Madopar) with a dopamine agonist (bromocriptine or lisuride).
- After long-term levodopa therapy, when the response becomes unreliable and on–off fluctuations and *dyskinesias* develop, the levodopa dosage needs to be modified, and various strategies for controlling these complications are introduced.

It is difficult to predict who will derive maximum benefit from a particular medication, because this changes with the stage of the illness and the severity of the symptoms. A degree of trial and error is involved in determining the optimal drug regimen, or drug dosage, for an individual patient. As a general rule, most medications start with the lowest possible dosage, which is then gradually increased to determine the optimal therapeutic dosage that will effectively control the symptoms without major side-effects. When a drug is no longer effective in controlling the symptoms, it should be stopped. However, medication taken to treat Parkinson's disease, particularly levodopa, should not be stopped suddenly, but gradually withdrawn under medical supervision.

Although a variety of drugs is available to treat the disease, the aim is to achieve maximum control of symptoms and prevention of disability with the smallest possible number of drugs and the lowest dosages. Some people with Parkinson's may be taking more than one type of medication, but the number of tablets a person is taking is not an indication of the severity of the illness. Each individual has a set of specific symptoms that require treatment with particular types of medication. The medications that are prescribed for treating Parkinson's disease do not usually produce adverse reactions when taken together, and doctors are aware of those that might and so take it into account when prescribing. You should always inform doctors and dentists about the types of medication you are taking.

Levodopa Therapy

When it first became widely available as a treatment for Parkinson's disease in the 1970s, levodopa produced such profound changes in symptoms that it was seen as a miracle drug. Even today, it is still the most effective drug available. In fact, it is so effective that one of the criteria for diagnosis of idiopathic Parkinson's, as mentioned earlier, is that the symptoms improve with levodopa.

Levodopa treatment is a replacement therapy that aims to achieve symptomatic improvement by compensating for the dopamine deficiency. Only certain substances can get from the bloodstream into the brain, because the so-called blood–brain barrier acts as a selective filter, and dopamine is one of those substances that cannot cross it. For this reason it cannot be directly used in the treatment of Parkinson's disease, but levodopa, or L-dopa, is used instead, which *can* cross the blood–brain barrier, then to be converted into dopamine in the brain. The dopa molecule exists in two forms that are mirror images of each other in three-dimensional space: an L-form (laevo, meaning left) and a D (dextro, meaning right) form. Only the L-form of dopa, or levodopa, occurs naturally and is effective in the treatment of Parkinson's. The full chemical name of L-dopa is L-3,4-dihydroxyphenylalanine. It is made up of hydrogen, oxygen, carbon and nitrogen atoms. Levodopa is changed to dopamine by the action of dopa-decarboxylase, which is an enzyme (a substance that regulates chemical changes in the body). This conversion is not rate-controlled, which means that it is possible to increase the amount of dopamine in the brain by taking more L-dopa. L-dopa is an amino acid first discovered in the broad bean. It is also present in other plants, as well as in animal tissues. An amino acid called tyrosine, found in protein-rich foods, can be used in conjunction with the enzyme tyrosine hydroxylase to make L-dopa in the body. This mechanism is very strictly rate-controlled, so that eating more dietary tyrosine will not increase the amount of dopamine in the brain.

When levodopa is taken orally it passes from the mouth to the stomach and then to the small intestine. Dopa-decarboxylase, the enzyme that converts levodopa to dopamine, is present in the gut, liver, kidneys and blood vessels as well as in the brain. Levodopa is absorbed in the bloodstream from the lining of the intestines, then circulates around the body in the blood. Some of it is changed to dopamine and broken down in the kidneys, then excreted in the urine. Only about 1 to 10 per cent of it reaches the brain. To prevent levodopa being converted into dopamine peripherally—that is, outside the brain—with the consequence that much of the resulting dopamine is wasted—the levodopa is combined with a dopa-decarboxylase inhibitor (a substance that inhibits the action of dopa-decarboxylase and thus the conversion process) that itself cannot get into the brain. In this way the amount of dopamine available to the brain is multiplied by a factor of ten, which in turn reduces the required oral dosage of levodopa. Also, side-effects due to the action of dopamine outside the brain are reduced. Carbidopa and benserazide, peripheral inhibitors of dopa-decarboxylase, are combined with levodopa in the ratio of 10 to 1 or 4 to 1. Sinemet and Madopar contain levodopa and dopa-decarboxylase inhibitors, and are the medications most frequently used to treat Parkinson's disease.

When levodopa was first introduced, the general practice was to use the maximal tolerated dosage. Now, 25 years later, the experience gained from observing the effects of long-term treatment with levodopa has led to the minimal effective daily dosage being recommended; in other words, the optimal dosage is the smallest that will control the symptoms and the associated disability. Most doctors recommend that levodopa therapy is started with Sinemet LS or Madopar 62.5, twice or three times a day, each tablet taken with or after a meal to minimise nausea, which is a common side-effect. The dosage is then gradually increased to a 100mg pill, taken three times a day. The patient should avoid the temptation to increase the dose in order to achieve complete relief of symptoms.

In 85 per cent of those with idiopathic Parkinson's disease, a marked alleviation of disability occurs with the start of levodopa therapy. All the main symptoms are relieved, with rigidity and bradykinesia responding the most. Tremor is less alleviated and, together with postural instability, may take some time to respond to the therapy. When levodopa treatment is first started, people with Parkinson's report that they are more alert and attentive, and can both move and perform daily activities more rapidly. But a feeling of restlessness and some problems in falling asleep may also be experienced. The period of action of the combined levodopa/decarboxylase inhibitor pills is about four hours.

In the initial phases of treatment, a relatively even response to levodopa therapy throughout the day is obtained. Some take their first dose of the day early, before getting washed or dressed. The best strategy is to try to time the doses so that the best benefit is obtained at times when it is important to be most mobile and physically active. For example, there is usually no point in taking one before going to bed or, for most people, in the evening, when they are most likely to be relaxing at home.

After taking a pill, there is a delay in the appearance of the benefits of levodopa because of the time-consuming digestive process that it undergoes when taken by mouth. It takes about twenty minutes for the drug to cross the barrier between the blood stream and the brain. Acidity, or other factors that may delay the emptying of the stomach, can further delay the absorption of dopamine. Although, in order to reduce nausea, it is recommended that levodopa medication be taken with food to begin with, meals, particularly those with a high protein content, may delay its absorption and its peak concentration in the blood. The precise amount of daily protein that will interfere with levodopa absorption is not clear. Current opinion is that, in those with advanced Parkinson's disease, a daily protein intake in excess of the recommended daily allowance of 0.8g per kilogram of body weight would diminish the response to levodopa. Furthermore, the closer the high-protein meal is to the time of taking the tablets, the greater the interference caused with the absorption of levodopa. A 'protein redistribution diet' is a simple procedure that can significantly prolong the efficacy of levodopa therapy, particularly in those who have developed fluctuations in their response to levodopa. In this approach to the problem, daytime protein intake is limited to less than 10g, and most of the daily allowance of protein is restricted to the evening meal.

It is safe to take levodopa with most other medications. The exception is that antidepressants of the monoamine oxidase inhibitor-A type (MAOI-A) such as phenelzine (Nardil) and tranylcypromine (Parnate) should be discontinued for at least three weeks before starting levodopa. Large quantities of vitamin B6 (pyridoxine) can accelerate the conversion of dopamine in such a way that little reaches the brain, though this is less of a problem with the combined pills containing a peripheral decarboxylase inhibitor. The major tranquillisers used to treat psychotic symptoms such as hallucinations and delusions act by blocking dopamine and consequently produce Parkinsonism. This medication should not be taken concurrently with levodopa.

The immediate and short-term side-effects of levodopa therapy

Although levodopa therapy is very effective in controlling the symptoms of Parkinson's disease, most people experience a number of undesirable side-effects immediately or shortly after starting the treatment. These side-effects differ in terms of how serious or bothersome they are, and include the following:

- Nausea and vomiting can occur, and are due to dopamine stimulating the vomiting centre in the brainstem. With prolonged treatment, the vomiting centre usually becomes habituated to the presence of dopamine and no longer responds to it. Because the stimulation of the vomiting centre is most likely to occur when the amount of levodopa in the blood increases rapidly, one solution is to take your levodopa dose after a meal, as mentioned above, so that its absorption is slowed down. Another solution is to increase the dose of decarboxylase inhibitor, thus preventing the peripheral synthesis of dopamine. Alternatively, you might have to take additional medicine such as domperidone, to overcome the nausea.
- Levodopa therapy can affect the sympathetic nervous system, which controls the heart and blood vessels. As a result postural hypotension—that is, a drop in blood pressure when you stand up—can develop. In fact, blood pressure could fall so low that you might feel dizzy and faint. These problems can be partly overcome by taking salt tablets, or wearing elastic stockings to constrict the blood vessels of the legs.
- Psychotic symptoms such as hallucinations, delusions and confusion are experienced by about 20 per cent of people taking levodopa. Psychotic symptoms occur more frequently in older people with a later onset of the disease. Other possible mental effects include restlessness during sleep, vivid dreams and nightmares. Depression may be made worse by levodopa therapy. These problems can be partly overcome by reducing the total dosage, and by taking the last dose before going to bed.
- Sleep disturbance is a side-effect of levodopa therapy that can be troublesome both to the person with the illness and to his or her spouse or partner. Sleep problems, which tend to increase with the length of treatment, are mainly caused by the alerting effect of levodopa. Insomnia, a common complaint, can be partly overcome by not taking any medication after the evening meal. Another common side-effect is sleep fragmentation, in which the patient experiences many brief awakenings throughout the night. As well as more vivid dreaming, jerky movements during sleep can be problematic.
- Another side-effect of levodopa treatment is the discoloration of urine and sweat. Before the kidneys eliminate the levodopa absorbed in the intestine, it is broken down into dopamine and then into a series of inert substances, one of which is melanin, a pigment that varies in colour from orange to red to brown. When melanin is discharged into the urine it gives it a reddish colour that can leave

stains on underwear—but this should not cause alarm. Similarly, when a small amount of levodopa is secreted through the sweat glands, the sweat too can occasionally be of a dark colour and discolour clothes.

The long-term complications of levodopa therapy

Levodopa has proved not to be the miracle drug it promised to be. With long-term use adverse reactions develop. After three to five years of levodopa therapy, the majority of people with Parkinson's disease experience some loss of benefit as well as medication-induced complications. These complications, which affect 90 per cent of those treated for ten or more years, include unwanted involuntary movements, or *dyskinesias*, and *response fluctuations*. Response fluctuations include the 'wearing-off' effect, a gradual loss of benefit at the end of the dose, and 'on–off fluctuations', which are more abrupt episodes of loss of benefit. We will discuss these long-term side-effects at some length, as they influence the patient's quality of life later on in the illness and become a main focus of medical management.

Dyskinesias The dyskinesias, or involuntary movements, induced by levodopa are commonly *chorea* (dance-like writhing movements) and *dystonia* (involuntary muscle contractions or spasms producing abnormal postures). They can also take the form of jerks or muscle twitches, and may affect a variety of muscle groups in the face, neck, trunk and limbs, and sometimes the chest or diaphragm. Dyskinesias occur either at the peak or at the end of the dose. In his book, Ivan Vaughan graphically describes his experience:

> My body is possessed of two demons. Off the drugs, with too little dopamine in the system, I suffer the three classic symptoms of Parkinson's disease: trembling, rigidity and slowness of movement . . . With surplus drugs swilling around in my bloodstream, another demon takes over and my body begins to writhe to a different tune. My arms seem double-jointed as they snake up to my face, the hands bending grotesquely at right-angles . . . Of the two demons, I prefer the drugless rather than the drugged.

Sidney Dorros, who described his experiences of the illness in his book *Parkinson's Disease: A Patient's View*, also gives a vivid description of dyskinesias—in contrast to Vaughan, he states a preference for the 'overdosed, dyskinetic' state:

> At times, though, the dyskinesia was so extreme that I felt as if I was spinning in a centrifuge. My arms and legs seemed to be

pulling from their sockets, my inner organs seemed to be pressing to get outside my body or to turn themselves inside out. My muscles, particularly in my arms and around my shoulders, developed very sharp pains and cramps. The dyskinesia could be almost entirely eliminated by reducing the dosage of medication to the point of slight underdose, but underdosage was so disabling, depressing, and frightening that I preferred to be slightly over-dosed even at the cost of involuntary movements.

Dyskinesias may develop as a result of dopamine receptors (see p. 73) becoming supersensitive over time. Once these involuntary movements have developed, they can be induced by even very small doses of levodopa—clear evidence of intolerance and receptor-supersensitivity. It is not clear what determines when the dyskinesias develop, but there is some evidence that both the likelihood of developing them and their severity increase with higher dosages and the length of the therapy.

Gradual 'wearing-off' effect, or end-of-dose deterioration   After some years of levodopa therapy, a proportion of patients become aware of the effect of individual doses: that is, they know when the medication has 'taken' and is working, and when it is not. After six years of the therapy, about two-thirds of people with Parkinson's develop 'end-of-dose akinesia', or the 'wearing-off' effect. The individual complains that the beneficial effect of the drug wears off two or three hours after the last dose. And with continued treatment, the degree of benefit from each dose lasts for a yet shorter period. While initially the benefits of a dose would last from six to eight hours, later on they may disappear after half an hour. The individual experiences this as a gradual slowing down. An analogy has been drawn with a clock or a mechanical toy that requires winding up. It is not known what precisely it is that causes this wearing-off effect, but it may be related to a reduced capacity of the remaining neurones in the substantia nigra to synthesise, take up and store dopamine.

Rapid on–off fluctuations   With long-term levodopa therapy, periods of slowness, immobility, stiffness or tremor, sometimes com-bined with depression, may occur. These 'off' episodes alternate with 'on' periods when the medication is working effectively and the indi-vidual is mobile, relatively symptom-free, alert and able to work. The 'off' periods occur mainly in the afternoon and evening and last several hours, and once these fluctuations start the duration of benefit from each dose may be reduced to two or three hours. In addition, during the 'on' periods involuntary movements, or dyskinesias, may develop. The term 'on–off fluctuations' to describe these rapid and sudden swings in efficacy of levodopa therapy during the day was first used by a patient of Dr Roger Duvoisin's, who compared the alerting and mobilising effect of the drug to the switching-on of a light and the sudden return of the Parkinsonian symptoms to the light going off. Such fluctuations in the psychomotor state of the individual with Parkinson's first appear two to five years after starting levodopa therapy, and occur several times a day. Each swing in mobility and mood lasts from one to three hours. Initially the fluctuations may be relatively regular and predictable, but later they may occur relatively randomly so that planning work-related, social and leisure activities becomes impossible.

In his book *A Shadow over My Brain: My Struggle with Parkinson's Disease*, child psychiatrist Cecil Todes describes his experience of on–off fluctuations:

> How often did I find myself in my dinner suit, all primed for a party, sitting in the car or driving about outside, waiting for the drug to come through. Life with Parkinson's disease was a continual personal battle of trying to gain stability on drugs. The precarious balance between being Off and being On and moving into dyskinesia (grimaces) was very difficult to achieve.

The exact mechanisms of these long-term complications are not fully understood, but three main factors may play a role in their development.

1   It is possible that these side-effects are related to the by-products of breaking down dopamine. Long-term dopamine replacement therapy may contribute to the pathogenesis of the disorder, as it increases the production of toxic free radicals (see p. 26) resulting from the breakdown of dopamine. These substances could speed up the degeneration of dopamine-producing neurones in the substantia nigra. Research suggests that the incidence and development time of these levodopa-induced complications correlates with the duration of levodopa therapy and the cumulative dosage taken by the patient over many years.

2   However, levodopa therapy cannot be the only factor responsible for the development of fluctuations, because before it was introduced as a treatment for Parkinson's disease, fluctuations in motor function were already noted. In other words, the variability in motor function occurs with the progression of the illness, with or without levodopa therapy. Progression itself, then, is another important factor that results in the loss of dopaminergic neurones and terminals. The loss of dopaminergic terminals in the striatum means that the storage and regulation of the activity of dopamine in this area are also

impaired. As the illness progresses, levodopa can no longer compensate for the dopamine deficiency in the striatum because there are too few neurones remaining in the substantia nigra to synthesise enough dopamine to stimulate the dopamine receptors in the striatum.

3 Most importantly, perhaps, the reduced levodopa benefit after long-term therapy may partly result from a change in the brain's sensitivity to dopamine, whereby a process of 'down regulation', or subsensitivity, of striatal dopamine receptors develops.

The management of the long-term complications of levodopa therapy

As already noted, after ten years of treatment 90 per cent of people with Parkinson's who are on levodopa are affected by response fluctuations, and these fluctuations constitute one of the major therapeutic challenges facing doctors in the management of the illness. A number of strategies, already mentioned, are used to prevent or delay the development of the response fluctuations. The overall aim is to minimise the cumulative amount of levodopa that people take over the course of their illness:

- delaying the start of levodopa therapy until it is indicated by moderate to severe disability in daily activities
- using the lowest dose of levodopa that will control the symptoms
- combining levodopa therapy with a dopamine agonist that will permit the use of a smaller dosage of levodopa.

To minimise these fluctuations and dyskinesias once they have developed, a number of strategies, some of them already mentioned, are employed:

- The dosage of levodopa is fractionated, so that smaller doses are taken more frequently during the day.
- A dopamine agonist such as bromocriptine or pergolide is added to levodopa—again, to permit the levodopa dosage to be reduced.
- A low-protein diet is recommended, or protein intake is rescheduled, so that amino acids in the diet do not interfere with levodopa absorption and entry to the brain.
- Brief 'drug holidays' for a day or so are considered, to allow the resetting of dopamine receptors which have been overworked during levodopa therapy.
- Methods of continuous dopaminergic stimulation are introduced to

prevent the rises and falls of the levodopa level in the blood, which are partly responsible for the fluctuations in mobility and the dyskinesias.

Several methods for continuous dopaminergic stimulation have been developed and used.

- The standard Sinemet and Madopar tablets are absorbed in about 30 minutes. Sinemet CR (controlled release) and Madopar CR are special preparations that allow the gradual and controlled release of levodopa into the stomach over four to five hours, thereby maintaining adequate drug levels in the blood for about eight hours. In effect, instead of a sharp rise and fall, the CR tablets allow a steadier level of levodopa in the bloodstream over a longer period. As a result, the CR preparations produce longer 'on' and shorter 'off' periods, smooth the wearing-off response and reduce the number of tablets that have to be taken each day; in fact, they can effectively control on–off fluctuations in a proportion of cases. They are more effective in those who have had the disease for a shorter time, and who have also been on levodopa therapy for a shorter time. The tablets must be swallowed whole with a glass of water.
- A small battery-operated mobile pump system, which includes a needle for insertion into the side of the abdomen, is used for continuous subcutaneous delivery of dopamine agonists. The pump itself can be carried in a pocket or attached to a belt. Subcutaneous delivery of lisuride controls motor fluctuations in many people, but it can also produce psychiatric side-effects. Continuous subcutaneous injection of apomorphine, another dopamine agonist, has been more successful. The only drawback with this method is that many people find the pump too difficult to cope with. An easier alternative is the Penject system, which provides a single-shot subcutaneous injection of apomorphine.
- Continuous delivery of levodopa into the duodenum (a part of the small intestine) has been used to overcome the possibility that irregular emptying of the stomach may be partly responsible for unpredictable absorption of levodopa into the bloodstream. At the moment, the procedure is too complicated to be generally applicable.
- Intravenous injections are another way of reducing fluctuations, but this is not a particularly practical method.

When should levodopa therapy be started?

Because of the disabling nature of the long-term complications associated with levodopa therapy, medical opinion is divided about when it should be started. Those who believe that the optimal period of therapy lasts for about two to five years, recommend withholding treatment until it is absolutely necessary and then using as small a dose as possible for as long as possible. Others believe that the development of levodopa response complications is a function of the progression of the disease and disease severity rather than of treatment duration. These, therefore, consider that to withhold levodopa therapy is inappropriate.

There is also evidence that by delaying the complications of immobility, treatment with levodopa increases life expectancy. As already noted, therapy has not altered the rate of progression of the underlying disease pathology, but the symptomatic deterioration has been slowed down. Before the levodopa era, within five years of onset 28 per cent of people with Parkinson's disease were severely disabled (as measured on the Hoehn and Yahr scale, stages 4 or 5; see p. 53) or had died. In the post-levodopa era, only 9 per cent of people treated with the drug reach the stage of severe disability within the first five years. Before the introduction of levodopa, mean life expectancy was ten years after onset, and slightly higher with a younger age of onset. Since the use of levodopa, 60 per cent of people with the illness live to the age of 75, compared to 25 per cent previously.

These various considerations need to be weighed against each other when deciding when to start levodopa therapy. Since the circumstances and needs of each person are unique, a doctor can only inform the individual and the family concerned of the available options and their likely benefits and side-effects, then in light of his or her expertise make recommendations in the individual case. This advice depends on the age of the person as well as on his or her personal circumstances. For example, for someone with young-onset Parkinson's, who will have to live and cope with the disease for 30 to 40 years, consideration of the present quality of life needs to be balanced against long-term future prospects. Here it might be best to postpone levodopa medication for as long as possible. In contrast, for a 75-year old with Parkinson's disease, the quality of life in the short term should be made a priority, and levodopa introduced when disability first appears.

Ultimately, doctors can only inform and offer expert recommendations. The decision about whether or not to take levodopa medication and when to start it should always be taken by the patient. Ivan Vaughan states his personal preference clearly:

Of the two demons, I prefer the drugless rather than the drugged
... Yet there can be massive pressure from doctors (who should
know better) and people around me to take as many drugs as are
necessary to mask the symptoms of Parkinson's—but these
people do not fully admit the consequences and discomfort of
L-dopa's side-effects. You can manage more easily on the drugs;
you are less of a burden on those around you; but the social
consequences of the writhing side-effects can be as daunting to
the sufferer as the symptoms they 'cure' ... I am not saying that
being on the drug, even with side-effects of dyskinesia, is worse
or that people are daft for taking the drugs. But, given my personality, I prefer the non-drug state. In a strange way I feel more in
control, even though I have less control in a motor sense.

Dopamine Agonists

Dopamine agonists are another class of medication used in the treatment
of Parkinson's disease.

As described in Chapter 1, neurotransmitters are chemical messengers of the brain that allow the transmission of information between
neurones, which are separated from each other by clefts called synapses.
One neurone releases its neurotransmitter, which then acts on receptors
on the next neurone, and so on. The information is transmitted across
the synapse by a neurotransmitter stimulating the post-synaptic receptors—that is, the receptors of the second neurone on the other side of
the synapse. In the brain each neurotransmitter—such as dopamine,
acetylcholine or noradrenaline—has special receptor cells that selectively respond only to neurotransmitters of its own kind. The lock-and-
key analogy is often used here: each neurotransmitter is like a key that
opens only the door to its own lock, or receptor.

Besides the naturally occurring neurotransmitters, there are synthetic
substances, called *receptor agonists*, that are similar enough in their
chemical structure to fool the receptors into accepting and responding
to them. The several types of dopamine receptors that exist in the brain
are known as D1, D2, D3, D4 and D5 receptors. Dopamine itself can
act on all of these receptors; stimulation of D2 receptors is most important for the relief of the symptoms of Parkinson's.

Bromocriptine (brand name, Parlodel), lisuride (brand name,
Dopergine), pergolide (brand name, Permax) and apomorphine are synthetic dopamine receptor agonists (Table 3). Each drug operates by
directly stimulating post-synaptic dopamine receptors. As described
on p. 71, apomorphine is currently given by injection using a small
battery-operated pump or by means of the Penject system. When tremor

is severe, the patient may need help in operating either of these.

Although generally less effective than levodopa, dopamine agonists have several advantages. Unlike levodopa, these substances do not have to be converted to dopamine in order to be effective, and the absence of a conversion process alleviates some of the side-effects of levodopa. In addition, by directly stimulating dopamine receptors, dopamine agonists lower the rate of dopamine turnover in the brain and thereby reduce the toxic by-products of breaking down and metabolising dopamine. Because of this they may do less damage to dopaminergic neurones. Moreover, they do not compete with other amino acids for absorption, and so neither the amount of proteins in the diet nor the time of eating proteins affects dopamine agonist medication.

It was originally hoped that dopamine agonists would replace levodopa, and thus eliminate or reduce its associated complications as well. But long-term experience has shown that their efficacy is limited. This is partly because whereas there are several types of dopamine agonist in the brain, the currently available agonists mainly stimulate D2, receptors, and it may be that the stimulation of all types of dopamine receptors is necessary for maximum effect. Furthermore, although for the first few months of treatment dopamine agonists such as bromocriptine can be as effective as levodopa, in the long term they are not.

The short-term side-effects of dopamine agonists are similar to those produced by levodopa, but more noticeable and distressing. They include nausea and vomiting, loss of weight, hypotension, sleep disturbance, depression and agitation, confusion, hallucination, dyskinesias, cardiac arrhythmias, nasal stuffiness, dry mouth and headache.

Each of the various types of dopamine agonist that are currently available alleviate the symptoms of Parkinson's disease to a similar extent. But particular individuals may respond better to a particular one. Absence of effect or intolerance of one dopamine agonist does not mean that others will not be effective: sometimes when one loses its efficacy, its replacement by another dopamine agonist restores the benefit. Dopamine agonists are mainly used in conjunction with levodopa therapy. To reduce or postpone the long-term complications of levodopa therapy it is recommended that pharmacotherapy is initially started with a combination of levodopa and dopamine agonists.

Anticholinergics

As long ago as 1869, extracts of the plants *Hyoscyamus niger* and belladonna, which have anticholinergic effects, were used by the French neurologist Jean-Martin Charcot in the treatment of Parkinson's disease.

As is evident from their name, anticholinergics are a class of drugs that operate by blocking the action of the neurotransmitter acetylcholine in the brain. This blocking action has beneficial effects on the symptoms of Parkinson's disease, but also produces side-effects.

Benzhexol/trihexyphenidyl (Artane), orphenadrine (Disipal), benztropine (Cogentin) and procyclidine (Kemadrin) are anticholinergics used in the treatment of early and mild Parkinson's disease (Table 3), mainly to postpone the introduction of levodopa therapy. As these drugs have a period of action of four to six hours, doses are taken three or four times daily. The main benefit of anticholinergics is in reducing tremor, excessive salivation and dysphagia. They also alleviate rigidity, or muscle stiffness. Bradykinesia, and balance and walking problems, are not so well alleviated. Anticholinergics, also called cholinergic antagonists, are not as effective as levodopa.

Besides the concern inherent in giving cholinergic antagonists to people with Parkinson's disease, a disorder with some cortical cholinergic deficit, there is the problem of the side-effects. These include blurred vision, constipation, dry mouth, urinary retention, reduced sweating, and a number of mental and cognitive side-effects. Particularly problematic in the elderly person with Parkinson's may be forgetfulness and memory loss, depression, confusion and hallucinations. The older patient with signs of dementia is specially at risk to the negative effects of anticholinergics. Treatment with these drugs is not advisable if the patient has glaucoma or prostate problems.

Anticholinergics should be withdrawn gradually—sudden withdrawal can result in the return of the symptoms and produce anxiety.

Amantadine

Amantadine (Symmetrel) was initially introduced as an antiviral agent. It was by chance that it was first found to have some anti-Parkinsonian effect. A 58-year-old woman with Parkinson's disease, under the care of the American neurologist Dr Schwab, was taking amantadine as a prevention against the flu when she noticed that her rigidity, akinesia and tremor were unexpectedly alleviated. This beneficial effect was later replicated in wider-scale clinical studies. The precise mechanism of action of Amantadine is unknown, but it seems to have some anticholinergic properties as well as enhancing dopaminergic transmission by increasing the release of dopamine or blocking dopamine re-uptake.

Amantadine alleviates slowness of movements, particularly fine movements, and improves posture and facial mobility. It also has some beneficial effects on akinesia and rigidity, but tremor is not much relieved. The improvements are noticeable after two weeks of first starting the drug. A daily dose of 200–300mg is usual, and is well tolerated by younger people with Parkinson's. Its benefit usually wears off after three to four months. The side-effects of amantadine are blurred vision, dry mouth, constipation, confusion, hallucinations, an unusual rash on the lower limbs called livedo reticularis, and oedema (accumulation of fluid in spaces between cells), all of which disappear when the drug is discontinued.

When directly compared to other anti-Parkinsonian medication, amantadine has been found to be less effective than levodopa but better than anticholinergics. It is primarily used as the sole medication for short-term therapy (six to twelve months) in people with mild to moderately severe symptoms. It helps to postpone levodopa therapy.

Selegiline

Monoamine oxidase (MAO) is the enzyme that breaks down dopamine, and it exists in two forms, A and B. MAO type A is found in the adrenal glands, heart, liver and other bodily organs; MAO type B is present in the brain. Substances that inhibit the action of MAO type A prevent the breakdown of dopamine as well as of adrenaline and of noradrenaline. MAO-A inhibitors are used as antidepressants. They should not be taken with food containing the amino acid tyramine, such as cheese, red wine, pickled herrings and Marmite, as they result in the so-called 'cheese effect'—that is, fluctuations in blood pressure and hypertensive crises.

Selegiline (Deprenyl, Eldepryl) is an MAO type B inhibitor, which has the unique feature of selectively blocking the action of MAO-B, so preventing the breakdown of dopamine in the brain, while allowing the normal degradation of other monoamines such as noradrenaline, adrenaline and serotonin. With selegiline no dietary restriction is required. Its mode of action is different from that of other medication.

The recommended daily dose of selegiline is between 5 and 10mg. As it may cause insomnia if taken at night, it is usually taken in the morning. There are two reasons why the daily dose of selegiline is kept low. First, 5mg inhibits MAO-B, the enzyme that breaks down dopamine in the brain, by 90 per cent. Second, with a daily dose higher than 20mg the selective action of selegiline on MAO-B is lost, and it also inhibits MAO-A so that the 'cheese effect' is more likely to occur.

Selegiline was first used as a treatment for Parkinson's disease by Dr Birkmayer and his colleagues in Vienna in the early 1980s. Subsequently, the demonstration that in laboratory animals the effects of

MPTP, the toxin that selectively destroys neurones in the substantia nigra, could be prevented by prior administration of selegiline further confirmed the potential value of selegiline. Clinical trials were restarted, in which Drs Tetrud and Langston demonstrated that for patients on selegiline the symptoms worsened at a rate that required the introduction of levodopa after 548 days. In contrast, for those on a placebo (not a drug, but an inert substance) the introduction of levodopa was required after 312 days. In other words, treatment with selegiline delayed the need to start levodopa therapy by about eight months. The larger multicentre DATATOP (Deprenyl and Tocopherol Antioxidant Therapy of Parkinsonism) study, in which the long-term effects of treatment with selegiline were examined, obtained similar results, showing that Deprenyl delayed the need for the introduction of levodopa by an average of 13 months. However, when people with Parkinson's disease who took part in the DATATOP study were followed up, the results suggested that the benefits of selegiline were short-lived. Another large-scale study by the Parkinson's Disease Research Group in the UK suggested that, in the long term, levodopa in combination with selegiline seemed to produce no clinical benefits over levodopa alone. The results of this study also suggested that the long-term mortality rates were higher for those taking levodopa with selegiline than for those taking levodopa alone. This is clearly an issue that requires further investigation.

For patients whose Parkinson's disease starts in their sixties, where short-term symptomatic control and enhanced quality of life may be a priority, the combined use of selegiline and levodopa may be appropriate. When taken with levodopa, selegiline increases the duration of action of levodopa and prolongs the benefit from each dose. But at the same time the side-effects of levodopa may be accentuated, and it may become necessary to reduce the levodopa dosage. Selegiline may also be useful for people with Parkinson's disease who have developed on–off fluctuations after long-term levodopa therapy.

In the short term selegiline has no major side-effects of its own except, sometimes, insomnia and nausea. The side-effects that patients experience are mainly those associated with levodopa. Selegiline is not recommended for people with peptic ulcer. It may have an antidepressant effect that can be helpful for those who have become depressed. An occasional side-effect of long-term levodopa therapy, or when selegiline is added, is hypomania—a sense of well-being, mild euphoria, enhanced ambition, increased talkativeness, increased sexual desire and excessive motor activity and agitation. To prevent hypomania, the dose may have to be reduced.

Other Medication

Besides the major classes of medication used in the treatment of Parkinson's disease, which are summarised in Table 3, other drugs are used to deal with specific problems.

When tremor is the main problem, it may not respond very well to levodopa therapy or to anticholinergics in small doses. Propanolol, which is a drug normally used to treat high blood pressure or an irregular pulse, often proves effective in suppressing tremor; it has no effect on the other symptoms of Parkinson's disease. Alternatively, low doses of the minor tranquilliser diazepam (Valium) may be used to control tremor. Painful rigidity of the muscles is treated with muscle relaxants.

Occasionally, minor tranquillisers such as Valium, lorazepam (Ativan) and oxazepam (Serax) are used to overcome the restlessness or insomnia that can sometimes accompany Parkinson's disease. The problem with the use of these drugs is that in Parkinson's disease they can produce drowsiness, dizziness and sometimes increased slowness. Also, with prolonged use physical and pyschological dependence may develop, such that their withdrawal will result in agitation and nervousness.

When it is severe, depression in Parkinson's disease needs to be treated directly with antidepressant medication. The tricyclic class of antidepressants is often used; these also have a mild anticholinergic action which can be beneficial in Parkinson's, and a mild sedative effect that can help with insomnia.

Constipation in Parkinson's disease is due to the reduced motility of the muscles of the bowel, and it is worsened by some types of anti-Parkinsonian medication. It is best treated by increasing the intake of water and dietary fibre, but if these are not effective, it may become necessary to use laxatives or enemas. Diuretics can be useful in relieving the swelling of the legs and feet that can occur in Parkinson's as a result of bradykinesia and the reduced muscular activity and mobility of the limbs. As mentioned earlier, akinesia results in reduced mobility and lubrication of the eyes, and soreness, redness and scaliness of the eyelids. Artificial tears that mimic the liquid and salt composition of natural tears can help to increase the eyes' lubrication. Seborrhoea, scaliness and oiliness of the skin and hair, can be reduced by levodopa treatment; frequent washing of the face with special oil-controlling soaps and the hair with dandruff-controlling shampoos can also help to deal with the problem.

Drug Holidays

At times it may become necessary to stop taking anti-Parkinsonian medication for a number of days, or even weeks. For instance, it may have to be stopped for a few days when the patient is undergoing surgery that involves a general anaesthetic, and for a few weeks before trying a new type of tablet. Sometimes, stopping medication for a few weeks can make the drugs more effective when they are restarted.

This period of being off all medication is called a 'drug holiday'. Withdrawal of medication can make the symptoms much worse, and the patient immobile. For these reasons drug holidays can be dangerous, and should always be medically supervised and ideally carried out during hospitalisation. The patient should never stop his or her medication without consultation. When surgery or treatment for other medical complaints is to be undertaken, it is important to inform the surgeon or other doctors concerned about the Parkinson's disease and the medication used to treat it.

SURGERY

Surgical treatment of Parkinson's disease has a history that goes back to the early 1900s. Those early surgical procedures involved *lesioning*—that is, cutting or destroying small areas of the brain that control movement. Complications were common, and success was very variable. A much safer technique, using *stereotaxic surgery*, was first developed in the United States in 1947 by Drs Spiegel and Wycis. It was applied to the treatment of Parkinson's disease in the 1950s by, among others, Professor Narabayashi in Tokyo and Dr Cooper in the United States. In stereotaxic surgery a special frame is fixed to the skull, then a hole is made in the skull and a needle-like electrical probe is inserted into the brain to produce a small focal lesion. The direction and depth of the probe insertion is determined with X-rays or scans, which are used to create a map of the various parts of the brain. This map then guides the surgeon during the operation. The procedure is carried out under local anaesthetic and sedation, so that the individual is alert and can co-operate in the placement of the probe.

Between 1957 and 1972 stereotaxic surgery, mainly thalamotomies and pallidotomies (see below), was used relatively frequently to treat Parkinson's disease in various centres across the world. Since the mid-1970s, the therapeutic management of the disorder has been dominated by levodopa therapy, but more recently the long-term complications of that therapy have regenerated the interest in surgical management.

Technological advances in brain scanning have improved the precision of both stereotaxic probe insertion and the focusing of the lesion in the target area of the brain. This in turn has enhanced the success and safety of surgery. Current surgical approaches to the treatment of Parkinson's disease are thalamotomy and pallidotomy, thalamic, pallidal and subthalamic nucleus stimulation, and brain implantation.

Thalamotomy

The thalamus consists of a group of neurones that connect the basal ganglia (see p. 21) to the frontal lobes (the front part of the brain). The thalamus acts as a relay station between these areas. Thalamotomy involves placing a stereotaxic lesion in a specific part of the thalamus, usually the ventrolateral nucleus. In the late 1950s and 1960s, before the introduction of levodopa therapy, many thalamotomies were carried out on people with Parkinson's disease. These were effective for controlling tremor and to some extent rigidity, but they were less effective with bradykinesia and akinesia. The mortality associated with the procedure was 1 per cent. The major complication following bilateral thalamotomy was dysarthria, or slurring of speech. Partial paralysis of one arm and/or leg, together with memory disturbance and impairment of judgement, were other short-term complications of the procedure in a minority of cases. Now thalamotomies are recommended in special cases only—those with severe, intractable unilateral tremor.

In his book *Parkinson's Disease: A Patient's View*, Sidney Dorros gives a detailed minute-by-minute description of his thalamotomy operation, from the fitting of the frame to his head, through the drilling of a small hole in his skull to the insertion of a surgical probe to 'freeze' the target neurones. In his case, the unilateral thalamotomy, undertaken before levodopa therapy became available, was successful in that it resulted in complete elimination of tremor and rigidity on the left side of his body. However, this was accompanied by increased tremor and stiffness on his previously 'normal' right side. With hindsight, he states:

> People often ask me if I would have chosen to have the operation
> ... knowing what I do now. The answer is, 'Of course not!' But
> neither I nor anyone else knew at the time how soon a new drug
> treatment would be available that for me would be more effective
> and safer than surgery. One can only act on the best information
> available at the time of decision. On that basis, I believe my wife
> and I made the right decision.

Thalamic Stimulation

This procedure allows long-term electrical stimulation of the same area of the thalamus that is removed in a thalamotomy, and is also most suitable for controlling severe tremor. It involves the surgical insertion of high-frequency electrodes into the ventralis intermedialis nucleus of the thalamus. The electrodes are connected to a programmable stimulator surgically placed under the skin, with which the electrical stimulation of the thalamus can be turned on or off and the intensity of stimulation controlled. During stimulation, tremor in the arms is controlled, tremor in the trunk and legs may be reduced, and balance may be improved. This procedure is less risky than thalamotomy, and may be preferable to it, especially when bilateral intervention is required.

Pallidotomy

Pallidotomy—that is, the placing of a lesion in the globus pallidus, the output gateway of the basal ganglia—is one of the older surgical procedures used to treat Parkinson's disease. When this operation was performed in the 1950s and 1960s, the lesion was placed in the anterior and dorsal parts of the globus pallidus (the procedure known as anterodorsal pallidotomy). This relieved rigidity, but not the other symptoms of the disease, and it was modified in the 1950s by a Swedish neurosurgeon, Lars Leksell. This modification, which involved placing lesions in more posterior and ventral sections of the globus pallidus (known as posteroventral pallidotomy), seemed more effective and resulted in alleviation of tremor and akinesia as well as of rigidity.

Leksell's modified pallidotomy procedure has recently been refined and carried out stereotaxically. The stereotaxic map guides the surgeon, who places the needle-like probe into the appropriate part of the globus pallidus, after which a brief current is passed through the needle to create a small lesion.

Since 1985 a number of people with Parkinson's have had Leksell's pallidotomy, carried out in Sweden by Professor Laitinen and his colleagues. The operation was reportedly of great benefit, allowing medication to be reduced by 50–75 per cent. In particular, levodopa-induced dyskinesias were considerably reduced on the opposite side of the body to which the surgery was carried out. Many more patients have now had this operation in Sweden, including Anne Marshall, whose experiences are described in an issue of *YAPmag* (the magazine of the Young Alert Parkinson's Partners and Relatives group, see p. 201). A made-to-measure frame was built to hold her head in position during surgery, which was conducted under local anaesthetic. She was awake during the operation, which produced no pain, and was asked to describe her experiences while the surgery was actually being performed. Immediately after the operation the tremor in her right limbs was much less, and she could move them more freely. Her medication, Madopar, worked much more effectively and she no longer needed apomorphine.

The new pallidotomy procedure has now been carried out worldwide, and many people with Parkinson's disease have had the operation in the USA and UK. It has been successful in relieving levodopa-induced dyskinesias as well as rigidity and akinesia.

Pallidal and Subthalamic Nucleus Stimulation

These procedures are similar to thalamic stimulation, except that a different site is selected for the stimulating electrodes. The fine electrodes are inserted into the internal segment of the globus pallidus—this is for pallidal stimulation—or into the subthalamic nucleus (for STN, or subthalamic nucleus stimulation), which is another relay station between the striatum and the frontal cortex. The electrodes are then connected to a programmable stimulator surgically placed under the skin. Both high-frequency pallidal and STN stimulation have been shown to be effective in reducing bradykinesia, rigidity, tremor and dyskinesias. Compared to pallidotomy these procedures have the advantage of not destroying the target brain areas, and of being reversible.

Brain Implantation

As already explained, in idiopathic Parkinson's disease the symptoms arise from the loss of dopamine-producing neurones in a relatively small area of the brain, the substantia nigra, which results in dopamine deficiency in the striatum (see p. 22). Because of the relatively confined nature of its pathophysiology, idiopathic Parkinson's has been at the forefront of the research into *brain implantation*—used here to refer to the implantation of dopamine-producing cells into the brains of people with Parkinson's disease. The rationale is this: if the implanted cells can survive, release the deficient neurotransmitter dopamine, and establish connections with the non-functioning neurones, then partial or complete reversal of the symptoms of the disorder may be possible.

Since the 1980s, after years of experimentation on animals, it has been possible to implant into the striatum of the patient, dopamine-producing cells from his or her adrenal glands—these are situated above the kidneys and have their own dopamine-producing cells—or from tissue obtained from aborted foetuses. The first implant of adrenal tissue into the brains of four people with Parkinson's were carried out at the Karrlinska Institute in Stockholm in the early 1980s. Adrenal autografts—that is, tissue taken from the adrenal glands of the patient—were used, in order to reduce the risk of rejection of the grafted tissue. The benefits obtained were not impressive, and it was concluded that the procedure held little promise. But at about the same time in Mexico, Dr Madrazo performed the same procedure and claimed better results. Over three hundred such operations have now been carried out, mainly in the United States.

From a review of the outcome of the surgery in these cases, a number of conclusions are possible:

- The benefits were usually minimal. People with Parkinson's disease who have undergone the adrenal autograft procedure continue to require levodopa therapy, although the duration of action of the drugs may be longer and the degree of disability during 'off' periods may be smaller after the implants.
- Both the abdominal surgery to remove adrenal tissue and the neuro-surgery carry the risk of complications, which occur in about 10–20 per cent of those operated on.
- PET scans (see p. 49) in life and post-mortem studies have shown that the transplanted adrenal tissue did not survive. Therefore, the benefits obtained may have been due to the release of growth factors produced by the damaged brain tissue—these stimulate the regeneration and growth of the surviving nigrostriatal nerve terminals in the damaged striatum.
- A number of symptoms, including disruption of the sleep/wake cycle, hallucinations, delusions, confusion and mood changes, may be experienced by some people after the operation, the majority of which disappear in a few months. In a few cases, depression and sleep problems may be longer-lasting.

The general consensus is that the modest benefits of these autografts of adrenal tissue do not justify the risks of the procedure.

Subsequently experimentation on laboratory animals moved on to using tissue obtained from animal foetuses. On the basis of the better results produced by these experiments, the implant work of the Swedish team was resumed in the late 1980s using neurones from the substantia nigra of aborted human foetuses. The technique was refined by using a stereotaxic procedure and a smaller needle to inject the implant tissue into the striatum. PET scans have demonstrated that the implanted tissue survives, and can develop a blood supply and new nerve connections in the receptor site. In general, implants of foetal nigral tissue have produced better results than adrenal autografts, and several hundred people with Parkinson's disease have had them. The benefits differ from person to person, but have mainly been to do with a longer duration of 'on' time, or response to levodopa. Rigidity and slowness are most alleviated, tremor least. However, truly impressive benefits, such as complete reversal of symptoms, have not been obtained in a single case, and only one person has been able to stop all anti-Parkinsonian medication after implantation.

Dr Cecil Todes was the fourth person with Parkinson's disease to undergo brain implantation of foetal tissue in Britain. He obtained relatively little benefit from the procedure, and describes his reactions and feelings about it in his book *A Shadow over My Brain*: he felt 'disappointment in the realisation that the operation [had] been of no benefit ... I felt that having the operation when I did was premature and an ill-considered risk.'

Brain implantation as a treatment for Parkinson's disease is still experimental, and many procedural questions and ethical issues remain to be addressed. Besides the moral objections of a minority, the ethical issue of using 8–12-week-old foetal tissue has been raised, and guidelines have been drawn up. The main concern has been that, to meet the demand for transplants, a black market may develop and foetuses may be conceived and aborted for the sole purpose of providing tissue for the transplants. However, these problems may be averted by the novel methods for producing implant tissues that are currently exploring the use of cultured cells, or tissues that have been genetically engineered, to produce the desired neurotransmitter.

Long-term suppression of the patient's immune system with appropriate medication may be necessary, in order to avoid rejection of the implanted foetal tissue by his or her brain. How long this immunosuppression should be continued, and the potential risks, are unknown. There is also the possibility that the implant may eventually be subject to the same degenerative process that produced the disease in the first place. Furthermore, the efficacy of the procedure may be limited by the fact that dopamine is not the only neurotransmitter system affected in Parkinson's disease, and that other affected neurotransmitters are *not* replaced by the implanted tissue. Other procedural questions that remain to be addressed are the age span and the amount of the human foetal nigral tissue necessary for a viable implant, and the best implantation site in the striatum. Much work remains to be done before brain implantation is firmly established as a treatment for Parkinson's disease.

Who Should Have Surgery for Parkinson's Disease?

Surgery does not aim to cure the illness. As with drug therapy, the aim of surgery is to control the symptoms and to prevent or reduce disability. The other similarity with medication is that although surgery may successfully control the symptoms for a while, with progression of the illness the old symptoms may become severe enough to re-emerge or new symptoms may develop. Most people with Parkinson's who have undergone one or other of the possible surgical interventions still need to take some medication afterwards, but perhaps at reduced dosages.

The decision to undergo surgical treatment is usually taken after discussion with a neurologist and/or a neurosurgeon, who provide full information about the likely benefits, side-effects and risks. These surgical procedures are now recommended for a minority of people with Parkinson's disease—those with unilateral symptoms, those with a predominance of tremor and rigidity but relatively little akinesia and bradykinesia, younger people, and those who have developed severe levodopa-induced dyskinesias.

Undergoing surgery is a major decision which should only be taken after finding out all the relevant facts. Once the decision is made, in addition to acquiring information about the likely outcome, the patient usually finds it reassuring to find out more about the practical aspects of surgery: the procedures of admission and information about the ward, what to expect on the day of surgery, how long the operation is likely to take, what sensations and experiences to expect during stereotaxic surgery, and the process of post-surgical recovery. To be well informed helps to alleviate anxiety and fear.

KEY FACTS 3

Is there a cure?
No, unfortunately there is no cure for Parkinson's disease yet.

How can Parkinson's disease be treated?
It can be treated with medication or with surgery. Compared to other neurological illnesses, many effective forms of medical treatment are available for Parkinson's.

What are the main types of medication used?
Various kinds. Levodopa therapy (Sinemet or Madopar), dopamine agonists (bromocriptine, lisuride, pergolide, apomorphine), anticholinergics (benzhexol, benztropine, orphenadrine, procyclidine), amantadine and selegiline are the main types of medication used in the various stages of the illness.

When does drug therapy start, and for how long do I have to continue taking medication?
The decision as to when to start drug therapy is dictated by the symptoms and the associated disability of each individual, together with his or her age and life circumstances. Once treatment is started, the patient needs to remain on medication for the foreseeable future. To achieve maximum benefit, the type and level of medication may have occasionally to be altered.

What are the main types of surgery?
Thalamotomy (cutting a specific section of the thalamus) and pallidotomy (cutting a specific section of the globus pallidus) are surgical procedures that have been used to treat Parkinson's disease since the 1950s. Thalamic stimulation through surgical insertion of electrodes, and thalamotomy, are methods of treating cases of severe tremor. Pallidotomy, and pallidal and subthalamic nucleus stimulation, are used for the treatment of cases with severe levodopa-induced dyskinesias and rigidity. Also current is the implantation of dopamine-producing

cells from the adrenal glands of the patient or from the nigral tissue of aborted foetuses into the patient's brain.

What are the pros and cons of each treatment?

Levodopa therapy is the most effective treatment for Parkinson's disease, particularly for the first five years after starting it. The short-term side-effects include vomiting and nausea, low blood pressure and postural hypotension, psychotic experiences and sleep disturbance. The major drawback of levodopa therapy is that after three to five years most people develop medication-related complications such as dyskinesias, wearing-off phenomena and on–off fluctuations. The advantage of dopamine agonists, used in the treatment of Parkinson's either in the early phases when the symptoms are mild, or after levodopa-related complications emerge, is that they produce fewer of the medication-related complications associated with levodopa. But they are not as effective as levodopa and their beneficial effects tend to wear off after 18–20 months of continued use.

In the early phases when symptoms are mild, anticholinergics may be prescribed. These mainly alleviate tremor and are not as effective as levodopa. Blurring of vision, constipation, dryness of mouth, urinary retention and memory problems are among their side-effects. To control stiffness or slowness in the early phases of the illness, amantadine is occasionally added to anticholinergics.

The advantages of the available surgical procedures are listed above. In addition, tremor and slowness can be alleviated by palidotomy. Partial paralysis and slurring of speech are complications that can occur with thalamotomy.

The implantation of foetal nigral tissue into the striatum has produced some beneficial effects on motor function, but brain implantation is still in the early phases of development and only time will tell whether it is a viable treatment. Unfortunately, even in the hands of the most expert surgeons all forms of surgery carry the risk of irreversible damage to the brain, or even death.

Part II
Living with Parkinson's Disease

4

Chronic Illness

Marjan Jahanshahi and Brigid MacCarthy

This chapter gives you background information about the general as well as the more specific ways in which a chronic illness such as Parkinson's disease can affect the lives of the individual concerned and of his or her family. Stress, and its effect on mental and physical well-being, has been a topic of intensive research. This research has increased our understanding of how people react to and cope with stressful life events, and of the factors that are important in determining good or poor coping. The onset of a chronic, progressive and disabling illness such as Parkinson's is undoubtedly a major life event.

We believe that knowing about the variety of reactions to stress and loss, and finding out which environmental and personal factors influence an individual's ability to face the challenge of stressful life events, can be helpful in several ways.

- It will prepare the person with Parkinson's disease, and his or her carer and family, for what to expect.
- It shows that a large proportion of those who experience stressful life events cope remarkably well.
- It gives insight into the personal and environmental resources that individuals need in order to arm themselves against the impact of stressful life events.

STRESS, APPRAISAL, SOCIAL SUPPORT AND COPING

To most of us, the concept of stress is a familiar one. The term entered common usage in the 1960s, and ever since then the public has been aware of stress as something to be avoided. From a commonsense understanding of stress we tend to assume that its effects are simple and obvious: that when something unpleasant or difficult to handle happens to them, people feel bad, either physically or mentally. However, most readers will recognise from their own experience that this straightforward equation—stressful event leads to adverse reaction—fails to describe the complex process of adjustment when they are 'under stress'. Research evidence has also clearly demonstrated that individuals show enormous variation in how they respond to basically similar stresses. This has led scientists to develop more subtle, complex descriptions, or 'models', of how people cope with stress.

Stress is difficult to define. In current thinking on stress and coping, it is defined in deliberately general terms, as changes in the relationship between a person and his or her environment. When some major change happens, whether pleasant or unpleasant, the individual has to make some effort to adjust to the new circumstances. This adjustment will draw on personal resources—physical, mental or social. A 'change' becomes a 'stress' when there is a marked imbalance between the effort required to adjust and the personal resources available.

Psychologists have studied the degree to which major life events such as the death of a loved one, marriage, divorce, the onset of a disabling illness, the birth of a child, the loss of one's job, moving house, children moving away from home, are perceived and experienced as stressful. Two main findings of this research are of interest:

1　There is general consensus about which life events are perceived and experienced as more or less stressful. For most people the death of a loved one such as a spouse or a child is the most stressful of all. In general, events that are unexpected and over which the individual has less control, such as death and illness, create most stress.
2　Apparently positive life events such as marriage, the birth of a child or promotion at work are also stressful. So it is obvious that stress is created by any change, whether positive or negative, that outstrips the individual's ability to cope.

The harmful effects of stress on physical and mental health are produced by various means. First, stress creates a biological and physiological imbalance in the body. Second, under stress people are more likely to engage in potentially harmful behaviours such as smoking, or excessive alcohol or food consumption. Harmful effects can be measured in terms of subjective feelings of well-being and physical health. However, these effects are never static. While individuals try to adjust to and cope with stressful life events, these coping efforts, in turn, influence and redefine the nature of the stressful event. So instead of coping with stress being a question of a few simple reactions, an adequate understanding of how individuals deal with it requires consideration of three sets of factors—what we might call antecedents, mediating factors, and outcomes.

Antecedents

The first set of factors to consider, present before the stressful event happens, can be summarised as *environmental conditions* and *personal characteristics*. By 'environmental conditions' we mean the social and economic resources and constraints to which all individuals are subject. These include the amount and quality of *social support* available—that is, people in the individual's environment on whom he or she can rely, to whom he or she can turn for practical support, and for emotional ventilation, sympathy and understanding. At times of stress or crisis, social support may be provided by family, friends or colleagues. Emotional support takes the form of gestures of understanding, caring, comfort and sympathy which help people to feel less isolated under stress.

When an individual is facing major changes, access to both kinds of support, practical and emotional, has been shown to contribute much to his or her eventual sense of well-being. To function as an effective buffer against stress, the quantity and quality of the social support provided must match the individual's needs. In the context of chronic disease, high levels of uncalled-for social support may at times constitute a threat to autonomy and independence, and in effect reduce his or her sense of self-worth. Ultimately, it is for the individual to perceive the amount and quality of social support available as satisfactory and matching his or her needs. For some people, a few intimate relationships are adequate, whereas for others a network of support from friends and family is required.

Financial security can also cushion the impact of many different kinds of stress. In the personal accounts given by people encountering stress there are many instances of households being better able to cope by having ready access to goods and services that can be bought.

Personal characteristics include individual motives and beliefs about the self and the world. Self-esteem (see p. 276), or the beliefs, attitudes and feelings that each of us has about our worth as a person, is a strong determinant of reactions to and coping with stress. Motives are shaped by the goals to which we have made a commitment, and by our value system. Personal goals and values tend to be formed in young adulthood and change little during adult life. They set our priorities for action and shape our emotional and practical responses when we are faced with stress. Beliefs concerning the degree to which events are perceived as personally controllable or due to chance affect our approach to coping with those events. In the case of a physical disorder, the degree to which symptoms are objectively controllable, the rate of progression of the disorder, and our beliefs about whether our health is under our own personal control or under external control by powerful others such as doctors, or chance factors, are all likely to be important in the choice of the strategies we use to cope with illness. These personal characteristics contribute to our perception of events in our lives and determine the way in which we eventually cope.

Mediating Factors

As we said before, the relationship between stress and coping is not direct or simple. In fact, it can be tracked along a number of complex routes. Thus the impact of stress on the individual is influenced or moderated by a number of mediating factors, the most important of which are personal appraisal and coping strategies.

It has been said that, like beauty, stress is in the eye of the beholder. Events are not inherently stressful—they are interpreted as so. To experience an event as stressful, a person has first to appraise or label it as such. The process of *appraisal*, which begins when an individual notices the onset of a stressful change, involves an evaluation of that change as either beneficial or harmful. The outcome of this judgement will depend on the external circumstances and personal beliefs and values described above, and will in turn determine how the individual chooses to cope. The concept of appraisal is central to the argument that personal perception and interpretation play a significant role in determining eventual well-being under stress. An event that fills one person with dread may strike another as an interesting challenge, an opportunity for personal development or the pursuit of important goals. Such non-threatening appraisals of potentially stressful life events can substantially diminish their negative impact on the individual. The importance of appraisal in determining the outcome of stressful events shows that we all have access to psychological mechanisms within ourselves that can help us combat stress.

The concept of *coping* is equally difficult to define. Coping is considered to refer to all the various ways in which an individual faced with a stress-inducing situation, or stressor, tries to deal with or overcome his or her problems. These include his or her practical efforts, as well as the mental and emotional strategies he or she uses to come to terms with or reduce the emotional impact of the stressor. In general, people try to cope in two main ways: either by actively trying to change some aspect of their environment or of events, referred to as problem-focused coping, or by controlling the negative emotions they experience as a result of the stressful change—referred to as emotion-focused coping. Health-related examples of problem-focused strategies include seeking information about alternative therapies, participating in a medical treatment, or finding a new job which minimises the impact of disability. The individual may also focus his or her coping efforts on changing the way that he or she interprets a specific stress, in order to change its emotional meaning. These efforts are not passive, but involve an active process of restructuring of goals and values in line with the limitations imposed by the event. Examples of such emotion-focused strategies are finding new interests, discovering new faith or a different philosophy of life, and changing priorities.

When faced with the stress of illness, besides using strategies for controlling the symptoms, most people look for social support and resort to emotion-focused coping. Research has shown that when people seek to combat the demands of chronic physical illness, certain sorts of coping strategy—such as information-seeking or action-taking— lead to positive well-being. In contrast, strategies involving avoidance, denial and blame are related to distress and a poorer overall adjustment to the illness. So coping strategies differ in terms of their effect on the individual's short-term or long-term adjustment, and can be either adaptive or maladaptive. Any coping strategies that improve people's adjustment to their new situation and enhance their sense of well-being are considered adaptive. Coping strategies that interfere with acceptance and adjustment are labelled maladaptive.

Clearly, not all coping strategies are equally effective, although research findings indicate that it is important to keep an open mind about what particular strategies are likely to be effective in particular circumstances. Misusing alcohol and drugs and unnecessary risk-taking are two prevalent strategies that seem rarely to have a positive effect. Denial and emotional distancing are less clearly maladaptive. In some circumstances—again, depending on the exact relationship between external circumstances and personal resources—they may be the only viable option.

Of course, no one relies exclusively on either problem-focused or emotion-focused efforts to cope. People who use a range of specific coping strategies have more positive outcomes, but it also seems that those who use systematically a limited number of ways of coping do better than those who grab randomly at a large number of strategies.

Efforts focused on changing emotions and personal interpretations are likely to be more effective in situations where the source of stress is relatively intractable, while problem-focused efforts have more impact when there is considerable scope for manipulating external circumstances. In Western societies, stoicism, bearing it all with a smile, the stiff upper lip, being in control—however it may be described—is a highly valued coping style. In practice, this idealistic but rather superficial means of coping can be kept up for only a short while, and usually at great emotional cost. More effective and realistic coping needs to incorporate and allow emotional expression, as well as more problem-focused ways of adjusting to illness.

Outcomes

Finally, and most importantly, it is worth taking a fresh look at the outcomes of coping. What do we mean by saying that an individual coped well with a stressful event? As we noted before, good and poor outcomes are defined in terms of the individual's adjustment to his or her circumstances and physical and psychological well-being. Satisfactory outcomes are associated with improved adjustment and physical and psychological well-being. Deterioration in adjustment and in physical and mental health are features of unsatisfactory outcomes. In the case of a chronic illness, we might also examine the effect of the patient's emotional state on his or her longer-term physical well-being. The significance of this latter factor has been harder to demonstrate clearly, perhaps because of the inevitable deterioration that is a feature of most chronic illnesses.

It is clear that many factors contribute to the way in which stressful events, such as the onset of a chronic illness, affect people. There is some evidence that the longer-term effects of stress are more closely related to an individual's expectations and aspirations than to external circumstances. Coping efforts bent on either meeting or changing personal agendas are likely, therefore, to be more successful. Indeed, personal accounts of coping with stress make it very clear that people are capable of infinitely flexible and courageous adaptations to very difficult circumstances.

In writing about his experiences of living with Parkinson's disease, Ivan Vaughan likens the stress of the illness to standing in front of a dam that is starting to leak. As a coping mechanism, he at first resorted to minimising the significance of the diagnosis:

I felt as though I were standing in front of a dam. The walls were springing leaks in different places one after another. I raced round frantically trying to patch them up, but with my eyes closed in case I caught sight of the flood of water that threatened to engulf me. I could not acknowledge the seriousness of the illness because if I did so fear and panic would undermine the self-confidence I was still able to generate. Can't you see, Jan? [his wife]—it's a race between my developing ways of coping and people finding out about the illness. I accept that I've got the illness, honest, but I've got to pretend that it is not too serious, otherwise I'll be too intimidated to deal with it.

The Objective Burden and the Subjective Burden

Adapting to any major crisis requires an effort to cope. But the consequences of an event, however traumatic, cannot be predicted simply by examining its basic features. As already suggested, individuals show an enormous range of reactions to essentially similar events, and vary as much in their ability to cope constructively. Also, as people *respond* to the threat or challenge that the stressful event poses, the nature of that event changes. They may manage practical consequences well or badly, so that the original event's impact is altered. Or they may alter the way they view it, so that it is perceived as more or less threatening. As we said before, the individual's appraisal of the stressful event and the particular coping strategies that he or she employs play a fundamental role in determining its physical and emotional impact.

Burden is a term that professionals use to help them think about the impact of a chronic disorder on the patient and on his or her carers. Distinctions are drawn between the visible difficulties and deficits to which a household with a chronically disabled member is prey—the so-called *objective burdens*—and the degree of *distress subjectively experienced* by the household members as a result of the objective burdens they face. With a chronic illness, the potential objective burdens, for patient and carer alike, may include the physical and social consequences of providing physical care, economic hardships, dwindling social networks and loss of autonomy. The subjective burden represents not only the degree to which specific objective burdens are experienced as distressing, but also the overall impact on mental health and well-being of coping with a chronic disease.

Studies of people coping with different disorders have confirmed that objective and subjective burdens do not always closely coincide. These findings emphasise the importance of appraisal, personal perceptions and interpretations in determining how stressful any one individual will find a particular set of circumstances. The levels of subjective burden, determined by personal agendas, expectations and aspirations, can exaggerate or reduce the impact of any single objective burden. This being so, helping people arrive at more realistic appraisals of stressful events can, to an extent, diminish their distress and their subjective burden. Personal perception and appraisal act like a filter that modulates the relationship between the objective and subjective burdens, either enhancing or diminishing the anxiety, distress and even depression experienced by the individual exposed to a stressful life event.

The Acute Illness and the Chronic Illness

The image that most people have of being ill is modelled on episodes of acute illness such as appendicitis. Injury or pain and suffering descend suddenly. There is a crisis; doctors are called or consulted; hospitals, nurses, maybe operations, are all part of the picture. For a short while everyone may feel extremely worried about the patient's chances of survival. But after the crisis is past the patient recovers and life eventually returns to normal. The essential priorities in the management of *acute illness* are getting medical attention and treatment quickly, speedy cure, and survival.

The picture with a *chronic illness* is quite different. The onset of most chronic illnesses is not marked by a sudden crisis, but more characteristically by a gradual decline in physical well-being. Sometimes the onset, as with Parkinson's disease, is so slow and unremarkable that the symptoms may be mistaken for several other, minor disorders before a correct diagnosis is reached. Even after diagnosis, the person with Parkinson's will usually have only occasional involvement with hospitals and doctors. Survival is not at issue in the early stages of most chronic illnesses, so people are spared that intense acute anxiety. But the lack of a definitive focus for concern, the absence of an immediate crisis that everyone can recognise, bring their own difficulties. Most problematically, the patient, the family and everyone else concerned have to come to terms with the fact that life will *not* shortly return to a familiar version of normality, that their expectations of the future must subtly change to accommodate a lifelong illness. The priorities for managing a chronic illness are very different: to delay deterioration, to limit discomfort and to maintain the best possible 'quality of life' whatever stage the disease has reached. These apparently modest aims are immensely challenging.

An episode of *acute illness* has a marked effect on the social status of its victim. For a limited time, the need for the patient to seek refuge in the role of sick person is fully recognised. This 'sick role' gives him or her time off from normal responsibilities, and grants him or her the right to be looked after, to be more dependent or helpless than at any time since young childhood. It also gives the the patient the space to concentrate on fighting the illness and recovering. Although many adults feel intensely frustrated by the temporary loss of personal autonomy that goes with being cast in the sick role, they recognise the advantages of complying, of being a 'good patient'. There is no lasting stigma attached to this temporary status—after recovery, the previously sick person resumes all his or her old social roles, as spouse or partner, parent, colleague, friend.

But the effect on the social status of a person with a *chronic disease* is significantly different: being cast in the sick role does *not* provide a welcome refuge that will facilitate a rapid recovery. Instead, it can be experienced as debilitating, threatening the individual's will to combat the disabling aspects of the disease, and ultimately promoting handicap. Loss of autonomy is an important issue for most people with chronic disorders, and successfully minimising that loss at every stage is a key factor in maintaining a reasonable quality of life. Adjusting to the consequences of the disease may entail either immediate or gradual surrender of some social roles—for example, the work role—and subtle changes in the responsibilities inherent in others, such as those of spouse or partner, father or mother. In addition, most Western societies, with the high value they attach to autonomy and free choice, have difficulty in responding positively to the diminished social participation of chronically ill people.

Future aspirations, expectations of oneself, of employment, of interaction with spouse or partner, with children, family and friends, are all altered by chronic illness. And the disability-associated loss of familiar social roles, activities and interactions in turn results in a sense of psychological and emotional loss, and diminished self-esteem.

Our reactions to loss of any sort, whether the death of a loved one or the loss of normal function and familiar roles brought on by chronic illness, are similar. All loss is associated with grieving, a process that often has four phases.

1   shock, disbelief and denial
2   anger
3   mourning and depression
4   acceptance and adjustment.

Different people pass through these four stages at different speeds. One individual may pass from the initial phase of shock to the fourth stage of acceptance and adjustment in a matter of months, or even weeks. In contrast, progressing through the four phases may take another person years. The fact is that despite the overall similarities in people's reactions to loss, the processes of *grieving*, *acceptance* and *adjustment* are very individual. In a sense, each person has to bear his or her own cross and come to terms with the loss in his or her own unique way.

Another characteristic of coping with loss is that the process is continuous and ongoing. Particularly with an illness such as Parkinson's, the nature and extent of the associated problems wax and wane over the years and people may find that they occasionally revert, emotionally, to an earlier phase, feeling angry, depressed or unable to accept the reality of the disease. This may happen, for example, when there is a sudden deterioration of symptoms after a period of relative stability both of the symptoms and of the associated disability.

THE 'PHASES' OF CHRONIC ILLNESS

One important determinant of how well people cope with a chronic progressive illness such as Parkinson's is, of course, the rate at which it progresses. For some luckier individuals, this will be a very slow process. For others, the symptoms will become worse very quickly. Four broad phases can be distinguished.

1 *Pre-diagnosis and immediate post-diagnosis phase* Symptoms develop gradually and become clinically manifest over time. This first phase is often marked by feelings of uncertainty and shock.
2 *Early phase* The period when the signs and symptoms are so mild that no treatment is yet required, or when changes are well controlled with treatment. Impairment and disability are either non-existent or mild.
3 *Middle phase* Usually the longest. As the disease progresses, impairment and disability will become greater. Treatment will still effectively control the symptoms, but they will show variations in severity during the day, with the wearing-off effects and on–off changes already described. Medication-related dyskinesias including dystonia (see p. 67) may cause additional problems.
4 *Late phase* By now the disease is producing severe symptoms. Medical treatment produces little relief, and the medication-related fluctuations and side-effects lead to marked disability.

Besides the variations in symptom severity and in disability, these four phases also differ in terms of the physical challenges that they present for both patient and carer, and in terms of the emotional challenges— the feelings of loss, depression and anxiety that may be associated with each phase. And although Parkinson's affects the life of each individual in a unique way, for the majority the early phase is probably the least stressful, while the other three may be times of intense upheaval, anxiety and depression.

The Pre-diagnosis Phase

As described earlier, the symptoms of the illness develop gradually over many years, and the length of the pre-diagnosis phase differs widely from person to person. For some time before the formal diagnosis, the individual will have been aware that something is wrong, without knowing exactly what, or its true significance. Even after the symptoms become clinically manifest, there may be a period of 'diagnostic uncertainty', when doctors are not sure how to label the illness. One patient wrote:

> It took about nine months from the first appearance of symptoms before I was diagnosed, and nobody seemed to know what was wrong.

This is also a period during which the symptoms may be noticed by the person concerned, but hidden from everyone else. This secrecy partly results from uncertainty about the meaning of the symptoms and partly from an unwillingness to be seen as complaining unnecessarily. One person with Parkinson's revealed:

> It took me almost six months to tell my friends and family.

So the pre-diagnosis phase is likely to be characterised by uncertainty and confusion, while the individual and those close to him or her struggle to make sense of rather vague or subtle changes in his or her physical and mental well-being. Typically in this phase, people search for ways of understanding any emerging disability, and may settle for explanations that are inaccurate or unhelpful.

The Immediate Post-diagnosis Phase

As already suggested, once given the diagnosis, people vary widely in their immediate reaction to being told that they have Parkinson's disease. Diagnosis may be associated with shock, confusion, anger, apprehension, resistance and denial; or acceptance, and relief that finally the symptoms that have been slowly creeping up have been labelled and are not of psychological origin or due to a tumour, but caused by a recognised disorder. In his book *The Spaces in Between* the graphic designer John Harris recalls:

> The shock had been profound, as much to the family as to me, and that should not be underestimated. The very name had conjured up images of some doddery old geriatric, dribbling at the mouth, shaking and staring into space. Was this going to be me in ten years' time?

This sense of shock is expressed by others.

> I was shattered, as I thought that they would not be able to do anything for me.

> I felt angry and sorry for myself.

> Two main reactions. Fear, because it is a progressive and incurable condition, but also relief that somebody had finally put a name to it and confirmed that it was not 'all in my mind'.

> I was shaken up, and it took me five weeks before I told my wife and later some friends that I had developed Parkinson's disease. I was scared of being disabled. Working in the hospital I knew the sequelae of Parkinson's disease.

> I was filled with disbelief for a few seconds, as during a career as a nurse I had met only elderly people with Parkinson's disease. I was only 43! Then the enormity of having Parkinson's disease hit me and I was devastated. All I could think of was that it was a life, if not a death, sentence ... My husband and I cried for two days, as did my daughter, aged 17 at that time.

When the child psychiatrist Dr Cecil Todes was told by his GP that he probably had Parkinson's disease, his reaction was, by contrast, one of relief. In *A Shadow over My Brain*, he writes:

> I was so relieved at not having a terminal brain tumour that anything less was welcome, especially as, in time and space, the end point seemed so far removed for the newly diagnosed sufferer.

The sense of relief following the diagnosis was expressed by another patient, too:

I was very afraid of what the diagnosis might prove to be. At one stage I guessed it was Parkinson's and was relieved when that was confirmed. I had imagined far worse scenarios, such as a brain tumour.

Just as in the pre-diagnostic phase, another early reaction to the diagnosis may be the desire to keep the illness a secret. Ivan Vaughan recalls:

I was absolutely determined to conceal from friends and colleagues that I was ill and, when I could no longer keep it secret, to minimise the seriousness of the illness ... I tried to avoid meeting people. I hid from friends I met in town and pretended I was not in when friends came round. Jan and I refused invitations to dinner parties or to visit friends. If I could not avoid seeing people, I would refrain from telling them what was wrong. I always preferred to be thought of as odd rather than as someone who was seriously ill.

The Early Phase

During the early phase, which, as already mentioned, may be quite prolonged for some people, disability may be minimal. Nevertheless, people with a chronic disease have to make a major psychological transition at this point. Both their self-image and their perception of their social status must adjust to the knowledge that they are no longer perfectly healthy, and never will be again. For some, this will entail little effort. If the individual is relatively elderly and perhaps does not place a high value on physical vigour, or if the level of disability progresses slowly enough to allow gradual adaptation, then this transitional phase may have little emotional impact. But old and young alike are confronted with the reality of coming to terms with the knowledge that they have Parkinson's disease. Feelings of loss are very common during this phase, when people recognise that they have permanently lost their sense of physical invulnerability, and that some of their plans for the future must be given up. There are likely to be numerous practical issues to sort out, some of which will be to do with employment and future finance.

The Middle Phase

In the middle phase, which is usually the longest, levels of disability are moderate but the impact of the disease will be extremely variable. When it progresses slowly, adaptations can be made to new impairments, and this will in turn reduce the degree of disability or handicap resulting from each deterioration. At this point, the main challenge for both patients and carers is to strike the right balance between health and illness. A major concern is to obtain the maximum relief from medication. Levodopa may remain effective for some, but for others a decrease in its effectiveness will mean that other medication will be tried. As a result, contact with health professionals may become more frequent.

Researchers have identified a style of coping with this stage of Parkinson's disease which they characterise as 'sanguine and engaged'. This is exemplified by patients actively trying to cope with altered circumstances and enjoying the challenge of managing the practical and emotional consequences of the disease. In this phase, those whose disabilities increase too fast, or for whom medication loses its efficacy too quickly to allow this continual process of minor adjustment, are most vulnerable to serious depression. People in this situation tend to feel they are engaged in an unsuccessful struggle, and they often become very worried about the future.

The Late Phase

By now the disease is giving rise to severe symptoms that are no longer responsive to medication. Medication-related fluctuations and side-effects are distressing in their own right. Now that disability has become severe, depression is much more common. Both patients and carers lose much of their ability to influence the course of events— the disease is more clearly in charge now, and a sense of helplessness may prevail. Physical demands become pressing. The patient gives up his or her active participation in a number of personal, family and social roles, and the loss of independent functioning in turn entails a loss of privacy and dignity, which places high demands on mutual trust between patient and carer. As the scope for practical action is severely curtailed, coping efforts at this stage tend to focus more on emotional responses.

From what we have said, it will be clear that adapting to a serious chronic illness is not a neat and tidy process, completed at or soon after the point of diagnosis. It involves a continual series of adjustments, the timing and outcome of which are determined both by aspects of the disease process and by the psychological and social resources on which the individual can draw. The relationship between the severity of the illness and the psychological well-being of individual patients is not as simple and direct as one might expect: people who are more disabled are not necessarily more unhappy than less disabled people.

What seems to happen is that psychological well-being ebbs and flows as the disease progresses, and this ebb and flow reflects the outcome of people's efforts to cope. Strategies that worked well at an earlier stage will not necessarily be adequate to deal with fresh challenges posed by a further deterioration, or a new combination of disabilities. While searching for new coping strategies the individual is likely to feel anxious or miserable, but once ways are found to manage the practical and emotional implications, he or she regains a psychological equilibrium.

IMPAIRMENT, DISABILITY AND HANDICAP

In these last few sections dealing with the effects of stress on health and well-being, we have largely ignored the *symptoms* of Parkinson's disease. No one would minimise the importance of tremor, akinesia, bradykinesia and rigidity—after all, the impact of a chronic illness on an individual's life is a consequence of the symptoms. But how do they translate into everyday life? A useful way of thinking about the consequences of the symptoms of Parkinson's is to use the distinction suggested by the World Health Organisation (WHO) between *impairment, disability* and *handicap*. In everyday language we tend to use these terms interchangeably. But let's clarify how they differ and why such a distinction may be helpful in understanding the effects of Parkinson's disease.

Impairment is most closely linked to the physical symptoms of the disorder. In a sense, impairment is the net result of the combined effects of the symptoms of tremor, rigidity, akinesia and so on. The term refers to deficits or the changes from normal function that occur as a result of the symptoms. In Parkinson's disease the most significant impairment is in motor function—in other words, the impairment relates to how the person starts and carries out all forms of movement, from the simplest to the most complex. This motor impairment is not limited to particular movements or to specific parts of the body. It affects all movements and all parts of the body to different extents. Movements of the hands and arms appear to be most severely impaired.

Disability is the way in which impairment affects daily activities or restricts the individual's behaviour. So in Parkinson's disease the motor impairment, when it becomes severe enough, leads to problems in getting dressed, drinking from a cup, using a knife and fork, writing, speech and non-verbal communication, walking, driving, and so forth. These are all forms of disability.

Handicap refers to the impact of the disease in its widest personal and social sense. The handicapping effects of illness are considered in relation to broad areas of life: mobility, work, social and leisure activities, relationships with others (colleagues, friends and family), physical independence and economic self-sufficiency. While impairment and disability are measured against some general notion of normality, handicap can be judged only in relation to each individual's life, his or her immediate social context and future expectations—that is, in terms of how he or she functioned, worked and played before the onset of the illness, or in terms of the life he or she would have been expected to be leading if the illness had not occurred. Loss of a job, marital breakdown and divorce or the inability to play the piano after the onset of the illness are handicaps for people who were working or married or who derived great pleasure from playing the piano. These things would not be at stake for those who are single or have never worked, or who have never played the piano. For this reason, the WHO definition of handicap is 'a disadvantage for a given individual, resulting from an impairment or disability, that limits or prevents fulfilment of a role that is normal (depending on age, sex, and cultural factors) for that individual'.

Social prejudice, legal restrictions and regulations, and environmental obstacles can magnify, or even cause, handicap. Most public places do not adequately cater for people with disability. Public transport, and most theatres and restaurants, are inaccessible to people with a motor impairment who are confined to a wheelchair, and fire regulations may restrict their use of public premises. Social prejudice can play a major role in creating handicap. Ignorance, fear and discomfort in the presence of disabled individuals lead people to treat them differently, to exclude them from ordinary social participation. Furthermore, the person with the illness may sometimes share some of these biases. For example, a sense of embarrassment or not wanting to be seen as different or odd can lead people to give up certain social roles or to restrict their social participation. Also, the degree of handicap depends on the individual's coping mechanisms and on how he or she adapts his or her lifestyle to accommodate the illness and the associated impairment and disability.

The WHO has summarised the relationship between impairment, disability and handicap in the following way:

$$Impairment \rightarrow Disability \rightarrow Handicap$$

But when looking at this simple equation it is important to remember that the link between impairment, disability and handicap is not always direct, or one-to-one. Not all impairments lead to disability, and not all disabilities are handicapping. Some people may be disabled with relatively little impairment, while others, despite having severe disabilities, may not be handicapped at all.

The degree of impairment and disability is undoubtedly important, but handicap depends on many other things as well. The life circumstances of the individual (age, marital status, job, financial security), the physical and social setting in which he or she lives (house or flat, with or without lift or facilities for wheelchair; whether or not he or she lives alone; whether there is a social support network available), his or her personal characteristics (self-esteem, beliefs, goals, motives, appraisal of the illness, and so on)—all play a part in preventing or producing handicap.

We have suggested in the preceding pages many intervening, or mediating, variables that determine the nature and severity of the disability and handicap experienced as the result of a given level of impairment. This complexity has an advantage—namely, that impairment and disability do not inevitably lead to handicap. Instead, individuals have the opportunity to make the most of their personal and social resources in order to prevent impairment and disability from producing handicap.

QUALITY OF LIFE

As we mentioned earlier, the traditional medical model of disease has been concerned with acute illness. Within this model, the individual falls ill, is treated, then recovers quickly, and contact with the medical profession ceases. Although this conventional picture does not fit well with chronic illness, here too medical management is often solely aimed at treatment of the symptoms, mainly through medication. The WHO considers this traditional approach to be inappropriate for chronic illness, in which the primary concern should be with 'quality of life'.

'Quality of life' is difficult to define, as it has many meanings. Under normal circumstances, a person's quality of life is related to how he or she functions and feels; it encompasses his or her physical and mental health, social activities and relationships, and economic, work and environmental circumstances. When an individual falls ill, 'quality of life' embraces the total effect of the illness, and its subsequent treatment, on physical, psychological, social and occupational function, as perceived by that individual. In relation to the chronically ill, 'quality of life' refers also to the personal and emotional reactions of individuals to the differences they perceive between their actual and their desired life.

Quality of life is influenced by three sets of factors:

1   the wishes and expectations of the individual and of his or her family
2   the limitations imposed by the illness on the individual's ability to fulfil his or her wishes and expectations
3   the individual's reactions to these limitations, which include both emotional reactions and behavioural changes, such as changing jobs or finding new hobbies.

Like handicap, quality of life is extremely individual, and this is why there are many factors determining how chronic illness impacts on it. Beliefs, desires and expectations, habits and living circumstances, culture and social milieu, are all important determining factors. Of course limitations are also largely dictated by the nature of the symptoms and the associated impairment, disability and handicap. The WHO recommends that in cases of chronic illness, instead of concentrating solely on medical treatment of the symptoms, doctors and health professionals should shift the emphasis to managing disability and handicap. The primary concern should be with promoting and maintaining a good quality of life for the ill person and his or her carer and family.

KEY FACTS 4

What is stress?

Any change, whether positive or negative, that creates an imbalance in a person's life and outstrips his or her ability to cope, becomes stressful. The most stressful life events are those that are unexpected and over which the individual has less control, such as the death of a loved one or the onset of an illness.

What factors determine the effects of stress on an individual?

People differ in their reactions to stress and in terms of how well they cope with it. The *outcome* of stress can be either an improvement or a worsening of adjustment and physical and emotional well-being. The effects of stress on the individual are not direct but, rather, are influenced by antecedent and mediating factors. *Antecedent factors* are present before the stressful encounter; they comprise the personal characteristics of the individual (such as his or her sense of self-esteem, motives, beliefs about personal control), and the environment in which he or she lives (which includes financial circumstances and the availability of social support). The features of the stressful event that he or she has to face (rate of progression and controllability of symptoms in chronic illness) are also important. *Social support*—that is, the availability of people on whom the individual can rely for sympathy, understanding, emotional and practical help—has been shown to protect individuals against the negative impact of stress. *Mediating factors* such as the individual's personal appraisal of the situation and his or her coping abilities moderate the effect of the stress—that is, either magnify or reduce its impact. *Appraisal*, or personal perception and interpretation of the stressful event as negative or positive, is a major determinant of reactions to it. The *coping strategies*—that is, the behavioural, practical and emotional methods used by the individual— can help him or her to come to terms with the change and reduce its impact on his or her life. So the effects of stress are not straightforward, but can be modified in many complex ways.

What are objective and subjective burdens?

The term 'burden' signifies here the impact of chronic illness on the individual and on his or her carer. *Objective burdens* are all the demands and restrictions imposed on the family's resources by chronic illness, such as the physical strain of caring, the shrinking of social networks, economic hardship, loss of independence or autonomy. *Subjective burden* is the distress experienced by the ill person, the carer and other family members as a result of the objective burdens. Objective and subjective burdens do not have a one-to-one relationship. Some experience very little subjective burden even when exposed to major objective burdens, while others feel greater subjective burden despite facing smaller objective ones. The distinction between objective and subjective burdens highlights the importance of personal appraisal, of the individual's perception of the stressful event and his or her circumstances, in determining the way in which he or she copes.

How do acute and chronic illness differ?

An acute illness such as appendicitis is associated with sudden pain and suffering followed by medical intervention and restoration to full health. During the usually short while that the person is ill, there may be anxiety, survival may be at stake, and he or she can adopt the 'sick role' and be exempt from normal responsibilities. Once cured, the individual resumes previous roles and returns to normal function. The onset of chronic illness is often much more gradual: usually there is no event clearly marking the transition from health to illness, other than diagnosis of the symptoms by a doctor. When chronic illness is progressive, the symptoms become worse over time: daily activities, and social and occupational functioning, will show a gradual decline. The chronically ill person gives up familiar roles at work, at home and socially. In the later phases, loss of autonomy and increasing dependence may occur. In chronic illness, survival is not an issue. The focus is on delaying deterioration, limiting discomfort and distress and ensuring the best 'quality of life' possible.

How does chronic illness create a sense of loss, and what are the related psychological stages?

The symptoms of chronic illness result in loss of normal function and disability in daily activities. The relinquishing, over time, of familiar personal, occupational and social roles, alterations in habitual ways of living and interacting, pose a threat to self-esteem. Future expectations and aspirations are fundamentally changed. All of this can create a sense of emotional loss in the chronically ill person. Reactions to loss, whether of a loved one through death or of normal function and roles through chronic illness, are similar. Loss, like grieving, has four phases: (1) shock, disbelief and denial, (2) anger, (3) mourning and depression, (4) acceptance and adjustment. The pace of psychological transition through these phases varies from person to person—a few months or many years. Also, as the nature and severity of problems posed by Parkinson's disease change over time, people may occasionally revert temporarily to an earlier phase of emotional reaction—for example, when new or more severe symptoms develop.

How do the demands and challenges posed by chronic illness change with the 'phase'?

Coping with a chronic illness is not a 'one-off' challenge, but a continuous and ongoing process with many ups and downs. The rate of progression plays a major part in determining the demands and challenges faced by the ill person, the carer and the family. In Parkinson's, four 'phases' can be distinguished:

1 *Pre-diagnosis phase*   Often marked by uncertainty and confusion; followed by the immediate post-diagnosis phase which may be associated with shock, anger, resistance and denial, as well as relief that the symptoms finally have a recognisable label.

2 *Early phase*   Symptoms are very mild, disability is non-existent or equally mild. Patients must now modify their self-image and future expectations to adjust to the knowledge that they have a progressive illness. Practical arrangements may be instigated to prepare for future unemployment, loss of earnings and disability.

3 *Middle phase* (usually the longest)   Moderately severe symptoms and disability. Medication is more or less effective in controlling the symptoms. Social and occupational roles may be relinquished. Much effort may centre on obtaining a combination of medications to produce maximal control of symptoms. Depression may ensue when a sudden or severe worsening of symptoms occurs.

4 *Late phase*   The illness is producing severe symptoms, no longer controlled by medication. Medication-related complications such as on−off fluctuations, wearing-off and dyskinesias add to the disability. Feelings of helplessness may set in, as the disease may seem to take over and physical dependence increases.

What are the differences between impairment, disability and handicap?

These terms differ in the extent to which they relate either more closely to the symptoms of the illness, or to the individual's characteristics and circumstances. *Impairment* relates most closely to the symptoms. In Parkinson's disease, motor impairment results from the combined effects of tremor, rigidity, bradykinesia, akinesia and postural instability. This gives rise to *disability* in daily activities. When impairment becomes severe, the individual has difficulty with daily activities such as dressing, bathing, shaving, cooking, eating with a knife and fork, drinking from a cup. *Handicap*, which has been defined as 'a disadvantage for a given individual, resulting from an impairment or disability that limits or prevents fulfilment of a role that is normal (depending on age, sex, and cultural factors) for that individual', relates more closely to the individual and his or her social circumstances than to the symptoms. Chronic illness can create restrictions to do with mobility, work, social and leisure activities, relations with others, physical independence and economic self-sufficiency. The association between impairment, disability and handicap is not direct: not all impairments lead to disability, not all disabilities are handicapping. Some people may be severely disabled despite only mild impairment; others may not be handicapped at all by severe impairment and disability. Social prejudice, legal restrictions, environmental obstacles, can all help create handicap. The individual's psychological make-up, appraisal of the situation and the coping strategies he or she uses are important in determining handicap. The complex route to handicap allows people ways of using their personal and social resources to prevent impairment and disability from creating handicap.

5

From the Perspective of the Person with the Illness

Richard Brown

This chapter considers the broader aspects of Parkinson's disease as seen from the patients' perspective, and the impact of the symptoms on their lives. As Chapter 4 has outlined, depending on their circumstances and their outlook on life, people react very differently to the problems and limitations imposed by chronic disease; some of these reactions can be positive and others negative.

I had two major problems in setting out to write this chapter. First, I do not have Parkinson's disease. I can only suppose, from my experience as a clinical psychologist and the knowledge I have acquired through talking to many people who have, what their lives must be like. I realise that I will be wide of the mark at times. Second, my experience has taught me that Parkinson's will not affect any two people in exactly the same way. Indeed, the main message of this chapter is that you cannot separate the disease from the person, and that you cannot separate the person from the world in which he or she lives. Even if I did have the illness, my experiences and thoughts about it would be very different from others' — what might be true or appropriate for me might have very little relevance for another person with Parkinson's.

For these reasons, I have tried to deal with the broad issues of living with Parkinson's disease. Where I can, I illustrate these issues with examples. Some of you may recognise yourself and your life in these descriptions, while others may find little that seems familiar. I hope, though, that you will all find something of value here, even if it is just an alternative way of looking at your situation.

First, I'll consider the impact of Parkinson's disease on various aspects of an individual's life. The categories that I have used—daily activities, mobility, leisure and so on—are, in some ways, artificial. Obviously there is often a close relationship between them. Factors that affect one area will also influence others; strategies for dealing with one aspect of handicap can be applied to others. However, there are also some important differences between them, which I will highlight as they arise.

DAILY ACTIVITIES AND SELF-CARE

Once we leave infancy behind us, we take responsibility for a number of key areas of our lives—we wash and toilet, dress and feed ourselves. These activities probably represent the most basic level of independence. They are things that we take for granted for most of our childhood, not just as adults. But there is obviously more to independence than this. It may also include, for instance, being able to do your own shopping, cooking and housework, turning on the television when you choose, reading a book or using the telephone. We all have a core of activities that form our lives as individuals, that constitute an important part of our sense of personal identity.

As described in Chapter 4, all of us at some time or other go through periods when we have to suspend these activities for a short time— for example, if we are taken ill, admitted to hospital for an operation, or if we break a limb. In such cases it is relatively easy to cope with the lack of independence, because we know that soon it will be regained. But in Parkinson's disease, the decrease in independence happens gradually. This has both positive and negative implications. On the positive side, it is possible to make adjustments, both practical and emotional, gradually, as the changes occur. There is no sudden, overnight loss of independence with which you and others have to cope. On the negative side, everyone with Parkinson's is aware of the progressive nature of the disorder. Although they will hope for a dramatic new treatment or even a miracle cure, most will be aware that the future holds the prospect of increased dependence on others.

Unlike some other aspects of handicap, problems with the *activities of daily living* shows a relatively predictable increase as the disease progresses from the early to middle and late phases. This is because these activities are amongst the most closely related to the physical symptoms of the disease.

In the earliest phase of Parkinson's, daily activities are largely unaffected. Some tasks you may be slightly slower at carrying out, but they can still be done independently. To some degree, the amount of difficulty experienced will depend upon the pattern of the symptoms. For example, Parkinson's always starts on one side of the body before progressing to the other. If the disorder starts on the right side rather than on the left, a right-handed person may have more early problems with simple tasks. The sort of difficulty that occurs in the earliest stage tends to be fast repetitive hand movements. For instance, you may notice that brushing your teeth or polishing shoes requires a bit more effort, and takes longer. Handwriting may be noticeably slower. It is sometimes this type of difficulty that is the first sign that an individual has Parkinson's disease. But although possibly annoying, such difficulties are going to have little impact on his or her ability to look after him- or herself.

As the disease progresses, problems with the activities of daily living become more marked, although the vast majority of everyday tasks are still achievable. They simply take a bit more time and effort. Previous difficulties may be more noticeable, and new problems may develop. For instance, slowness or tremor may make getting dressed a chore, particularly where buttons and other fasteners are concerned. Some of the problems will be associated with a general decrease in mobility (discussed below). For example, it may become more difficult to take a bath, if getting in and out is a problem; extra care may be needed to minimise the risk in potentially dangerous actions such as lifting a saucepan of boiling water.

However, although such everyday tasks are more difficult, or require extra attention in order to avoid accidents, it is still rare for independence to be seriously affected at this stage. This is mainly because there are many opportunities to work around any problems, such as:

- changing the time when you attempt a particular activity, so as to make the optimal use of your best time of day
- replacing old ways of doing things with new ways that are less problematical, such as showering rather than having a bath, or using zips or Velcro rather than buttons.
- using any of the many simple aids and tools that are available, such as a button-hook, or a handrail on the bath.

Of course, how helpful these strategies are depends on how willing the individual is to change and adapt. The person who rigidly tries to do the same things, in precisely the same way, at precisely the same time, will have many more problems than the person who is always ready to try out new ways of doing things. The subject of *strategies* for coping with some of the problems of living with Parkinson's disease is dealt with more fully in Chapter 9.

In the late stage of the illness, the physical symptoms have progressed so that many of the everyday tasks may be difficult or even impossible without help from someone else. For some, the early and middle stages of Parkinson's disease will last for seven or eight years, while others may continue to take care of themselves without major difficulty for twenty years or more. Indeed, a few people never seem to progress to the late stage. However, those who do, sooner or later, reach this stage may find themselves dependent on others for some activities. This will be particularly true when general mobility is severely affected, and the individual requires a wheelchair. He or she will often need help when moving from bed to wheelchair, or from wheelchair to toilet.

Other problems that severely limit self-care are severe tremor and abnormal involuntary movements. These may make *tasks requiring fine control* such as shaving, or eating, virtually impossible. However, there are still things that can be done. There will still be times of day when the individual has some mobility or when the symptoms are relatively mild. Making best use of these times will enable him or her to maintain some independence. Even when the symptoms are at their worst, there will always be something that the individual can do, whether alone or with someone else's help. These little acts, however insignificant they may seem at the time, are very important in maintaining self-esteem—as the following case illustrates:

John's Parkinson's disease had started 15 years earlier. Although still mobile about the house, he had problems with severe abnormal involuntary movements which made it difficult for him to do simple tasks such as making himself a cup of tea, shaving or dialling. He found that he either had to leave these things undone or call for help from his wife, both of which he found frustrating and sometimes demoralising. However, he enjoyed the challenge of thinking of ways around his problems, and attempted to treat it as a bit of a game. So he started making his tea when he was in a good phase and storing it in a thermos flask with a straw; he switched from a safety razor to an electric one, and bought a telephone with large buttons and a storing facility for frequently used numbers. He valued the opportunity to demonstrate his continued independence about the home, and the ability to use his brain in his battle with the 'dreaded movements'.

MOBILITY

Together with daily activities and self-care, mobility is probably the most significant aspect of life affected by Parkinson's disease. The ability to move around independently, in our homes or outside, is critical to us all. It enables us to carry out the many activities to do with work, leisure and day-to-day tasks that define much of our lives. Where mobility is reduced, the resultant handicap can be widespread. It is for this reason that so much of the clinical management of Parkinson's is concerned with maintaining mobility.

While walking is the most obvious aspect of mobility, there are many other actions and behaviours involved in moving our bodies from place to place. 'Mobility' includes climbing stairs, bending down, getting up from a chair, turning over in bed, as well as our ability to travel longer distances on bicycles, in wheelchairs, in cars and on public transport.

Moving Your Body

First, how is your ability to move your body 'under your own steam' affected when you have Parkinson's disease? In the early phase there will be little impact. You may notice some physical changes—your stride may be shorter and you may walk a little more slowly—but there is little handicap. Getting up out of a chair and turning over in bed will present no significant problems. In other words, you will still be able to do all the things you could do before, if sometimes a little more slowly. Any handicap will be slight.

Walking: a complex problem

As the disease progresses, problems with mobility begin to arise. In particular, difficulty with walking may become more obvious; this is due to a number of factors, which may develop at different rates and emerge at different stages:

- decreasing stride length
- increasing fatigue
- flexed posture
- problems with balance
- 'freezing'.

Stride length will continue to shorten, and walking may become more tiring. The person with Parkinson's may be able to walk only short distances before he or she needs to take a short rest. In addition, another set of symptoms starts to emerge—problems with *posture* and *balance*. The body starts to become flexed, with the knees bent and the head forward. There is an increasing tendency to walk with the weight forward, on the balls of the feet or on the toes, and with the heels off the ground. This posture is less stable, and the individual may feel uncomfortable and slightly off balance when walking. Unfortunately, the normal reflexes that we use to maintain balance cease to function properly in Parkinson's disease. An extra problem that develops later on in some people is 'freezing', as described in Chapter 1. When walking, taking the first step may be a problem—the feet may seem to be stuck to the ground. At other times, such as when going through a doorway, the feet may suddenly stop. In both cases, getting started again may take some time and effort.

Falls

One major problem when you have Parkinson's disease is falling. This is a result of the many factors described above—the change in stride pattern and posture, the loss of normal balance reflexes, and freezing. While problems with walking may be inconvenient and restrict your actions, falls present a real danger, with the risk of severe bruising or broken bones. The loss of postural reflexes tends to mean that when an individual falls, he or she falls more heavily than usual. So while anyone else may stumble and reach out a hand to steady him- or herself, the person with Parkinson's will fall like a felled tree.

Falls may occur through tripping over small obstacles, when attempting to stop suddenly, when changing direction, when trying to walk too fast, or through suddenly 'freezing' when on the move. Stepping backwards—for example, when opening a door—is also a problem in Parkinson's disease, and may lead to a fall.

While falls can be dangerous in themselves, they can also have a wider impact. Some people, although unsteady, may never fall but may be afraid of doing so. Others may fall once or twice, and become fearful. Such individuals may avoid walking, or stay within their own homes where they feel more confident. As a result, they suffer a severe loss of mobility. Clearly, this handicap is caused more by fear and loss of confidence than by the physical symptoms of Parkinson's disease.

Other mobility problems

As mentioned earlier, other actions such as rising from a chair or getting out of the bath may present problems as the disease progresses.

Penny had moderate Parkinson's disease, which had started about eight years earlier. Although quite capable of moving about the house on her own, and looking after herself, she found that she was always getting stuck in chairs, particularly the comfortable armchair that she most enjoyed sitting in. She would try to lean forward and push with her arms, but would be unable to shift herself more than a few inches before falling backwards. She would either have to call for help, or gradually shuffle forward to the edge before struggling to her feet.

Why should simple actions suddenly become so difficult? One reason is that they are not really so simple. They seem so because we have been practising them since early childhood, but in fact they require the precisely timed and co-ordinated movement of many different muscles. Parkinson's disease seems to interfere with carrying out such *automatic* actions. People who have it often report having to think about the individual components of an action, then having to carry out each one deliberately and consciously. Unfortunately, because we have never had to think about these actions before, it is not always obvious what we have to do to achieve them. As in the example above, it is common to see someone with Parkinson's disease struggling to get out of an armchair—pushing up with the arms and legs but unable to rise successfully to his or her feet. In fact, it is only by watching someone *without* Parkinson's that you can see how it should be done. First, he or she brings the feet in, as close as possible to the chair, or even slightly underneath it. Second, the upper body leans forward. These two actions serve to move the centre of gravity of the body over, and slightly in front of, the feet. Only then, with the upper body still moving forward, does the person push up, using arms and legs together. However, ask him or her how it's done, and he or she will probably be unable to tell you.

Cars and driving

Of all forms of transport, as a society we have grown to depend most upon the car. For many people with Parkinson's, the question of driving is a critical issue. Should they be driving? When should they stop? How will they manage if they do stop? And the emotional impact of giving up driving is likely to be as important as the practical consequences. For many, this signals the point at which the disorder is starting to have a real impact on their life. Depression is a common reaction.

It is required by law that you inform the Driver and Vehicle Licensing Agency in writing, immediately after diagnosis. Similarly, the car insurance company should be notified, as failure to do so may affect the validity of any subsequent claims. Notifying the DVLA does not necessarily mean that the individual in the early stages of Parkinson's disease, with no or only mild disability, has to quit driving completely. After notification, a DVLA form about your medical condition has to be completed, which together with information provided by your GP allows the medical officer of the DVLA to decide whether or not you can continue to drive. The licence may be reviewed every few years, to assess the extent of disability and your continued fitness to drive.

Slowness of movement initiation and execution, rigidity and dyskinesias are the symptoms that most affect driving. When the symptoms are mild, such as when the individual is slightly slower than before or has a slight tremor, he or she can continue to drive. But when disability becomes moderate or severe, it is safer to stop driving. Some people with Parkinson's give up driving before they need to, perhaps through lack of confidence. Others time their car journeys to coincide with their best 'on' periods and continue to drive safely for short distances for a number of years. If you do decide to give up driving, it is important to look at all the alternatives that are available, preferably before stopping. (This is dealt with more fully in Chapter 10.) Depending on where you live, there will probably be a whole range of options, from public transport, taxis and minicabs, *Dial-a-Ride* and *mobility buses* (see p. 251), to getting lifts from friends and members of local voluntary groups. Making full use of these options is critical, if stopping driving is not to mean that you feel housebound.

However, although alternative means of transport are available, they bring with them some new problems. There may be a long walk to a bus stop, for instance, and stairs or escalators to deal with. You may have to cope with crowds pushing on and off buses and trains, and the often unpredictable starts, stops and turns, which can be problematic when you are standing or walking towards the exit. All of these can be dealt with, though, and some suggestions are offered in Chapter 9.

WORK AND LEISURE

Why is mobility important? The main reason is that it allows us to get from A to B, either in the home or outside of it, and the reason for getting to B is usually in order to *do something*. Mobility, therefore, is a means to an end, not an end in itself. Besides self-care activities such as washing, dressing and going to the toilet, we spend most of our time resting, working—either at a formal job or doing household chores—or at some form of leisure or social activity. Occupying our time in a purposeful, productive and hopefully enjoyable manner is crucial to maintaining both our mental and our physical well-being.

Work

Parkinson's disease may appear after the individual has finished his or her normal working life and has retired. For such people, the main impact of the disease will be on their ability to engage in their usual leisure and social activities. For younger people, however, the impact of the illness on their work is an important concern. Apart from the obvious financial implications, a person's job often forms such an important part of his or her sense of personal identity that giving up work can leave a gap that is difficult to fill. Most people, therefore, will want to continue working for as long as they can.

However, the obvious question—'Will Parkinson's disease affect my ability to work?'—is an almost impossible one to answer in general terms. Happily, the immediate answer for most people is that there is no reason why they should not be able to continue working as effectively as before. In the early stage, when the symptoms are mild and well controlled by medication, it should be business as usual. With time, and progression of the disease, though, things may change. But even then no two people's situations will be the same. As we have already seen, individuals vary enormously in the rate of progression, their particular pattern of symptoms and their response to medication. People vary just as much, of course, in the kind of work they do. For those with active, physically demanding jobs, mobility may be a limiting factor in their ability to work. As noted in Chapter 1, writing is a major problem for many people with Parkinson's disease. Tremor and dyskinesias can make even the neatest handwriting illegible. Even when tremor and involuntary movements are not a problem, the legibility may still be reduced, particularly if the handwriting size decreases—so-called *micrographia*. And writing is not the only form of communication that may be affected: some people with Parkinson's find speech a problem (*dysphonia*). The voice may be softer and more monotonous—at worst it may be virtually inaudible.

Parkinson's Disease and Employment: The Experiences of Forty-three Patients is a booklet compiled by John Williams, detailing the individual work experiences of people with Parkinson's disease—from army colonel to housewife, from gardener to priest. One of the facts that emerge is that, when it comes to the influence of the disorder on the individual's ability to perform his or her job, what is critical is how the job and the disease 'fit' together. With luck, the person's job and his or her own 'personal' Parkinson's disease will be compatible, allowing him or her to continue working for many years, perhaps to normal retirement age. If the individual is unlucky, the symptoms will make it impossible for his or her usual work to be carried out, even early on. The choices may then be early retirement, a progressive reduction of working hours or, if possible, changing the nature of the job. These are reflected in the following varied experiences of three people with Parkinson's disease.

Dorothy worked as a registrar in a local registry office. An important aspect of her job was entering the details into the official registers of births, marriages and deaths. She had always taken pride in her handwriting. One of the first signs of her Parkinson's disease, even before it was diagnosed, was a gradual deterioration in the size and clarity of her writing. Things improved once she started taking levodopa, but soon started to deteriorate again. Although her other symptoms were still mild, and her handwriting was still legible and adequate by most people's standards, it was not good enough for her to continue her work as a registrar. She chose to retire a few years early and make the most of the time when her Parkinson's disease was still mild.

Tom worked from home as a freelance book editor. His job involved reading manuscripts, copyediting—that is, correcting typescripts before the publishers sent them for typesetting, and proofreading. After 16 years, his Parkinson's disease had made him largely housebound, and dependent upon his wife for much of his day-to-day care. However, he was still able to sit at his desk and read, and his handwriting, although slow, was still legible. He was not able to carry on for more than an hour or two without getting tired, but working from home, he could take a rest whenever he needed to. Although he knew that he might have to reduce his workload at some point in the future, he saw no reason why he should not continue working indefinitely.

David had been a taxi driver for 20 years before his Parkinson's disease was diagnosed. He continued working for five years, but found it increasingly difficult. He was uncomfortable sitting for long periods without being able to stretch his legs, and an increasing need to go to the toilet proved inconvenient. However, he was reluctant to give up work completely. His employers were sympathetic, and found him a position in the control room, taking calls and assigning fares to the other drivers. In this way he was able to maintain links with long-standing friends and colleagues, continue to use his local knowledge, and keep a wage coming in before he reached retirement age.

Early retirement or changing the nature of their work is perfectly acceptable to many people. For others, however, making such decisions is seen as a defeat. Rather than adapting their working life around the limitations of the disease, they try to carry on as before despite increasing difficulty.

The central role of *fatigue* as a factor limiting people's ability to continue to work was noted in most accounts in John Williams' *Parkinson's Disease and Employment*. Fatigue is a fact of life for many patients, and one for which they are not always prepared. Perhaps because even everyday tasks require more effort, they are liable to tire more easily, and require breaks to 'recharge their batteries'. Unfortunately, medication does not necessarily relieve this feature of the disease. As with symptoms such as tremor and freezing, rushing or working under pressure—which, sadly, are features of many people's jobs—is likely to make it worse.

Fatigue is not simply physical. Many people with Parkinson's report that they find it difficult to concentrate for long periods without a break. Depending on the nature of the job, it may be this mental fatigue that is the main limiting factor. One of the people who figured in Williams' booklet, a pharmacist, found that he had to concentrate so hard on manipulating the equipment and pouring medicines from one bottle to another that he was afraid of making a mistake in the prescriptions. In his case, lapses in concentration could have had serious consequences. At home, of course, it is possible to take things easy for a while, or schedule physically or mentally demanding tasks for the 'best' times of the day. At work this may be more difficult to arrange, and will depend on the nature of the job and whether employer and colleagues are understanding.

Another common theme in the accounts that Williams gives is the importance at work of other people—employers, colleagues, employees. This is dealt with more fully in Chapter 10, but it is important to introduce it here because it raises a crucial issue about living with Parkinson's disease—the willingness to be open and honest with others. Within the workplace it is commonly feared that *telling other people* about the illness will lead to the individual concerned being treated differently, and to his or her disadvantage. The ill person tends to expect people to feel sorry for him or her, to underestimate his or her capabilities, or feel embarrassed and steer clear. There may even be the fear that he or she will be made redundant, once management knows about the illness.

Robert worked as a salesman for a farm equipment manufacturer. He had always enjoyed his job, and had taken pride in the fact that his name was always near the top in the monthly sales figures. His job involved long hours and a lot of driving about the country. When he was 53 he discovered that he had Parkinson's. Although the disease was still mild and well controlled by medication, he was extremely worried about the impact that it would have on his work, and on his employer's attitude. Because the farm equipment market was sluggish at that time, and his work was judged on results, he was afraid that his employer would dismiss him and take on a younger and fitter salesperson. At his age, he was worried about his ability to find another job. As a result, he told no one about his Parkinson's disease. He kept his visits to the office to a minimum, and avoided meeting colleagues socially in case they noticed any of the symptoms.

In contrast to Robert's feeling that it was essential to maintain secrecy, the overwhelming message coming from the writings of those with Parkinson's disease is the exact opposite—they were amazed at how helpful and supportive everyone at work was, once they knew. Many, such as David, the taxi driver mentioned above, were able to continue working purely because of the support of others. It is encouraging to hear that people's fears about telling others are seldom realised.

Eventually Robert found that the pressure of work and the stress of keeping his Parkinson's disease a secret were too much. He went to his manager and told him that he wished to resign. Explaining about his illness, he was surprised to discover that his manager had suspected the truth for some time, as his own mother had it. He was also unwilling to accept Robert's resignation, saying that his experience and long-term contacts with clients were too valuable for the company to lose. He asked him to carry on, adding that the company would be willing to make some allowances if he found things too much, perhaps by reducing the size of his sales area. Robert accepted, and continued working productively for several years before choosing to take early retirement.

Leisure and Social Activities

Leisure and social activities form an important part of our lives. For the person who is working, they provide the opportunity to switch off the stress of work and to relax. Depending upon the activities concerned, they may provide either physical or mental exercise—which are important for everybody, but particularly for someone with an illness such as Parkinson's. And for retired people, such activities constitute a major way of occupying their time.

If anything, people's *hobbies* and other leisure pursuits are even more varied than the types of work they do, so it's difficult to generalise about how much of a problem in this area Parkinson's disease will be. Individual symptoms may interfere or not, depending on the nature of the activity, although factors such as fatigue may have a more general impact. Fortunately, we have far more flexibility in organising our leisure pursuits than we do our work. We have the freedom to choose what we do and when we do it. The danger, as will be discussed below, is that with Parkinson's disease the individual may take this freedom to an extreme and choose to do nothing for much of the time.

Hobbies and other leisure activities can be broken down into two broad areas—things that we do in our own homes and things that we do outside. Often, our home activities will be solitary, while those outside will involve other people. With Parkinson's disease, it is the latter, social, activities that are most at risk.

There are many reasons why people with Parkinson's may cut back on *social activities* outside the home. Often these will relate to problems of mobility: individuals may be unable to walk as far as they used to; they may have given up driving; public transport may be expensive, unreliable or inconvenient. All of these may make getting out more difficult. Fatigue may also play a role—the effort of getting to their destination may leave people with Parkinson's disease too tired to enjoy themselves once they get there. The result may be that, more and more, they spend time at home.

But psychological factors may be even more responsible for this reduction in social activities. Someone who is subject to falls, 'freezing' or unpredictable on–off fluctuations may lack the confidence to venture far from home. These, and many of the more visible signs of the illness such as tremor and dyskinesia, may be a source of embarrassment. Many of the accounts written by people with Parkinson's describe accidents or other incidents in public situations. This is from Sidney Dorros' book—*Parkinson's Disease: A Patient's View*:

Suddenly, as I got close to a crowd I froze in my tracks. I could not take a single step more, and had I not been supported by my wife and friend, I would have slipped to the floor. They practically carried me to a nearby couch and stretched me out on it. I had to rest there for over an hour before I could move.

Eating and drinking in public, whether in restaurants or at the homes of friends, is another important social activity that is often avoided, even in the early stages. Tremor or dyskinesia may make eating and drinking difficult or messy. Cutting food may be a problem, as may swallowing. Dorros describes a typical scene:

I remember how this 'on–off' effect affected me when my wife and I and another couple had dined at a fashionable restaurant in a hotel near our home. During dinner I was so dyskinetic I tipped over my water glass and scattered food off my plate in all directions.

Another example is provided by Dr F., a general practitioner, in another booklet compiled by John Williams, *Parkinson's Disease: Doctors as Patients: Eleven Autobiographical Accounts*:

My table manners have deteriorated and I sometimes need help with cutting up meat. Involuntary movements of my legs some-times cause trauma to those of adjacent guests. I try to avoid cocktail parties: I spill my drinks if standing up and if sitting tend to be treated as an ashtray or a social leper with whom the occasional guest will spend five minutes before 'circulating on'.

The social embarrassment associated with the symptoms and avoidance of social situations is also described by Dr J., a medical officer:

One of my biggest handicaps and fears is in being invited out to tea or any social gathering. I am fine for perhaps 20 minutes, then tremor takes over and I feel lost and miserable. I know I can avoid such gatherings, I don't go very often, but then one becomes a recluse and that is not good either.

It is easy to see how people may want to avoid such situations, perhaps from an early stage. From childhood, we are taught about the importance of 'behaving properly' in public. Society tends to dictate rules and standards that we expect of ourselves and of others. But it is those very rules and standards that make 'disabled' or 'handicapped' people withdraw, often voluntarily, from participating in a full and active social life.

Resting

While much of our time is spent working, looking after ourselves or our families, socialising and taking part in leisure activities, we all need time to unwind. 'Rest' includes such things as sleeping, sitting in a chair and looking out at the garden, reading a book, watching television. All involve little or no physical activity, and allow us to 'switch off'. Indeed, it is these very features that make resting so vital to people with Parkinson's disease, as a way of countering fatigue and 'recharging their batteries' before carrying on with more energetic activities.

However, these passive ways of passing the time are a double-edged sword. While resting is good, there is a real danger that it can become the main way in which those with Parkinson's spend their days. Because things are more difficult and more tiring, passive pastimes seem increasingly attractive. When combined with giving up work, a decreasing tendency to travel outside and a shrinking social network, the individual may find him- or herself spending more and more time indoors doing nothing in particular.

Even people who previously led remarkably full and active lives may fall prey to the temptation to do nothing. The eminent historian A. J. P. Taylor, who had Parkinson's disease, confessed:

> Gradually I get more reluctant to go out more than a few hundred yards. I can see that soon I shall be quite content to sit in the open air of my back yard or patio. I lose interest in what is happening further afield.

And again in an account by J.K., a psychotherapist, in John Williams' booklet *Parkinson's Disease and Employment: The Experiences of Forty-three Patients*:

> At such times I doubt my skills as a therapist and would like to contract out. How much easier to potter around in the garden. This tendency to avoid challenge is real and pervasive. I would like to avoid any social or professional encounter at which I may be viewed as less well than formerly.

Most people slow down, socially as well as physically, as they age. This process of cutting down on previous activities and on our social lives is sometimes referred to as 'disengagement'. But research has shown that it tends to happen at a younger age and to a greater degree in people with Parkinson's. In the findings of a study carried out in the USA, the author, Dr Singer, noted:

[people with Parkinson's disease] are less likely to engage in household tasks, or to have a close circle of friends; at the same time, they are more likely to engage in such solitary leisure activities as watching television and reading, and much more likely to report ways of spending time which are not 'activities' at all—namely, napping and idleness.

There is nothing abnormal in this pattern of behaviour. However, when comparing Parkinson's patients with different age groups in the general population, it was found that people under the age of 65 who had the disease were leading the lifestyle of others aged 80 or more. This led Singer to suggest that Parkinson's disease can lead to *premature social ageing*. Obviously, it is important to guard against this pattern setting in—suggestions for ways to keep active, physically, socially and mentally, are given in Chapter 10.

FINANCIAL INDEPENDENCE

All of us have a standard of living that we have grown used to. When something threatens our financial security and independence it can have a profound effect on many aspects of our lives, and on our self-respect. Parkinson's disease can have an effect on the financial status of the individual in two ways—if he or she has to give up work or accept a job with less pay, and through the extra costs of living incurred by having the illness. On the plus side, there are benefits that he or she may be able to obtain; the various kinds of benefit are described in some detail in Chapter 9.

As with employment itself, the impact of the illness on their finances is going to affect younger and older individuals differently. Those who have already reached retirement age and stopped working will suffer no change in their income—they will already have made the necessary adjustments to their lifestyle in order to accommodate any reduction in income associated with normal retirement. Such individuals will have their state pension and, probably, an occupational or a private pension. The major impact of Parkinson's disease will be on those younger people who are still of employment age; their particular financial problems are discussed in Chapter 8. Where the person with Parkinson's has been the sole or the main breadwinner, some couples choose for the other partner to start working, or to work more hours, to bring in extra income. This has obvious practical advantages for the finances, although the radical change in roles may have a wider impact on the relationship (see below).

Loss of financial independence can be a major source of stress for those who are unprepared, and who have not made the necessary adjustments. It should be remembered that people often retire or work shorter hours so as to reduce stress, but there is little point in this if work stress is replaced by financial stress. As discussed in Chapter 9, careful financial planning is important, to lessen the impact of any income loss.

RELATIONSHIPS

We human beings are social animals. The people around us often play central roles in our lives, be it at work or at home. They are vitally important to us, and the nature and quality of our interactions with them contribute to our sense of satisfaction and happiness.

We can think of our lives like the layers of an onion, with ourselves in the middle. Surrounding this core are our family or carers, friends and work colleagues, then health professionals and others that we may come across occasionally, and finally strangers. These various groups differ for us in both the amounts of time that we spend in contact with them and the intimacy of that contact—the extent to which we share our lives and our feelings with them. We can also think of this 'onion' in terms of the places or situations where we meet these various individuals—at home, at work or in social settings, in surgery or hospital, in shops, and in all the other places out there in the world. In each of these places and for each of these groups we can think of ourselves as having different roles. At home we may be husbands or wives, and parents; at work we are colleagues, while in a social setting we are friends. In hospital we are patients, while in shops we are customers. Even though the person inside is the same, we are viewed as different in each context and, to a degree, we act differently as we play our different roles.

Because of these multiple roles that we each have, and the many different kinds of people with whom we make daily contact, it is not possible to describe here every situation and every kind of encounter. But what we can do is consider in a more general way the different groups of people in turn, and how Parkinson's disease may affect the nature of our relationships with them.

The Immediate Family

There is no such thing as an 'average' family. For some, there may be a vast extended family of children, grandchildren and relatives of all kinds, who provide the main focus of their lives. For others there may be just a few people, some of whom they rarely see. For most, the immediate family of spouse or partner, and children, provides the most important and most intimate set of relationships. It is these people who will share, most closely, many of the ups and downs of Parkinson's disease.

For those with a spouse or partner, telling them about the illness is rarely a choice. Almost always, they will be fully involved in the processes leading up to and including the diagnosis. However, relationships will vary in the amount of openness and communication that is, or seems to be, appropriate.

One of the major stresses on a relationship is the effect that Parkinson's can have on established roles and patterns of behaviour. In any relationship, there is usually a division of labour and responsibility, built up over the years. One partner may be the main breadwinner and the other the main home-keeper. Care of children may be shared equally, or may be the main responsibility of one of the partners. One may take more initiative in organising and maintaining social contacts and recreation for the two of them, and so on. In the early stage of Parkinson's disease there are unlikely to be any changes to these established patterns. But in the middle stage, as symptoms become more evident and difficulties in various aspects of life may start to emerge, there is a tendency for previous roles to change or even to be reversed. If you are the one with the illness, and you have been the main breadwinner, your partner may choose, or need, to start bringing in more money. You may suddenly find yourself having to take on unaccustomed roles about the house so as to relieve the burden on your partner. Later on, if you become less capable of functioning independently, such flexibility may not be possible. This can bring with it another change—the role of partner becomes that of 'carer', perhaps full-time.

All of these changes can have their effect on a relationship. There may be dissatisfaction, at times, engendered by the loss of a previously valued role, or by the need to take on additional unwanted or unfamiliar roles. Also, certain roles may be psychologically incompatible—it may be difficult, for example, for a woman who has been in the carer role all day, and has just helped her partner to wash, undress and get into bed, to suddenly switch to the role of lover. The following case illustrates this:

Len had his Parkinson's disease diagnosed at the age of 48, and gave up his work as a car mechanic six years later. He had worked all his life, and found it difficult to adjust to the idea that he was no longer the main provider for the family. He continued to work on friends' cars for some of the time, but spent most of his day indoors at home doing nothing in particular. His wife, who had always taken care of all the household matters, found his presence an increasing irritation. To help with the finances she took on a part-time job. But Len was unwilling to do any of the day-to-day jobs such as shopping or cleaning. If he did do them, after persuasion, his half-hearted efforts tended to cause more arguments. After a time, his wife was offered a full-time job which she decided to accept, and she derived considerable satisfaction from the challenges and stimulation of her new career. Len, of necessity now, took on many of the household jobs. To his surprise he learned that he enjoyed cooking, and took particular pride in devising special surprises for supper when his wife returned from work. She, in turn, lowered some of her high standards and worried less if the carpets were not vacuumed every day.

A common problem is not knowing how much to do for the person who has the disease. Where is the line to be drawn between helping that person but not depriving him or her of independence? Pat talks here about her husband:

He is incredibly kind, but he seems to think that he has to do everything for me. If he sees me trying to get up from a chair he rushes over to help me up. If I even move towards the kitchen he tells me to sit down and asks me what I want. I know I shouldn't, but sometimes I want to scream: 'I may have Parkinson's disease but I'm not totally useless!' I really wish he would find some other interest and give me a bit of space, but I don't know how to tell him—he would be so upset. I really am very lucky, but sometimes I want to hit him I feel so frustrated.

And Edward, about his wife:

She is marvellous the way she copes with the Parkinson's disease—I wouldn't be able to be as brave as she is. After all these years, I feel that it's the least I can do to look after her, she deserves it. I can't say that it isn't a strain, physically and mentally. She doesn't demand help but I know that's just her—she has never asked for things, but I know she would be upset if I didn't offer. I must confess that there are times when I would just like to go out to the pub and have a game of darts like I used to, but I couldn't leave her on her own—it wouldn't be fair.

These examples illustrate the importance of striking the right balance between helping the patient and not taking away his or her autonomy and independence by being there at all times. This balance can only be established by honest communication of needs, and by flexibility to the changing demands of the illness.

The Sexual Relationship

One aspect of a couple's relationship that may be affected by Parkinson's disease is their sex life. Whatever their ages, an active sex life can form an important part of the relationship, even if they make love less frequently and the physical passion diminishes over the years. Unfortunately, sexual problems are common where one partner has Parkinson's.

What sort of problems can occur? Sexual problems are often classified as problems of arousal—men find it difficult to achieve or maintain an erection (impotence), while women fail to lubricate, making penetration uncomfortable, or they may suffer an involuntary contraction of the vagina making penetration impossible or painful (vaginismus). Many people, however, become aroused normally but have problems with orgasm. Men may ejaculate too soon (premature ejaculation) or are unable to do so (retarded ejaculation). Women too may have difficulty in achieving orgasm (anorgasmia). As important as these physical signs of sex is the question of satisfaction. Some people find that they enjoy sex less, and therefore want it less often, even if the physical 'machinery' is still working.

All of these problems are found in couples where one partner has Parkinson's disease. In a recent study of younger couples, about 80 per cent reported that they were having sex less often. In terms of the nature of the sexual problem, about 60 per cent of men reported erectile dysfunction or impotence, and 65 per cent had a problem with premature ejaculation. Among women with Parkinson's, 55 per cent reported lack of sexual arousal. Of course, the difficulties were not restricted to the person with the illness: partners, too, reported the same types of problems. This study revealed important differences between couples where the patient was the man, and those where it was the woman. Many more problems were reported by both partners where the man was the one with Parkinson's. This gender difference probably reflects the fact that, traditionally, men play the active role in the sexual relationship.

Exactly how may Parkinson's disease affect the sexual relationship? First, there are the physical symptoms. Unfortunately, many of these, such as fatigue, difficulty in sustaining repetitive movements, freezing, tremor and abnormal movements, can potentially interfere with the act of sex itself. And increased physical tiredness may also be a problem for the partner. Sidney Dorros, in *Parkinson's Disease: A Patient's View*, describes his, and his wife's, problem:

> Sexual relations presented the greatest challenge to timing. My peak period of mobility was so short that if I started to get amorous towards the end of the drug cycle, I would run out of energy at a most crucial point in the love-making cycle. It didn't increase Debbie's libido for me to say, 'Excuse me, I've got to take my pills now,' and then wait half an hour before continuing. She would usually fall asleep before the half-hour was up.

Obviously, the more physically active the individual's normal role in sex, the more handicapped he or she is likely to be by the physical symptoms of the disorder. And while the physical limitations of Parkinson's may be important, the *psychological* aspects are probably even more significant, involving both the individual *and* his or her partner. Unfortunately, particularly in the later stage, physical attractiveness may be diminished by some of the symptoms. These may include the involuntary movements, excessive salivation and sweating experienced by some, and there is the added possibility that limited facial expression and a monotonous voice may make it more difficult to effectively communicate interest or excitement. Furthermore, as noted above, some partners may find it difficult to switch from the role of carer to that of lover. Perhaps most damaging to a couple's sex life, though, is stress. Anyone's interest in sex, and their capacity to perform, can be seriously affected by stress and worry, whether deriving from outside or from within the home. If there is a general tension in the relationship, then it is unlikely that the couple's sex life will escape unaffected. If either partner has worries about work, finances or the future in general, this too will have an adverse effect.

Unfortunately, if problems start, sex itself can become a source of stress, and a vicious circle may develop.

> Mark's Parkinson's disease started nine years ago when he was 47. Both he and his wife worked, although he had recently started working part-time. Financially, they were finding things more difficult. Although Mark had always played an active role in the home, he was recently finding it more difficult to make a full contribution, placing more responsibility on his wife. This was a subject of concern for him. The marriage had been a happy one, and both he and his wife had always enjoyed their sex life. Gradually, however, they were having sex less and less often, and when they

did it was not always as satisfying as before. For Mark, this was a particular worry, because he felt that his illness was removing an important aspect of his relationship with his wife. He attempted to initiate sex more often, but she was frequently too tired. When they did have sex, Mark worried that he was forcing her to do something that she would rather not be doing. On occasion he was unable to obtain a full erection—which added even more to his worry. His erection problems became worse, so that both of them suffered increasing disappointment and frustration. The worry was there not just during sex, but beforehand, too. Would they be able to have sex tonight, or would there be another 'failure'? Despite persevering for some time, their attempts became less and less frequent, until sex essentially stopped altogether.

As in this account, problems with sex, if permitted to continue, can lead to a situation where it is avoided altogether—it is either too stressful or it requires too much effort, and both partners eventually give up trying. Before this point is reached, there may be an extended period when the couple continue to struggle to maintain some level of sexual relationship. Most problematic is when there is a difference in the two partners' desire for sex—in the amount of sex that they want, for instance. Although it happens rarely, a few people experience an enhanced desire for sex as a result of taking levodopa. More commonly, the imbalance will be caused by one of the partners losing interest. Whatever the cause, one may feel that he or she is giving in to pressure from the other, while the other may feel guilty for asking him or her to do something for which he or she has no enthusiasm. Emotions such as guilt and resentment are a poor foundation for a sexual relationship, and there is always a danger that the effects may spill over into other aspects of the couple's life. Even when sex has stopped, there may still be lingering negative emotions, particularly if it has ceased by neglect rather than by a spoken agreement between the two of them.

Many of these difficulties can be dealt with through honest and open discussion or, perhaps, with the help of an experienced therapist. The subject of how to deal with problems in the sexual relationship and how to seek professional help is covered in some detail in Chapter 8.

Other Family Members and Friends

Besides your spouse or partner, other family members may be involved in your life—children, grandchildren, brothers and sisters, and so on. Most important are probably any children who still live at home with you, but family members and friends too may be affected to some degree by your illness, whether you live in the same house or just meet them socially.

It is a common fear for people to think, when told that they have Parkinson's disease, that others will avoid or reject them if they know the truth. As already noted, this leads to the decision to make it the Big Secret—the assumption is that, if no one knows about it, life can go on as before. And, of course, it may work to some degree in the early stages when the signs are mild; but, clearly, it will not work for ever. Some people worry in particular about telling their children, for fear of frightening or worrying them. Unfortunately, this approach can have the opposite effect to that intended. All children, whatever their ages, are observant and they have fertile imaginations. If not kept informed it is likely that they will develop their own ideas about what is going on, and these versions may be far more frightening than the reality.

> Louise had her Parkinson's disease diagnosed when she was only 45. She and her husband had three children, two teenage daughters and one son aged seven. The diagnosis came as a severe blow to Louise. She decided that she wanted to carry on as before, and she was particularly concerned that the children should not know until it was absolutely necessary. Her daughters were studying for exams, and she was afraid that the news could be too upsetting for them. Her son, she thought, was too young to understand and would be frightened.
>
> However, it was increasingly difficult to maintain this situation. Her symptoms, although mild, were noticeable. Tablets had to be hidden and taken in secret, and one excuse after another had to be given for the GP and hospital appointments. Eventually, Louise's son asked her when she was going to die. He had seen the tablets and heard about the appointments, as well as over-hearing vague 'coded' adult talk about the illness, and had come to his own conclusions. Louise and her husband decided immediately to tell their children the truth. Not surprisingly, their daughters too had noticed that something was wrong, but because their parents clearly wanted it to be a secret they had felt unable to raise the subject. They too had formed their own conclusions. Talking together, and with friends, they had been through all possibilities from multiple sclerosis to cancer.

There are also risks in not telling children who have left home, or other relatives. The Big Secret approach, although rarely successful in hiding the truth from anyone for long, can lead to reduced contact. You may avoid seeing them, particularly in social situations, and they may feel embarrassed or awkward coming to see you. Familiarity and knowledge demystify illness, and turn it into an everyday fact of life. Your family should be informed so that they know as much as you do about Parkinson's disease, what its symptoms are, and what you can and cannot do.

The same advice applies to friends. As already discussed, there is a real tendency for many people with Parkinson's, and their partners, to withdraw from social contact and avoid social situations. The importantce of maintaining a network of friends and a social life cannot be overemphasised, particularly if other aspects of your life such as work or hobbies have been restricted by the disorder. Trying to keep the Big Secret will almost certainly lead to turning down invitations. Eventually the excuses will wear thin, and the invitations are likely to stop coming; contact, once lost, is almost impossible to re-establish. Even if maintaining the same level of social life as in the past may be neither physically nor financially possible, it is important to keep up the contacts. Keeping in contact with old-established friends will inevitably involve letting them know that you have Parkinson's disease and explaining the symptoms and its treatment. Friends, just as much as strangers or work colleagues, can misinterpret some of the signs and symptoms.

Peter had decided not to tell his work colleagues about his Parkinson's disease. But despite his efforts to act as normal, he was aware that others were treating him differently. In one-to-one situations, they seemed somehow less chatty and friendly than before. Eventually he asked a friend what was wrong. His friend was unable to be specific, but told Peter that he seemed more reserved; he laughed and smiled less, and seemed to be a bit depressed. Although Peter was not depressed, he realised that his facial expressiveness had subtly changed, and had taken on more of the mask-like expression characteristic of Parkinson's disease. His friends had been picking up these signals and interpreting them as boredom or depression.

It is possible that some old friends *will* be unable to cope with the reality, or with their perceptions of Parkinson's disease. Some people, for reasons of their own, feel acutely awkward or embarrassed around people with physical disorders. In such cases, no amount of information will help, and contact *may* be lost. While regrettable, this will emphasise the importance of those friends who remain close. Finally, there is no reason why the person with Parkinson's should not make new friends—indeed, the illness may bring about a broadening of social life rather than a restriction. If the individual has given up work, the extra time may allow him or her to meet new people and develop new interests better suited to his or her current situation. New friends will come to accept the whole person—Parkinson's disease and all.

MOOD

I have left this section until last because it is so intimately bound up with what has been discussed so far. Up to now we have been considering the impact of Parkinson's disease on specific aspects of life. Most of our discussion has been in terms of practical constraints or the effects on relationships with other people. But in addition, of course, Parkinson's can have a profound impact on a person's general outlook on life, on mood and on sense of well-being. Our opinions about ourselves, both good and bad, are very important when it comes to how we view the world and how we interpret things that happen to us. This sense of personal identity and 'self-concept' is partly a function of the many facets that make up our life—work and family, hobbies and interests, relationships with friends and colleagues. It follows that when an important aspect of our life is threatened, or is taken away, it can have a marked effect on our sense of personal identity. For example, people who have worked all of their adult life, will almost inevitably feel diminished if they have to stop working through illness.

Perhaps the first challenge that Parkinson's disease offers to the individual's sense of identity is the very knowledge of having it. You may feel that you have stopped being a 'person' and started being a 'patient'; that you have changed from being 'normal' to being 'disabled'. Later there may come times when you are unable to do something that you particularly value, such as participating in a sport or other leisure activity, or driving your car. For some people this can threaten, if only temporarily, their sense of self-worth. Potentially most threatening is becoming dependent upon other people for help in basic self-care. People will react in very different ways to these challenges to their sense of identity. Some seem able to keep a core sense of themselves as a person, as separate from the things that they can and cannot do. Others may become angry with themselves and with those around them, while yet others may become withdrawn. In any event, a large number will show signs of depression, some for a short period, some for many years.

Depression: a Broad Spectrum

Mood problems are common in people with Parkinson's disease. Perhaps as many as one-third may experience some degree of depression at any one time. But what is meant by the term 'depression'? For many it's simply 'feeling blue' or 'down in the dumps'. Hearing a particularly good joke or doing something enjoyable may enable these individuals to 'snap out of it'. In other cases, the mood change may be more fundamental and long-lasting. There may be a general sense of sadness and pessimism that is more difficult to shake off. The individual may be tearful, and derive less enjoyment from things going on around. He or she will tend to be passive and unmotivated, as well as worried, tense or irritable. But with severe depression there is more than just sadness and mood change. Individuals become preoccupied with depressive thoughts. Everything they see and hear will tend to be viewed negatively—the world, their situation and the future. They may feel guilt or self-blame, or feel that they are being punished. This negative outlook on everything may even lead the individual to attempt suicide. Other symptoms of depression are sleep disturbance, loss of appetite and weight, a sense of lethargy and lack of interest in anything at all.

Where, along this broad spectrum, is the person with Parkinson's likely to lie? In principle, he or she may experience depression from its mildest to its severest form, but the evidence suggests that depression in Parkinson's disease has some particular characteristics. Most typically, it shows itself as *depressed mood*. The person feels sad and tearful and may be pessimistic about the future, and these feelings may be prolonged and difficult to shake off. However, other features of depression appear to be far less common. For instance, very few people with the illness who are depressed express thoughts of self-blame or guilt, or feel that they are being punished. While they may think about death and even wish, at times, that they were dead, suicide and attempted suicide are very rare.

Why is depression common in Parkinson's disease?

There are two contrasting views on this matter. One is that depression in Parkinson's disease is a direct result of the biological changes in the brain—many of the brain chemicals affected by the illness are also implicated in mood change and depression. This can be termed the *biological approach*. The alternative view, which may be called the *psychological approach*, is that depression in Parkinson's is a reaction to the disabling and handicapping nature of the disorder; that it is the loss of important roles, the restriction of activities and the increased dependence on others that are the key factors in causing the depression.

Which is likely to be correct—the biological or the psychological view? The answer is probably both. Both are likely to play a role, although from one individual to the next the relative importance of one or the other will vary. It is my view, though, that biological factors account for only a small proportion of the depressive symptoms of Parkinson's disease, and are significant in only a minority of cases. I consider that in most people psychological factors are the most important cause.

Are some individuals vulnerable to depression?

Although depressed mood is common in Parkinson's disease, it is by no means certain that everyone with the illness will become depressed, nor that the individual who becomes depressed will stay depressed. Some people with severe Parkinson's will remain cheerful and optimistic, while others, who have only the mildest of symptoms, may become severely depressed. This begs the question, 'Why do some people with Parkinson's disease get depressed and not others?'

A related question is 'Who is vulnerable to depression?' Although anyone can become depressed, it does seem that some are more prone to than others. One important predictor is whether they have had periods of depression in the past, before the onset of their illness. A previous history of depression seems to greatly increase the chance that an individual will become depressed at some time during the course of his or her Parkinson's disease. Reasons for this increased risk are probably complex. The individual may have some biological predisposition to depression, or he or she may be the type of person who reacts to any stressful event or loss by becoming depressed.

Taking the psychological approach, we can suggest that depression will be more likely, the more the illness interferes with the individual's life. As we have seen, Parkinson's *can* (but need not) affect a person's ability to carry out everyday activities—to participate in hobbies and other forms of recreation and social life, to work and to maintain financial independence, to engage in relationships with other people. As discussed in Chapter 4, it is the interaction between the disease symptoms, the individual and his or her normal lifestyle that defines handicap, not the symptoms alone. So someone who suffers handicap, or the threat of handicap, will be more vulnerable to depression than another individual with the same symptoms who experiences little change in his or her normal pattern of life.

Perhaps the group under the greatest threat of handicap are the young.

In the context of Parkinson's disease, by 'young' I mean those between the ages of 40 and 60–65. It is known from research that this group is also the most likely to become depressed. People in this age group are likely to be still working, any children they may have are growing up or already adult, and they are passing through the stage of their lives when their peers may be enjoying the period of greatest financial and personal freedom. People in this age range may find themselves with spare money and time to enjoy themselves for the first time in many years. Parkinson's disease may directly challenge this freedom, and the threat of losing it may be difficult for some people to cope with.

> Barbara was diagnosed as having Parkinson's disease when she was in her early fifties. Despite coping well for a while, she developed severe on–off fluctuations, and her husband eventually gave up work to care for her. Their children had left home, and together they had been planning a long trip, touring India in a camper van. This adventure had been an ambition of theirs for years, throughout the time when their children had been growing up. They now realised that they would never be able to make this journey. This, perhaps more than the Parkinson's disease itself, was a source of great regret.

In contrast, when Parkinson's starts later in life, particularly after normal retirement age, the individual may feel that his or her chances of living a full life have been more or less fulfilled. Furthermore, as noted earlier, many of the necessary adjustments for retirement may have already been made. Older people probably have fewer financial commitments, and have already learned to get by on less money. Also, it is usual for older people to have less active social lives and to enjoy more leisurely and less physically demanding pastimes. For all these reasons, Parkinson's disease has less opportunity to cause severe handicap in them than in younger individuals. I am not suggesting that older people do not suffer handicap or depression—they do—but that younger individuals, or those with more active lifestyles, are going to have the greatest relative handicap and to be most at risk of becoming depressed.

When are the vulnerable times for developing depression?
Why do people get depressed at some times yet remain cheerful at others? A simple account might suggest that you are more likely to become depressed as the disease progresses. In fact, depression seems to show two peaks, one in the early stage and one in the late stage.

One critical period is the time immediately after diagnosis. As suggested earlier, for some people, being told that they have Parkinson's disease comes as a relief, particularly if they have feared something worse; reassurance and information from their doctor, combined with prompt and effective treatment, may allay fears and obviate any emotional reaction. However, for others the news can be devastating, particularly if they have a distorted view of the illness, such as distant memories of an aunt or grandparent in the late stages. Although such individuals may be perfectly able to carry on as before, fear of the future and the threat of having to let go of important aspects of their lives can cause depression. In cases like these, the depression can sometimes become more of a handicap than the disease itself.

Most people will eventually come to terms with their illness, particularly once they realise it need not stop them working or enjoying themselves. However, as the disease progresses and begins to have more of an impact, there may be times when an individual again becomes depressed. When new symptoms start to emerge or the medication ceases to be as effective, he or she may be required to make new adjustments, both practical and emotional. Some particularly stressful change or life event may happen, leading to a long-term loss of some valued role or opportunity. Major events such as giving up work or giving up driving can have wide-ranging consequences in people's lives, as well as threatening their self-esteem and sense of identity.

Except for such periods of change, depression is typically less of a problem in the middle stage of Parkinson's disease. It is only in the late stage, when the illness may have the greatest impact on the most basic abilities required for mobility and self-care, that depression becomes more common again. And again, it is independence and self-esteem that are being challenged.

Anxiety

Depression is not the only emotional problem experienced by those with Parkinson's disease. Although less common, anxiety may also be a feature. As with depression, anxiety ranges from the mild to the severe. Some may experience a general restlessness and sense of unease, accompanied by general worry about life and the future. At the other extreme, the anxiety may be quite disabling, taking the form of panic attacks in which the person feels acute fear, with breathing problems, rapid heartbeat, nausea, and even the fear that he or she is going to die.

To a degree, some anxiety may be a natural reaction to the challenges of living with Parkinson's disease. If the individual has had a fall, he or she may be anxious when walking for fear of falling again. He or she may have stopped work, and have real worries about managing financially. Although any anxiety is unwelcome, it can become a real problem when the individual starts to avoid the things that are causing the anxiety. The person who has fallen may avoid crowded places or public transport. Someone who feels anxious in front of friends or family members because of symptoms that (to him or her) are embarrassing may start to steer clear of social contacts.

Teresa describes herself:

I have always been a 'nervy' sort of person, but it never really affected my life. When I developed Parkinson's disease, however, I found myself worrying more and more about little things. When my balance began to be affected it really started to get worse. If I felt a bit wobbly I would immediately get anxious. Even though I had never fallen, I was afraid that I would fall and hurt myself. If anything, the anxiety made my unsteadiness worse. When at last I did fall it seemed to confirm my worst fears. I was in a supermarket. I tried to stop suddenly and crashed forward, bringing down a load of packets from a shelf. Although I wasn't badly hurt, I was terribly embarrassed. My Parkinson's was really bad for several hours afterwards, and I had to take some extra medication. A few days later I tried to go into the same shop, but I suddenly felt terrible. I was sweaty and shaky, and my heart was pounding in my throat. I sat down, but I still felt awful. After a while I had to go home. That was weeks ago, and I still haven't plucked up the courage to go back. Just thinking about it makes me feel sick. What is worse is that I am starting to feel nervous about going into any place where there are lots of people. If I am not careful, home will be the only place where I feel safe, which is silly. After all, I've only fallen once, but I can't stop worrying that I might fall again.

Anxiety, then, may serve to restrict a person's life, perhaps even more than the disease itself. The panic attacks experienced by some are the most severe form of anxiety. As we see here, even one attack in a particular location may lead to the individual avoiding the situation in the future. There is some suggestion that such panic attacks are somehow related to the disease itself, or to its treatment. A significant number of people feel a growing sense of panic during 'off' periods, often fearing that they will stop breathing or die. Once they come 'on' again, these fears disappear completely. One person with Parkinson's disease put it this way:

> When I am 'off', problems can often become mountainous. But when I come 'on', these problems fade away and the tasks appear quite feasible.

Fortunately, depression and anxiety are not inevitable, and even if the individual *is* depressed or anxious there is plenty that can be done. Chapter 11 deals with ways of avoiding these problems, and of coping with them if they do occur.

KEY FACTS 5

How will the symptoms of Parkinson's disease affect my life?

Parkinson's is much more than the sum of the symptoms. Because people lead such different lives, the impact of the illness can be very different from one person to the next, even if the symptoms seem similar.

Will there be changes in my ability to do everyday things?

As the disease progresses, there is usually a steady decline in the individual's capacity to carry out ordinary everyday activities as well, or as easily, as before. This is because many of these tasks are highly dependent on the aspects of movement directly influenced by the disease. Such changes, however, tend to take place relatively slowly, which permits the individual to adjust his or her life, to learn new skills, or to make use of special aids and equipment. However, just as important as the practical side of these activities is the psychological side. Being able to look after ourselves is very important for our self-esteem, and for our sense of personal identity. Maintaining as much independence as possible for as long as possible is probably the number one priority for all those with Parkinson's disease. When an individual is largely dependent on another, even small acts of independence are vitally important.

What about mobility?

As it progresses, the illness may influence walking and balance. Difficulty in walking can have a dramatic effect on other aspects of our lives, both inside and outside of the home. One of the major problems is balance: falls can occur, particularly in the late stage of the disease. Other aspects of mobility affected include apparently simple tasks such as getting up from a chair or turning over in bed; in Parkinson's disease, these actions are no longer carried out automatically, but often require conscious thought. But although walking and other actions may prove difficult, physiotherapy and special aids can be helpful, and there are many tricks and tips that can be learned. All of these can contribute substantially to maintaining mobility, allowing you to continue to lead an active life.

How are work, leisure and social activities likely to be affected?

For those of us below retirement age, work is probably the most important way in which we occupy our time. Perhaps here more than in any other aspect of life, the impact that Parkinson's disease is going to have will depend on the 'fit' between your symptoms and the nature of your work. Some people will be able to continue working until late into the disease, while others will already be finding it very difficult even in the early stages. As in other aspects of life, flexibility is important, as is your willingness to discuss your problems with those around you, particularly your employer. For those still working, leisure and social activities arc important for relaxation, whereas for those who have retired, such activities may be their main way of spending time productively. Fortunately, people can be more flexible in choosing their leisure activities to suit their situation than they can be in choosing their work. Everyone, however severe his or her illness, can find relaxing, enjoyable and rewarding pastimes. Although solitary activities are important, social contacts are vital for a sense of well-being. Unfortunately there is a real tendency for those with Parkinson's to withdraw from social contact and to lose touch with friends and relatives. Avoiding this should be a major priority for all of those with the disease.

Will my financial independence be threatened?

Parkinson's disease can be expensive. The impact of the costs, however, will depend upon your previous circumstances. Obviously, retiring early can have a major impact on income, although this may be offset by savings such as giving up the use of your car and eligibility for benefits. One danger of decreased income is a reduction in 'luxuries', which tend to include socialising and getting out and about.

How will my relationships with others be affected?

We all have people in our lives that we see more or less often, in different settings. Family, close friends and work colleagues are probably the most important. All of these will be affected in some way by your illness. Clearly, the closer the relationship, the greater the impact, and it is to be expected that any relationship will have to go through periods of adjustment and change as the disease progresses. For this reason, it is essential that others are involved as much as is necessary at all stages.

What about the psychological aspect?

The knowledge that you have Parkinson's disease can be a major blow, even before there are any problems. For some people, it may mean the loss of a particular role or activity that they greatly valued; sometimes, even apparently small losses can take on major significance. It is perhaps not surprising that depression is common in Parkinson's disease. Although some of the problem may relate to the nature of the disease itself, most is probably related to the handicap that it brings with it. Minimising handicap, therefore, is probably the best way of safeguarding against depression. Anxiety, too, can be a problem—worry can stop an individual doing things that he or she is perfectly capable of doing.

6

From the Primary Carer's Perspective

Brigid MacCarthy

This chapter is about what it is like to be a 'carer' or to live with someone who has Parkinson's disease; the challenges, the difficulties and the rewards. The first assumption here is that most people with Parkinson's have a carer—that is, someone involved in helping with daily activities, looking after him or her when the illness progresses and moderate to severe disability develops, and providing emotional support. Of course, this is not true of all individuals with the illness, some of whom live alone, without a full-time carer. Nevertheless, some of these probably have relatives or friends who to some extent have become involved in their care since the onset of the illness. The second assumption in much of this chapter is that, in the majority of cases, the spouse or partner is the primary carer. But although this seems to be borne out by statistics, we recognise that younger children, grown-up sons and daughters, sisters and brothers, and occasionally parents, friends, neighbours and professionals may also fill the carer's role.

Relatives often say that it is really difficult for them to understand what having and living with Parkinson's disease is like, as these comments reveal:

I often try to imagine what she feels like but I can't—it must be horrible.

We accepted from the start that there is nobody except the person who is ill who knows what it's like. Unless you've got it yourself you can't really appreciate it. I will look at it from a different point of view.

And just as relatives often feel that it's difficult to enter into the experience of the person they are caring for, so too they often feel that it's hard for outsiders to understand what it's like for carers—which is 'living with Parkinson's disease' in another sense. This perceived lack of understanding and appreciation of the impact of the illness on the carer can sometimes add to his or her sense of burden and of being cut off from others. Hearing and reading about the experiences of other people coping with similar situations can help carers to feel rather less isolated, to realise that their efforts to cope are not so solitary. If others have found different ways of dealing with the problems, maybe their tactics are worth a try. Also, the accounts of people who have found a way of coming to terms with their situation, however grave, show that there is hope even in the most distressing circumstances, and can be enormously encouraging.

In the course of our work with people with Parkinson's disease, we have talked to a large number of their relatives. We wanted to get their perspective on what was important to them in their efforts to cope with the illness. What follows summarises the insights gained from those conversations and interviews. As far as possible we have used people's own words or summarised their stories, changing minor details only, so as to protect their confidentiality. Not all the experiences described here are positive or encouraging—that would be unrealistic. Instead, the different stages of adapting to living with the disease are described, through the carers' eyes; the issues that arise in each phase are outlined, and the problems that have to be dealt with and the emotional cost those problems can bring are acknowledged.

The chapter is organised according to stage of illness.

BEFORE DIAGNOSIS

As you will have gathered from earlier chapters, the first signs of the disease often seem rather trivial. A barely noticeable tremor, for example, rarely leads people to guess that an individual may have Parkinson's disease. Usually, the first visit to the doctor is prompted by such relatively minor problems starting to interfere with work or leisure activities. For instance, one man whose trade involved using a high-speed saw had to change the way he did his job after one arm became stiff. The need to find a cure for such difficulties can speed up the process of diagnosis, and put an end to a troubling period of uncertainty. But for many relatives, as for the patients, the time between the onset of these niggling problems and receiving the final diagnosis can be extremely stressful.

The changes can be hard to pin down, or difficult to understand, and do not necessarily announce themselves as a physical illness:

> I found the way he spoke to me very upsetting, because I found the tone of his voice was hostile to me, but in fact it was the illness and I didn't realise.

Often doctors, too, are puzzled or uncertain, or go along willingly with attempts to minimise symptoms:

> It started with a slight tremor, and he put the words into the doctor's mouth, saying, 'I suppose it's old age, one shakes.'

Or, doctors may try to treat a completely different illness, so that when distressing symptoms are not alleviated by apparently appropriate treatment, both patient and relatives begin to feel helpless—not a strong position from which to hear a diagnosis which may at first seem very shocking.

> She had very bad arthritis, then she had the hip operation done, and she was getting on fine. Then all of a sudden, just like that, she couldn't walk. Their attitude was, 'Well, the operation was perfect, we've done the legs', so they put her onto another depart-ment and then they diagnosed Parkinson's disease.

During this early phase, the person concerned may become less active and unable to find anything of interest in activities that were previously central to his or her pleasure in life. This may lead relatives and friends to misinterpret the first symptoms as signs that he or she is profoundly unhappy. Sometimes both relatives and professionals may perceive this as malingering—which may leave the individual feeling blamed at a time when he or she is feeling particularly helpless. In the absence of a correct diagnosis, these changes can be very destruc-tive to vital relationships:

> We all thought he was swinging it, and that was a very difficult time for everybody. He sort of withdrew into himself completely.

Mutual trust and support, which will be so important in future years, can be severely eroded during the search for an appropriate explanation of the symptoms.

Alternatively, because of the apparent similarity of some of the early manifestations of Parkinson's disease to depression—for example, slowness, lethargy, changed tone of voice and lack of facial expression—the individual's symptoms may be diagnosed and treated as depression. Then, a referral to a psychiatrist may lead to the kind of frustration that was experienced when the wrong physical diagnosis was given. Time and emotional energy are lost in attempting to accept the distressing idea that the patient has a psychological problem, only to discover that another wrong diagnosis has been made:

> He went through all the paraphernalia of the psychiatrists and they found nothing at all wrong with him, nothing at all, and the doctor we saw looked at his hand and said, 'Well, it's only a slight tremor', and no treatment was suggested.

Sometimes family members suspect that the problem is Parkinson's disease, because they have known other people with the illness or because they have some relevant professional background. This can be particularly stressful if they remember people in the more severe stages of the disorder. But more difficult still is the situation in which the family try to keep their suspicions from the ill person, so that husbands, wives or children feel that they have to deal with the implications of their worries alone. This means carrying uncertainty and anxiety without support, and with the additional strain of having to hide thoughts and feelings from the person with whom they are usually closest.

THE DIAGNOSIS

Occasionally, relatives are not present when the diagnosis is made, so they may hear it directly from the patient. Not many of the relatives we talked to recalled that it had been personally traumatic at the time. For some it legitimised unexplained symptoms, and usually it heralded a period—years, in many cases—when life returned to normal, with symptoms at last being alleviated by the right medication. Generally the diagnosis was easier to accept if the individual concerned was already elderly. Where both carer and patient were already about retirement age or beyond and the impairments were still fairly mild, many families took the view that it was only an aspect of ageing, and that they and their contemporaries should expect to experience ill-health in some form.

Simply being given a name for puzzling changes can be enormously helpful for people with Parkinson's disease and their relatives alike. Once the problems they face have been identified, they can begin to adjust. They must now make choices about the balance they want to strike between making concessions to the illness and carrying on as normal. In these early stages, all concerned have to make practical and emotional decisions about how much in their lives has to change. Do jobs, houses, favourite activities have to be changed? Must household roles be modified? What about plans for the future? Is there bound to be a change in the quality of relationships? Will the carer be able to hold on to the same image of the person now under the spotlight as before the diagnosis? The relatives we talked to in the course of our work reacted with widely different ideas, attitudes and coping strategies. Not all of these were helpful to them, but they were what they felt were called for at the time.

For many who had feared a more threatening diagnosis, knowing brought relief and a feeling of 'Thank God, it could have been worse.' This was particularly likely if the individual was not significantly disabled at the time and the illness was progressing only slowly. Others felt fearful, particularly if they had known someone in the final stages of the disease, before today's sophisticated drug regimes were in general use, or if they assumed that dementia was an inevitable part of its course. These relatives were enormously reassured by seeing the remarkable effects of appropriate medication, and discovering that dementia only rarely occurs in Parkinson's disease. Others were very concerned for their children—worrying, unjustifiably, that the illness might be hereditary.

Couples dealt with the acknowledgement of the diagnosis in a variety of ways. But what was universally clear was that the sooner they could arrive at a shared perspective and a way of dealing with the news that was comfortable for both, the better. Often one or other partner found it very hard to accept the news initially. The wife of one patient reported that she had been unable to go home and face her husband until she had visited a close friend to talk over her own feelings. Only then could she prepare herself to be supportive. Uncertainty before the diagnosis, and the perceived need for secrecy in the early post-diagnosis phase, can add an extra burden that makes the situation intolerable. With secrecy, barriers get set up between individuals who are desperate for support and the very people who are their potential sources of that support. One wife describes how relieved she was when she finally let out the Big Secret.

It's much better now because our friends know and they make allowances. When you're trying to hide something, it's not actually that you're ashamed, but you don't want people to see it. I don't want sympathy, but now it doesn't matter because it's out.

Another woman spoke of being unable to reverse the feelings of isolation she suffered when her husband insisted that no one else should know his diagnosis:

I couldn't really face up to it. I couldn't cope with it, so I just sort of withdrew. When my husband first had it he didn't want me to tell anyone, and I found that very difficult. I would really have liked to tell someone, just to share the fact, and I think that's probably driven me too far within myself about it now.

THE PHASE OF MILD-TO-MODERATE DISABILITY

Once the diagnosis has been made and a treatment plan defined, the family and the patient have to arrive at a way of living with the associated disabilities. As already noted, usually there is a period, often several years long, where the consequences of having the illness are barely noticeable. Once he or she has been stabilised on the appropriate medication, the individual may even be more mobile and feel in better health than for some time. The slow and gradual decline in physical ability experienced by most patients, with long periods of equilibrium in between, allows everyone concerned to make gradual adjustments to daily routines, so that the emotional impact of inevitable changes is minimised. Those individuals whose decline is more abrupt tend to find the necessary adjustments more upsetting and difficult to make.

At this point, although the picture varies enormously from one patient to the next, carers report little observable difference in their relative's ability to look after him- or herself and to cope with daily routines. In the very early stages, changes in self-care and in other activities, if they are apparent at all, are likely only to affect the time that ordinary chores take to complete. It is easy to misconstrue such changes in pace as laziness or lethargy. Carers have described the difficulty they have had in adjusting the pace of their own schedules to match the patient's slowing-down, particularly before they have realised that it was an inevitable aspect of the illness. Mild occasional clumsiness can also be a problem. One woman described her anxiety each evening when her husband wiped the dishes, a task he insisted on doing. She recognised his need to make a contribution to the running of the household, but couldn't disregard the frequent breakages.

Loss of balance or falling over occurs relatively rarely at the stage of moderate disability, but its unpredictability and high public profile make it particularly difficult to adjust to. One woman reported that a couple of very public falls at the office had cost her husband his job long before he ceased being able to do the tasks the job required. Another felt she had to supervise her husband constantly at his favourite hobby which was gardening, after he had been injured by becoming entangled with garden tools when he fell. Sometimes carers reported feeling irritated by the symptoms, but were reluctant to mention this to the individual concerned. Cognitive difficulties such as absent-mindedness, where they were a feature of a person's illness, were problematic because they were unpredictable, and peculiarly disruptive to the quality of the relationship between carer and patient. More than any other disabling feature of the illness, cognitive problems seemed to lead to changes in the balance of dependency within relationships. A few carers whose relative had developed a blank face, having lost his or her full range of facial expressions, commented on how puzzling and distressing this symptom was. One thought her relative was feeling permanently hostile, while another had constantly to challenge her assumption that her husband was bored with what she was saying.

'On–off' periods also raised particular dilemmas for carers. Unpredictability made the scheduling of activities problematic, and they experienced special difficulties in matching their own pace to the much more erratic one of the person with the illness:

> When he comes on he gets super-energetic: it's as if he's missed something and he's trying to make up for it now. He even avoids sitting down. I think he's frightened in case he can't get up and get going again.

Carers felt forced to go at the pace of the patient, so that leaving the house on time or trying to keep to a timetable became highly stressful. This in turn made some carers feel inclined to abandon interests and activities of their own, to avoid the conflict or impatience triggered by thwarted efforts to keep some time for themselves.

In the phase of mild to moderate disability, it was not the physical or mental burdens of supporting someone through their daily routines that were the source of difficulty, but having to cope with subtle shifts in the balance of responsibility and initiative-taking. More specifically, concerns fell into three common categories: functional unpredictability, role reversal, and reduction of outside social contact.

Dealing with Functional Unpredictability and Erratic Performance

At this stage, many people with Parkinson's become rather erratic in the pattern of their activities. Lack of confidence and anxiety may often be greater obstacles in this respect than the individual's actual level of disability. This is partly caused by the 'on–off' element of the disease, which undermines confidence and motivation. Carers reported that they initially misread this loss of confidence and motivation as shirking, and had been impatient of it when it first appeared. The person with the illness can also miscalculate his or her ability to do familiar tasks; both underestimating and overestimating his or her disabilities can be peculiarly burdensome for the carer. One woman reported that her husband would regularly promise to go out and look for work in the morning, but by the afternoon felt incapable of helping with even the lightest domestic chores. She felt that her husband was equally unrealistic in the morning and in the afternoon, and she longed for him to settle for a realistic appraisal of his abilities, and stick to it. Carers reported that they found themselves constantly checking up on what had been done—some found it distressing when household chores were unexpectedly left half-finished. Predictability seems to make even major burdens easier to deal with.

As with daily activities, at this stage changes in mobility are likely to be more a question of subtle, qualitative differences rather than marked decline. Slowness and hesitancy are characteristic, and are much easier to deal with if both patient and carer are elderly, when rushing about is no longer the norm. Again, if the person with the illness is getting about less at this stage, it is more likely to be due to loss of confidence than to physical limitations. The carers that we spoke to often described their impatience both at the slow or irregular pace they had to match and at the need to encourage the person to undertake seemingly ordinary outdoor expeditions. However, as one man remarked:

I just have to bite my tongue, no matter how desperate I am to get a move on. Rushing her makes her go to pieces completely.

The performance of apparently simple tasks may by now have become difficult for the patient, particularly those that involve the complex co-ordinated actions that are carried out rather automatically by most of us, such as walking. As explained earlier, it is because these skills are performed automatically, and without any apparent effort, that carers find it very difficult to understand why the tasks that involve them are so hard for the patient to perform:

He looks just like a normal person when he walks down the stairs. Then he gets to the bottom and he can't walk along the hall.

There may be a big difference at this stage between the level of obvious impairment, which can be quite slight, and the degree to which people with Parkinson's disease feel they are handicapped. This discrepancy can test carers' sympathy to its limits:

He says, 'You ought to have it for just one day and then you'd realise what a struggle it is.' He's right, but all I see is him doddering about.

Role Reversal

Carers found they had to take on different practical and emotional roles within their relationship with the individual concerned. For wives this often meant assuming responsibility for managing family affairs, and taking major decisions, sometimes for the first time. Male carers had to learn domestic skills—again, sometimes for the first time. Subtle changes in the relationship can occur in the effort to cope with the patient's emotional needs, as he or she struggles with loss of confidence and occasionally depression:

> He was always the strong one, now I feel I have to be strong for both of us.

As discussed earlier, the point at which an individual has to give up work depends on a complex combination of factors, such as the nature of his or her job and the supportiveness of employers. And the consequences for a household of one of its members giving up paid employment are equally varied. Some couples or families reported that giving up work had been a welcome release; others saw it as a major step downwards, and postponed it for as long as possible:

> I think once he stops work, it will be the finish of him. I think it's because he fights to go to work every day that he keeps going.

Leaving work affects not only the financial status of the household, but also the amount of time family members spend in each other's company and, sometimes, the allocation of status. One barrier to the carer taking on full-time employment in order to make up the deficit in the household income is the uncertainty caused by the need to rush home to deal with emergencies. When the individual with the illness has been the main wage-earner, being reliant on his or her partner for money is a source of tension for some couples.

The carers we spoke to who worked full-time were sometimes annoyed to discover that no housework had been done by their husbands, who were unaccustomed to thinking of domestic chores as their responsibility and, possibly, lacked both the skills and the energy to contribute. A further source of irritation was dissatisfaction with how the task had been done, or being criticised for doing it differently. These problems cropped up during transitionary periods, and tended to persist if not dealt with by open discussion. One husband reported

having fallen victim to chronic nagging, which he now felt too demoral-
ised to attempt to confront.

Withdrawal from Outside Contact

The unpredictability of the symptoms, which can be detrimental to
self-confidence, seems to be an important factor in some individuals'
gradual withdrawal from social contact, and even from old levels of
intimacy within their family. Undoubtedly, reduced mobility also plays
a vital role. We found that those families that were able to carry on
running a car were much more able to maintain outside contacts when
the individual's disability increased (see p. 125). As he or she chose
to make less and less contact with the outside world, some relationships
were tested to breaking-point when partners were thrown together more
than they ever had been before, with little or no option for spending
time apart. For hard-pressed carers coping with a full-time job and
some degree of physical dependency, social life and non-essential
leisure activities are likely to be seen as dispensable:

> We do watch a lot of TV and nothing else, but I tend to ignore
> that, because I've worked all day and have to run a house. I'm
> wrong really. But she never suggests we should do anything else
> and I just sort of let it happen.

Other problems

While the *objective burdens* may be quite limited, the *subjective
burdens* (see p. 97) experienced by carers at this stage can be very
variable indeed. The subtle shifts in the balance of the relationships
described above may be felt very keenly by individual carers. Others
experience the changes as fairly trivial, or even welcome:

> His illness, although it's had its bad effects, has also brought
> some good effects in that he is a nicer person—he is not so
> go-getting, he values our quality of life more.

The burden was felt more acutely if the carers were ill themselves,
or emotionally vulnerable for reasons unrelated to the onset of the
Parkinson's disease. Then difficulties were more likely to be experienced as an enormous strain. Additionally, carers who were young,
and supporting someone who had contracted the disease relatively early,
seemed to have a harder time. Sometimes this was because there were
children involved, who also had to be looked after by the carer, so that
their resources were stretched to breaking-point.

THE PHASE OF SEVERE DISABILITY

The exact symptoms associated with this stage of the disease are fully described in Part 1. From the carers' point of view, they are now living with a person whose most basic abilities to care for him- or herself day by day are interfered with by the disease. For some patients, the most severely handicapping aspects will be intermittent during any given day, while others will have become almost totally dependent on other people's efforts to help them cope, with just a few precious opportunities to preserve mutuality in their relationships. As noted earlier, generally this stage is reached after a long period of slowly progressive illness, but in a few cases it arrives rapidly and abruptly, leaving everyone in the family with little opportunity to make the gradual adjustments that seem to aid adaptation over time. At this stage, the carers that we spoke to tended to express much more resignation to their situation, and concern and sympathy for the plight of the patient.

Falling (see p. 118) caused major anxieties, and efforts to be vigilant became very restrictive. Carers felt they could not leave the individual alone in the house for more than a few minutes, and often preferred to keep him or her in sight even within the house. This obviously intensified the sense of being thrown together unavoidably, and made organising practical tasks such as shopping or cooking very complex. 'Freezing', although less of a hazard, could place couples in awkward situations, particularly in public places. Some couples had worked out ways of 'unfreezing' the patient—for instance, one man found that laying a stick in front of his wife's toes could help her move forward. Such ingenious, shared solutions were much appreciated by both. The involuntary movements were very disruptive, and cut off the less resilient individuals and their carers from important sources of interest and satisfaction, such as trips to theatres and restaurants.

Besides major practical problems, in the more severe phase of the illness the symptoms that carers were most aware of, and felt most burdened by, were not necessarily the core symptoms. For instance, few carers focused specifically on difficulties arising directly from mobility, rigidity or tremor. Usually by this stage they had developed adequate strategies to deal with their immediate effects, and adopted a matter-of-fact attitude to them. Issues of greater concern were signs and symptoms that are perhaps less obviously part of the core problems, and are less easily managed by medication. It was the *mental and cognitive problems* of the individual, when they were a part of the illness, that were experienced as particularly distressing: memory lapses and paranoid ideas were upsetting to all parties, and often changed the quality of the relationship by undermining trust. *Sleep difficulties* also presented major problems: the individual's sleep was often very restless and disturbed by nightmares, leaving carers feeling anxious about his or her welfare round the clock, and sometimes guilty if they slept through the night themselves.

Practical Difficulties to do with Physical Dependence

Carers also reported a number of difficulties that were the consequences of the sheer severity of the disease. All sorts of practical problems arose from extreme physical dependence. When patients become severely impaired they may have difficulty in performing independently the most basic self-care skills. Carers may become involved in helping with *toileting* and *feeding*, work that can be very demanding, both physically and psychologically. Having to be responsive to another person's biological rhythms can be inordinately tiring, and the actual tasks may involve some heavy lifting and manoeuvring. But carers commented more often on the emotional strain of being engulfed by the physical needs of another adult. Trying to do practical tasks in or out of the house accompanied by the ill person could be overwhelmingly difficult.

Transport posed major dilemmas. By this stage, most people had stopped driving because of severe disability (see p. 119), and many were very reluctant to use public transport. Lapses in concentration, uncertainty in making choices and general loss of confidence added to the physical difficulties of getting on and off buses and trains. Carers who were able to drive found having a car a lifeline. However, manoeuvring someone who is stiff or jerky in and out of a car can be a physically taxing chore. Some carers spoke of the difficulty of pushing a heavy person in a wheelchair in public spaces, particularly if they had to cope with sudden and expansive involuntary movements. Also, who drives in a household can be a loaded issue. Some carers reported that their taking over the driving had caused subtle changes in the balance of relationships which needed tactful handling:

> Everywhere we go I have to drive. That's something else I do now which I've never done before. I think he misses the fact that we haven't even got him on the insurance now, and he's driven all his adult life. It's been a real blow to his self-esteem.

Carers also found it hard to tolerate the mess that occurred at mealtimes, and complained about an enormous increase in mess generally. This was particularly the case for the few people with Parkinson's disease who had problems with incontinence of the bowels. The main issue that carers commented on was the change in the level of intimacy entailed by having to help an adult with toileting.

When the Carer Falls Ill

Sometimes the patient or the carer contracts another major illness— for example, has a stroke or develops severe arthritis—whose consequences become completely unmanageable in combination with the problems of coping with severe Parkinson's disease. In *Parkinson's Disease: A Patient's View*, Sidney Dorros describes his increased dependence on his wife Debbie, and the necessity of role reversal brought on her by her developing breast cancer:

> For over a dozen years I had been receiving a great amount of physical and emotional support from Debbie. By 1976, I had become very dependent on her to run our household, solve family problems, maintain social relationships, transport me around, and cope with the many problems of my illness. Then a sudden collapse of Debbie's health and strength reversed our roles within a few weeks: she became the patient and I the nurse. The small improvement in my mobility induced by bromocriptine coupled with a strong motivation to help Debbie enabled me to return a little of the aid and comfort she had given me for so long. First she developed severe back pain which confined her to bed for two weeks. But shortly after she resumed normal activities, a much greater tragedy struck—belated discovery of breast cancer.

When the disability became severe, and individuals became dependent on their carers for most of their needs, the physical demands of looking after an ill person could be difficult for the carers, who were often elderly and disabled themselves. This is reflected in the remarks of some of the people with Parkinson's.

> My husband aged 62 looks after me. However, he has chronic diabetes and is at times quite ill himself. Things can be very hard, especially if we are both not well at the same time.

> My wife is my primary carer. She has osteoporosis of the spine, and also suffers from irritable bowel syndrome and hypertension.

> My husband is 73 but he is doing all the housework, assisting me to walk by helping me to keep my balance, dressing me and getting me in and out of the bath.

Some carers we spoke to, who were severely ill themselves, were desperately concerned about what would happen to the person with Parkinson's if they themselves became too ill to cope.

Difficulties in the Relationship

At a time when good communication is essential, both speech difficulties and lack of facial expression, mentioned earlier (see pp. 14, 15), are often obstacles to easy communication and shared understanding. Carers reported that they tended to give up trying to confide because it was difficult to gauge how the individual felt about what was being said. Carers also spoke of concealing their own worries because they recognised that worry of any kind increased the physical problems of their relative—who, on the other hand, often worried about the carer's well-being and quality of life.

Dilemmas in relationships which at earlier stages had reflected subtle shifts in the balance between partners, now developed into resigned tolerance of the status quo. Being thrown together for most of their waking hours imposed a severe strain on relationships that had never been based on shared interests. One man spoke with feeling of his and his wife's mutual frustration at having to go on shopping expeditions together—he simply hated shopping, and she felt inhibited in her enjoyment of looking around the shops, knowing his discomfort. This increase in daily contact was often imposed at a point when the possibility of reciprocity or meaningful communication was much reduced, which was an additional and severe burden.

> I see the expressionless face and the slowness in responding as a kind of veil over her. Trying to push my way through this veil is frustrating, and I'm inclined to feel a bit angry.

At this point, carers began to describe the person with Parkinson's as nothing like the person they first knew. Conversation can grow very limited, particularly if the household has few outside contacts. The carer's sense of isolation can be intensified when there is little mutual support available within the relationship. Carers commented that they had learned not to expect any support in a crisis.

> I can only describe it as having to have a complete sense of responsibility for him. If I feel unwell he seems to need much more from me.

Personal Grief

The subjective difficulties that carers described, unlike in the earlier stages, arose more directly from the physical problems imposed by the disease. They spoke of how upsetting it was to have to stand by helplessly and watch suffering—for instance, during periods of prolonged stiffness or uncontrollable dyskinesias. Several spoke of feelings of sorrow, concern and sympathy for the afflicted person. Carers who were unable to help their partner, because the main difficulties seemed intractable, found their situation hard to bear—they reported feeling totally helpless.

> I cry, but it's no use crying. My mind just goes blank. If I could help him, it would be much easier for me.

There were also many expressions of admiration for the patient's endurance. A few patients who were severely disabled actively considered suicide, and all carers faced with this problem found the distress and anxiety it caused insufferable. At this stage, also, carers have accepted, not only that the joint future they had planned together has been lost, but also that their futures are significantly different. This alteration of expectations was also associated with the carers' sense of loss.

Mixed Feelings and a Sense of Isolation

Of the toll taken on themselves individually, carers reported feeling that their physical and emotional resources were stretched to the limit by the length of time they had been struggling with a progressively deteriorating situation:

> They're only niggly things, but when you've had it week after week, year after year, it becomes difficult. Most days I'm all right, but I do lose patience. I suppose it's because now I am old and not so well myself.

It was more common for carers to speak of feeling irritable, and yet very guilty about getting angry with someone so obviously helpless. The carers' own opportunities for involvement with outside activities were severely limited by the consequences of the disease, which seemed to contribute, in turn, to the loss of alternative sources of informal support. Feelings of extreme isolation were quite common:

> Neighbours are for emergencies only now. No one wants you when there is illness about.

I would say it's purgatory. Half an hour is the most I go out for, and yesterday it seemed like ten years since I had last been out.

OTHER PEOPLE AS CARERS

This chapter has mainly reflected the experiences of those carers who are spouses or partners and who share a household with the person with the disease. There are, of course, other groups of relatives and friends who become closely involved in providing support, and most of the points made so far apply to all carers. However, coping with Parkinson's does present each kind of relationship with some unique issues. I shall now deal with specific problems confronted by parents, grown-up children and more distant friends or relatives who do not live with the patient; and finally, with the problems encountered by those who do not have a main carer.

Parents

When the well-being or life of a child is threatened, parents are faced with peculiarly painful emotions. This is true even if the child has reached adulthood. These emotional challenges are common to all severe disorders, and Parkinson's disease is no exception.

Primary threats to a child's well-being cannot but strike parents as untimely. It is just not part of the ordinary pattern of events for parents to survive their children, or to be fitter and healthier. Also, people who have contracted the disease in their parents' lifetime are likely to be younger than average at the age of onset. As was discussed earlier, those who are elderly when they become ill find the disabilities easier to accept, partly because they can be labelled as an ordinary part of old age. So parents seeing their adult children becoming disabled have to deal with this double issue of untimeliness plus the particular burden of grief about the loss of future hopes and expectations.

If parents are sharing a household with the ill person, roles and boundaries have to be renegotiated just as they do between spouses. Parents may find themselves resuming caring roles, with the grown child returning to a relationship of dependence long since outgrown. Negotiating these changes can be very stressful, and may rekindle conflicts dating from adolescence if the adult child's need for independence is not carefully respected.

Parents may feel very anxious about how their child will manage after their death—an issue of great concern for parents caring for children with lifelong disabilities. Support groups for carers, such as the Carers'

National Association, discussed in Chapter 9, are invaluable sources of information and practical help. Most boroughs have such organisations, which welcome any member, irrespective of the nature of the disability. Parents coping with other sorts of disorders, too, find that looking carefully at available residential or sheltered accommodation and planning for an eventual move allays some of their worst anxieties. Similarly, establishing good working relationships with homecare or respite services also proves helpful in reducing future uncertainties.

Grown-up Children

Some adult children sharing a household with a parent who has Parkinson's find that he or she becomes much bossier, playing the role of authoritarian parent and insisting that the household conform to his or her preferred regime.

> She asks us to do something and if we don't do it straight away, then she gets super-irritable, because her life is revolving around her routine.

The problem seems much more common among this group of carers than among spouses or partners. In an effort to keep on top of their disease, some parent-patients fall back on old ways of relating to their children that are no longer appropriate, either to the age of the children or to the shift in dependency.

Adult children reported much concern for their own future, including fears that they would not be able to develop their own independent life. At the stage when young adults would normally be struggling to shake off old patterns of dependency, they are forced to recognise that they will be providing care and support for some indefinite period. This raises concerns about studying, housing, having a family of their own. One such carer put it this way:

> I worry about the future more than the present. Say I was to get married—well, I couldn't move away. I would have to live upstairs.

Alternatively, when adult children have already moved away and have families of their own, caring for the parent with Parkinson's was sometimes an additional burden—albeit often willingly taken on:

> My mum has now had Parkinson's disease for ten years, and I have been most involved in looking after her since my dad died. My brother lives too far away to help on a day-to-day basis, but she spends all holidays with his family. I come over most days after picking up my children from school. I do all her shopping

and major cleaning. It is an added strain, but I see it as my duty as her daughter to do as much as I can to help.

Friends and More Distant Relatives

For those who are closely involved in providing support for someone with Parkinson's but who do not actually live with him or her, many of the same issues arise, but usually with less urgency. But although the burdens may be less pressing because fewer daily activities are shared, an alternative source of stress is the lack of control over certain aspects of living that can have an impact on the quality of life of a disabled person. Carers report finding it frustrating and additionally worrying not to be on the spot for much of the time. The unpredictability that is a feature of the disease and that tends to make carers who do share a household overvigilant, can be particularly problematic for carers who live separately. The solution in these circumstances is for carers to become effective *care-managers* rather than care-providers. Their main role then is to co-ordinate other agencies to provide the hands-on-care that they themselves are unable to give. Sometimes, feelings of guilt and uncertainty about where to draw the line as far as disrupting their own lives is concerned, can make it difficult for relatives and friends to perform this function as efficiently as they might.

PEOPLE WITHOUT A CARER

In a study of Parkinson's disease in Aberdeen conducted by Dr William Mutch and his colleagues, 19 per cent of people with the illness lived alone. Clearly, this group of people inevitably have the same physical needs as those with carers close at hand, and having to do things independently can often delay the disabling effects of the symptoms. However, this group has to find practical help eventually, and when they do they rely on formal, professional carers such as *community nurses* (see p. 222), or on individuals with whom they may not have long-standing relationships. The expectations and obligations within such relationships are likely to be relatively clear-cut, and many people are more comfortable with that. Certainly, negotiating complex emotional issues such as balancing dependence and autonomy is easier and can be dealt with more concretely. The down side of this kind of arrangement, for more vulnerable individuals, can be a sense of being intruded upon or forced into a level of intimacy and dependence with a stranger that is quite unwelcome. It is vital that people in this position feel able to state their needs explicitly.

KEY FACTS 6

In Britain, one in every five households contains a carer. In the case of the person with Parkinson's disease, the carer is most often the spouse or partner, although other relatives such as grown-up children, siblings or parents may also take on the role. Frequently, only one person acts as the primary carer, and he or she may have to combine this with other duties such as earning a living and running a household. Parkinson's disease in a close relative changes the life of the carer in fundamental ways; the adjustments involved change according to the phase of the illness.

Before diagnosis
Changes are slight or subtle, requiring little practical adjustment, but they can create tension and confusion while the diagnosis is still unknown. In some cases, the ill person may be blamed for behavioural changes over which he or she has no control. Particular strain is caused if anxieties and uncertainties are not discussed.

The diagnosis
Being given a label for puzzling changes can bring enormous relief. Reactions to hearing the diagnosis for the first time are determined by knowledge and by any previous experience of the disease: some see Parkinson's as part of normal ageing, while others are influenced by memories of people in advanced stages of the illness, before effective drugs were available. Best outcomes occur when carer and patient arrive quickly at an open and shared perspective on the news.

The phase of mild to moderate disability
This period is characterised by gradual adjustment to living with dis-ability. Abrupt deteriorations and rapid decline are more difficult to tolerate. People with Parkinson's have not lost their functions, but they may do things significantly more slowly and their ability to carry out tasks varies unpredictably. Carers find that they struggle with a tend-ency to be impatient, and need to be wary of taking over prematurely.

Many couples report that shifts in responsibility and some role reversal occur at this phase. With the individual's increasing disability, social contact may be gradually reduced.

The phase of severe disability

Carers' attitudes tend by now to be characterised by resignation and/ or sympathy. Usually the core symptoms are not the source of greatest distress, because strategies for dealing with the challenges they present have evolved gradually during the previous stage. Cognitive problems, if present, do cause distress. Falls make carers increasingly vigilant. This need for vigilance can create a sense of being thrown together too much, make organising domestic routines difficult, and may encourage carers to impose unnecessary restrictions on themselves and on the other person. It also increases the sense of isolation, as the outside world becomes less and less accessible. Relationships can be radically changed by the patient's need for help with basic functions such as toileting and feeding. Carers' own ill-health may be an additional burden. Loss is a dominating theme: carers recognise they have lost their old relationship with the patient, as well as their vision of the future. A sense of personal grief may be associated with witnessing the increasing disability and dependence of the patient.

Carers other than spouse or partner

Despite the common ground of shared experiences, carers who are looking after not a husband or wife, but another relative or friend, do have specific issues to deal with. When it is the *parents* who are the carers, the main issue is the untimeliness of Parkinson's disease, normally held to be a disorder of old age, hitting a young adult. Parents may find it difficult to acknowledge their adult child's continuing need for independence when they have to return to their long-outgrown role of providing a high level of physical care. Parents also worry about the child's future after their own death; those who make detailed practical plans seem to find this issue easier to deal with. When *adult children* are the carers, there are often conflicts over the degree of separation the child can achieve, and parental attempts to reassert old power structures, preventing the child from developing as much autonomy as he or she might. When *friends or relatives* do not share the household but have a major caring role, there may be worries about their lack of control over the situation. Carers who are able to co-ordinate a network of formal and informal care have much to contribute, though some are hampered in this respect because they feel guilty about not performing the tasks themselves.

7

Parkinson's Disease and Dementia

Dementia is a progressive loss of intellectual abilities and impairment of memory to the degree that the individual can no longer perform his or her usual social and occupational duties. Memory is impaired in a specific way: short-term memory—that is, memory for new events or items of information—is lost, but memory for events that occurred in the more distant past may be preserved. For example, the person with dementia may not remember what they had for breakfast half an hour ago, but be able to recall experiences during childhood. Other symptoms may include impaired judgement, inability to think or to learn, and changes in personality. The individual may be disorientated, not remembering the date or time or where they are, and engage in restless wandering. Simple tasks such as dressing and feeding, cooking a meal or finding the way to a local shop become impossible to do. In the later stages of the illness, the person may not recognise even his or her closest relatives or friends.

In most people, Parkinson's disease is not associated with dementia. In fact, dementia occurs in 15–20 per cent of cases. Inevitably, the co-occurrence of dementia poses additional challenges for the person with Parkinson's disease and for his or her carer and family.

THE NATURE OF DEMENTIA IN PARKINSON'S DISEASE

It is estimated that there are about 600,000 people with dementia in the United Kingdom. Dementia affects all groups in society about equally, and is not limited to a particular sex, social class, ethnic group or geographical location.

Dementia is primarily a disease of old age; although it occasionally occurs in middle age, the risk of it developing increases with age.

About 5 per cent of people aged 60 or over become demented. Among those aged 90 or more, the rate rises to 30 per cent. Alzheimer's disease is the most common type of dementia, and about half or two-thirds of people with dementia have Alzheimer's. It is named after Alois Alzheimer, the German neurologist who first described the disease in 1907.

The cause of Alzheimer's disease is not known. Its symptoms are associated with abnormalities in brain cells. At post-mortem examination under the microscope, the brain of a person suffering from Alzheimer's has a number of characteristic features called 'tangles', which are abnormal fibrous tissues in the brain cells, and 'plaques', abnormal deposits of a protein called amyloid. In Alzheimer's, tangles prevent the transport of chemicals in the brain cells, and plaques interfere with the transmission of signals between them; in addition, *acetylcholine*, one of the major neurotransmitters of the brain that plays a fundamental role in memory and other cognitive functions, is in short supply.

Other forms of dementia exist, besides Alzheimer's; multi-infarct dementia accounts for about 25 per cent of cases. As mentioned earlier, an infarct is a small area of dead tissue. In multi-infarct dementia, a blood vessel is burst or blocked by a blood clot, so that the blood supply to an area of the brain is cut off, the cells are deprived of oxygen and nutrients, and consequently die. With the death of a large number of brain cells, their functions are lost and dementia develops.

The risk of dementia in Parkinson's disease is 10–15 per cent higher than in the general population of the same age. An outstanding question is whether dementia in Parkinson's is simply Alzheimer's disease co-occurring with Parkinson's, or whether there is a Parkinsonian dementia that is quite a separate disease. At least in the early stages, the picture of dementia in Parkinson's is somewhat different from the profound loss of memory and intellectual abilities seen in Alzheimer's. The Parkinson's dementia is marked by forgetfulness, slowness of thought processes, loss of 'executive functions'—decision-making, planning, reasoning, coping with novelty—and lethargy.

Some scientists propose that 'cortical Lewy-body disease' may be the basis of dementia in Parkinson's. This condition is marked by the occurrence of abnormal deposits of a protein called *ubiquitin* that result in the appearance of Lewy bodies (see p. 23) in the cerebral cortex and elsewhere. Some investigators have argued that the nature of dementia in Alzheimer's disease is qualitatively different from that in Parkinson's. Others believe that there is no justification for such a distinction, in terms either of the pathological changes in the brain or of the nature of the cognitive deficits associated with them. These scientists consider Alzheimer's to be simply more severe than the dementia seen in Parkinson's. The debate, of both theoretical and practical interest, remains unsettled. The fact that cognitive function, particularly language and memory, is generally not as severely or comprehensively impaired in the person with Parkinson's who has dementia as it is in someone with Alzheimer's, at least in the early stages, has implications for the management of the illness, in that caring for the person with Parkinson's and dementia may be less demanding in those early stages. Later on in the illness, the dementia may be as severe as that seen in Alzheimer's disease and require similar amounts of caring.

THE SPECIAL NEEDS OF THE PARKINSON'S DISEASE PATIENT WITH DEMENTIA

In the following sections, we suggest ways of dealing with some of the special needs of the person with Parkinson's disease and dementia. More thorough coverage of the special needs of people with dementia can be obtained from many other sources. In particular, we recommend R. T. Woods' *Alzheimer's Disease: Coping with a Living Death* as well as the information and self-help pamphlets sent out by the Alzheimer's Disease Society.

Getting help from others

The GP is usually the first person to be consulted when loss of memory and intellectual functions becomes severe enough for the person with Parkinson's or a relative to become concerned. The GP may refer the patient to the consultant neurologist, or sometimes to a geriatrician or psychiatrist. After history-taking, followed by examination and referral for laboratory tests including a neuropsychological assessment, the doctor will diagnose—if the patient or carer is correct in his or her suspicions—the early signs of dementia. Change in the person's intellectual abilities and memory can be evaluated adequately if previous baseline assessments are available for comparison. This is one of the reasons why continuity of care from a single hospital or specialist centre is advisable, since the hospital notes will contain all records of such assessments and reflect the changes that have occurred over time.

Once dementia has been diagnosed, unfortunately there is not much that can be done in the way of medical treatment of the condition, and contact with the neurologist, geriatrician or psychiatrist may cease, or become less frequent. But the particular circumstances and needs of the person with dementia and his or her carer are now assessed, and other professionals such as clinical psychologists, social workers, occupational therapists and community nurses may become involved in the management of the case. The primary role of these professionals is to provide advice and emotional support. They can also arrange for practical help to be provided, such as help with the day-to-day care—bathing, dressing, feeding, day and night sitting services—as well as with tasks such as shopping, cleaning and cooking. Unsurprisingly, the burden of caring for a person with dementia is more likely to lead to strain and trauma when borne alone by the carer than when shared with others. Sharing the caring is not an admission of failure, rather an acceptance of the fact that it is impossible for a single person to deal with all the demands that caring for someone with dementia presents.

Medication

As already suggested, there is no cure for dementia, and there is no medication that can slow down the process of mental deterioration. When dementia is present in Parkinson's disease, the mental state of the person is often given priority over the physical state and mobility. *Neuroleptics*, or the 'major tranquillisers', are the type of medication normally used to treat disruptive behaviour in the demented person, but they are contra-indicated in those with Parkinson's and dementia, because they would worsen their motor symptoms. When neuroleptics are absolutely necessary, those that are least likely to exacerbate the symptoms of Parkinson's, such as thioridazine and clozapine, are used. When the person is agitated, minor tranquillisers such as lorazepam or oxazepam can be prescribed by the doctor. But these drugs are addictive, and cause sedation, further confusion and amnesia. Antidepressants such as trazodone (Molipaxin) and fluoxetine (Prozac) can have a general calming effect, improve sleep, and alleviate repetitive behaviour, tearfulness and depressed mood.

As far as the medication taken to control the symptoms of Parkinson's disease is concerned, dementia may limit the value of levodopa therapy. Side-effects such as hallucinations and confusional states are more likely, and will probably necessitate lowering the dosage of levodopa—the person may not be able to tolerate higher dosages. Some of the medication given for controlling the symptoms of Parkinson's, such as anticholinergics, may have to be discontinued, since forgetfulness and confusion, which are side-effects of these drugs too, can exacerbate the problems of the person with dementia.

The presence of dementia affects not only the choice of medication to be used to treat the individual, but also his or her ability to take the medication without supervision. Because of memory impairment, he or she may not remember to take the medication, or may be unable to take the appropriate dose at the correct time. It may be necessary for the carers to supervise this, or to set out the required number of pills in separate containers that are clearly marked with the time at which they are to be taken. Alternatively, the time of taking the medication can be tied in with mealtimes, to make it more memorable, or a timer can be set to go off when the dose is due.

A 60-year-old man who has had Parkinson's disease for ten years recently developed some memory problems. Together with his wife, he has developed ways of reminding himself to take his medication on time:

> Until recently I took responsibility for taking the pills myself and often forgot, so I got slowed down so much I was staying in bed all the time. I have a kitchen timer set at three-hour intervals which I carry around with me to remind me to take my medication. We have a white board in the kitchen set with medication times, which I tick off when I take my medication, so my wife can check I haven't forgotten to set the timer or take the pills.

Difficulties in persuading the person with dementia to take his or her medication may also occur. Gentle persuasion, combined with strategies such as disguising soluble medicine in drinks or using smaller pills that can be more easily swallowed, may overcome this problem. To ensure safety, it is important to discard unused supplies and to keep current medication locked away.

Coping with Dementia-associated Problems

The specific set of symptoms associated with dementia differs from person to person. This, together with the immense variability in the nature and severity of the symptoms of Parkinson's disease, means that no two people with Parkinson's *and* dementia pose the same problems in terms of their care and management. The major difficulties engendered by dementia result from the loss of memory and intellectual functions, which also affects people's ability to look after themselves, to communicate and to socialise. Wandering, agitation and aggression, mood disorders and incontinence, are other problems.

Forgetfulness

Forgetfulness is at the root of many of the other problems of the person with dementia. There are certain aids that can be used to supplement memory and improve orientation, such as a clock with large numbers and hands or a calendar clearly displaying the date each day, or a checklist of things to pick up (handbag, money, keys) or make safe (gas, windows, doors) before leaving the house. Having prominent, set places by the door for keys and handbags, or on a shelf in the living-room for spectacles, can prevent mislaying and save hours of searching. The best memory aids are those that are familiar, with a simple message that is easily absorbed. Simplifying procedures, breaking tasks down into a number of easily identifiable sequential steps, sticking to routines, repetition—all of these can help to minimise the problem of forget-fulness.

Self-care problems

This is one of the aspects of behaviour that deteriorate with dementia. Because of the memory problems, people with dementia forget whether they have bathed or eaten. They need to be tactfully reminded about personal hygiene, and may need supervision during bathing, dressing and feeding. Nevertheless, it is important to continue to encourage independence and allow them to carry out whatever aspects of self-care they can still manage alone. Simplifying each task, and introducing a series of clear steps, can help. For example, dirty clothes can be removed from sight and clean clothes laid out in the order that they are to be put on. Talking the individual through a procedure can also help. Replacing buttons and zips with pieces of Velcro, and using slip-on shoes, can make dressing easier. A variety of aids for bathing and feeding are available, details of which are given in Chapter 9.

Incontinence, which is most humiliating for the individual and unpleasant for the carer, is a problem in a proportion of those with dementia. It may become necessary to remind the individual to visit the toilet at intervals during the day. At night, cutting down on liquids just before bedtime, and the use of continence devices such as dispos-able pads and a waterproof cover over the bed, will minimise the incontinence problem and the carer's workload.

Language and communication problems

Initially, the person with Parkinson's disease and dementia may have only mild communication difficulties. *Dysarthria* —slurring of speech because of problems with articulation—may make his or her speech less easily understood, and there may be difficulty in finding the correct words. As the disease progresses, the individual will find it increasingly hard to communicate: to say what he or she feels and wants, and to make sense of what is being said. He or she may forget the drift of the conversation midway and start talking about a totally unrelated issue; a nonsensical phrase or a single question may be continuously repeated. All this can be very unnerving for the carer, and patience and tact may be required to deal with it.

Occasionally, the individual may be completely confused and disorientated, and mentally regress in time. For example, he or she may want to take the children to school although they are now grown up and married, or ask for someone who died many years ago. Because of the cognitive deficits, communication needs to be kept simple. It is important to speak clearly and slowly, using short sentences. To facilitate communication, if the individual uses sensory aids such as a hearing aid or glasses, these should be worn and kept in good working order. Since memories of the past are often better preserved, they can be more reliable topics of conversation. The carer may find that body language such as facial expression, eye contact and touching may enhance communication. When speech becomes very incoherent, holding the person's hands, or a hug or a cuddle, can convey warmth. Music and dance can sometimes be alternative means of contact and communication.

A number of ways have been developed of enhancing communication between the person with dementia and the carer or other family members. The aim of *reality orientation* is to help the person, who is continually making mistakes with the date, time, places, names and so on, to obtain as good an awareness as possible of his or her surroundings. This is achieved by using memory aids such as clocks and calendars and correcting the individual when places, times or names are misperceived, keeping him or her informed about things that are going on in the house or about major world events, and repeating the information several times. When appropriately phrased and delivered with sympathy, to emphasise strengths rather than highlighting weaknesses, such correcting can help to preserve the individual's remaining abilities. However, it's important not to correct whenever a mistake occurs—this may be perceived as too confrontational. Correcting should be done and information given in a sensitive manner to coincide with times when the person is most receptive and more likely to absorb and benefit from it.

Another approach, developed in the United States, is *validation therapy*, which aims to help the carer or other companion to understand what the person with dementia is trying to express. Gaining a sense of his or her feelings and experiences can open up a channel for communication. *Reminiscence therapy* is another technique. Here, photographs, music, accounts of everyday or historical events, are used as a basis from which to reminisce about the past, of which the person with dementia has a better-preserved memory.

Dealing with potential hazards

As the individual's memory, judgement and reasoning ability deteriorate, everyday situations may become potential hazards. So it may become necessary, for instance, to place medicines, bleach and other cleaning fluids out of reach, to put guards over open fires and electric heaters with exposed elements. The house also needs to be made safe as far as access to gas or electrical appliances is concerned, and trailing wires or other obstacles that may cause accidents. The stairs can be made safer with good lighting, and handrails on either side. Boiling water in the kitchen and bathroom can be hazardous. Get an electric kettle with an automatic cut-out and lower the temperature of the thermostat on the boiler. Handrails and a plastic mat in the bath will help prevent slipping and falls. If the individual smokes, have plenty of ashtrays around and use fireproof material for bedding and armchairs, to reduce the risk of fire. Locks on bathroom and bedroom doors may need to be removed, if he or she is likely to lock him- or herself in. Driving should by now be a thing of the past.

While it is essential to take sensible precautions, whether the individual lives at home or in residential care, some risks will inevitably remain. Minute-to-minute supervision would entail restricting the individual's freedom, and is impossible, anyway.

Mood and emotional problems

Although it is generally maintained that people with dementia have no insight into or awareness of their condition, for a significant number the gradual deterioration of their mental faculties is a source of anxiety and depression, at least in the early phases. Witnessing the disintegration of one's abilities can only be painful. It has been estimated that about 50 per cent of people with dementia experience mood disorder. Disorientation, forgetting where things are when in new surroundings, or forgetting the identity of new people, can lead to panic attacks. Some people with dementia are emotionally unpredictable, breaking down and crying uncontrollably over trivial matters. Sympathetic listening and comforting can help them to vent their feelings, no matter how confused. Some individuals become suspicious, accusing others of stealing their handbag or wallet, of trying to harm them or impersonating their husband or wife. Loss of inhibition is another common problem—they may undress in public or make sexual advances to strangers. Accusations and loss of inhibition are very upsetting for the carer, but remembering that it is the disease, not the individual, who should be blamed for these behaviours will promote better coping. Confusion and hallucinations may also be experienced—the person may see things that are not there, such as someone sitting in an armchair. Reality orientation advocates that he or she be orientated towards reality and corrected when making such errors. Going along with hallucinations is likely to exacerbate them.

Agitation, overreaction and aggression

Restlessness, agitation and aggression can sometimes become problems with the person who has become demented. Agitation and overreaction may be associated with being in unfamiliar surroundings, with disorientation, disruption of daily routines, physical discomfort or overstimulation. The person's anger may be magnified if the carer tries to interrupt or responds to it angrily. Since he or she has lost the ability to reason, attempts at reasoning are unlikely to be effective. Although it's not easy, it is often best to keep calm and let the angry outburst run its course. Forgetfulness means that the individual will usually forget the angry episode, once it is over. It may be possible to prevent these bouts of aggression by avoiding touchy subjects or confrontation, and reducing the demands made on him or her. If specific environmental contingencies that cause or contribute to agitation or aggression can be identified, it may be possible to prevent or control these behaviours. If problems of this sort occur frequently, it may become necessary to seek professional advice and help.

Aimless wandering

Among people who have become demented, wandering is relatively common. It results from disorientation, confusion and perhaps partly from excess energy and a lack of stimulation. Day and night may be reversed, so that the individual gets up to go shopping in the middle of the night. Once outside, he or she may walk for miles in the hope of coming across a place that looks familiar. Installing locks to prevent wandering, getting him or her to wear an identity bracelet with a contact name and telephone number, may prove effective means of dealing with the problem. It has been recently suggested that the risks of wandering may be reduced by using electronic tagging devices. But while this may improve the safety of the person with dementia and reduce the inconvenience created for the carer, it also raises ethical questions to do with restricting the individual's freedom.

Financial and legal matters

In the later phases of the illness, the person with dementia will no longer be able to look after his or her financial interests, and it will become necessary for a relative to take over the decision-making on his or her behalf. For this reason, it may be appropriate to ask the individual to appoint the spouse or partner, or other relative or friend, as his or her *agent* or to give the chosen person an enduring *power of attorney*. This is best done soon after the first symptoms of dementia develop, when the individual is able to understand what it implies. This will make management of affairs, such as picking up pensions and benefits, overseeing any investments or sale of property, easier to carry out. It is also sensible to encourage the individual to make *a will* early on, and select a relative or a solicitor as the executor. This can prevent much confusion later on and make it easier for the spouse and family to manage the estate after he or she dies. Information about appointing an agent, giving power of attorney, and making a will can be obtained from Citizens' Advice Bureaux or from any solicitor.

Strategies for preventing problems

Each person with dementia is an individual and should be treated as such. Eventually, he or she may reach the stage of being unable to communicate needs and preferences. However, conversations with him or her in the early phases of dementia, as well as with members of the family, can help to build a picture of current needs and preferences within the context of his or her previous life history and style. There are a number of strategies that may prove valuable when it comes to minimising problems:

- structuring the individual's daily routine so as to maintain a sense of familiarity and prevent confusion
- allowing him or her to engage as much as possible in enjoyable activities, such as listening to favourite music or talking about the past
- arranging visits from family and friends and outings to shops or pubs or drives in the countryside
- avoiding fatigue and reducing stress
- ensuring that he or she gets regular exercise
- encouraging self-expression through painting and dancing
- at the first signs of disruptive behaviour, resorting to distraction or talking to the individual in a soothing voice and making physical contact.

Moving in with Relatives or into a Nursing Home

Maintaining familiar routines and relationships is an important aim in the management of people with dementia. So living at home should be encouraged for as long as practically feasible. In the initial phases, the memory loss and impaired judgement may be mild enough to allow the individual to continue living alone. At this stage, a daily visit from a member of the local Social Services department or of a local voluntary organisation may be sufficient to ensure that he or she is bathed, dressed and fed adequately. Like Parkinson's disease, dementia is progressive and likely to get worse over time. The person with Parkinson's disease and dementia will eventually reach a stage when the physical and psychological symptoms are so severe that independent living is no longer feasible.

It is when the individual develops problems with self-care, is not eating properly, or is becoming a threat to his or her own safety or the safety of others that moving in with relatives or going into residential care may become necessary. The timing of such a move is of the utmost importance. It should not be left so late that the individual becomes completely dependent on others for care and requires full-time super-vision. On the other hand, a move that occurs too early may result in the loss of what remains of his or her capacity for independent function, as well as generating frustration and promoting dependence. Infor-mation about nursing homes and residential care can be obtained from Carematch, Counsel and Care for the Elderly, the Elderly Accommoda-tion Council and Grace Link. As the nature and quality of care provided vary, a personal visit may be a good idea when it comes to choosing the most appropriate residential placement.

With the deterioration of the person's condition, admission to resi-dential care becomes more or less inevitable. Such a move is invariably associated with experiences of guilt on the part of the carer, who may feel that it constitutes a betrayal of the loved one or be unable to reconcile the current situation with the memory of the personal dignity and personality that characterised him or her in healthier times. It is important to remember that the person with dementia is an individual, with the same needs and the same rights as any other citizen. Residential care should therefore be of a kind that safeguards the individual's right of privacy and choice, his or her friendships and links with the outside world, and engagement in activities and entertainment. With increasing age, people tend to become more rigid, less able to cope with change. This lack of adaptability is magnified in dementia, so that frequent changes of surroundings are not ideal. Once a move to residential care has taken place, the surroundings should be made more welcoming by the addition of a few familiar items of furniture, a lamp, a favourite chair, framed photographs and so on. Individuals should be allowed to wear their own clothing.

The Care of the Carer

Dementia not only causes profound changes in people with Parkinson's disease, but it also alters in many fundamental ways the life of the spouse or others living with them. Besides the psychological trauma of witnessing the gradual disintegration of a loved one, and the major changes that occur in the nature of his or her relationship with that person, the carer has to cope with the numerous additional daily demands that dementia presents. In addition to the practical issues, he or she may feel a sense of bereavement over the loss of companionship. There may be times when the person with dementia does not recognise the carer at all. Looking after someone with dementia can be physically, mentally and emotionally exhausting. Surveys suggest that about 40 per cent of carers experience depression. Care of the carer, looking after his or her physical and emotional health, is a major concern.

Given the virtual dependence of the person with dementia on the carer in the later stages of the illness, he or she may spend every hour of the day looking after that individual. So it is important that the carer has frequent breaks from the task of caring so as to devote time to relaxing and pursuing personal interests. Each day a short time can be allocated to just being alone, to sit quietly, read, watch TV or engage in whatever else may help him or her to unwind. For longer breaks, a relative or friend may be willing to look after the person with dementia, or a 'sitter' can be arranged through Social Services. Social ties should be maintained and strengthened—occasional venting of one's feelings to a friend or acquaintance can relieve the tension. Joining a self-help group, such as the Alzheimer's Disease Society which has many local branches throughout the United Kingdom, can provide access to a group of people with similar problems. Most of the other strategies proposed for the care of the carer in Chapter 12 also apply to the carer of the person with Parkinson's disease who has developed dementia.

KEY FACTS 7

What is dementia?

Dementia is a progressive loss of intellectual abilities and impairment of memory to the extent that the individual can no longer engage in the usual social and occupational activities or, later on, even the basic activities of daily living. When present alongside Parkinson's disease, dementia is initially mild, taking the form of forgetfulness, cognitive sluggishness, lethargy and emotional apathy.

What percentage of people with Parkinson's become demented?

About 15–20 per cent. The risk of dementia in Parkinson's disease is greater for people who are older.

What are the special problems of dementia in Parkinson's disease?

Initially forgetfulness, and later on severe memory difficulties, are major problems associated with dementia. Individuals become disorientated, and may fail to recognise their relatives and friends, and even regress in time. They will become unable to look after themselves—to feed themselves, bath or dress. Incontinence may be a problem in the later stages. Their speech may be slurred and they may be unable to express what they want or how they feel, and may forget the drift of conversations in mid-course. Boredom, confusion and disorientation may result in aimless wandering. The person with dementia may become unduly suspicious and make accusations, or become agitated and aggressive.

Can dementia be cured or treated?

Unfortunately, there is no cure for dementia, and not much in the way of medical treatment at the moment. When dementia is present, the mental state of the person with Parkinson's disease is often given priority, as far as medical treatment is concerned, over the physical state. Levodopa therapy can continue, but it may prove less effective, or only lower dosages may be tolerated.

What strategies are there for managing people with Parkinson's and dementia?

The management of dementia concentrates on overcoming practical problems, minimising risk and ensuring the comfort and well-being of both patient and carer.

- In the early and milder stages of dementia, the individual may be able to continue living alone. In the later and more severe stages, moving in with relatives or going into residential care may become necessary.
- When dementia becomes more severe, the individual may need help in performing most daily activities; supervision and some help may be required when taking medication, bathing, dressing and eating. He or she may need to be reminded to visit the toilet regularly during the day so as to reduce the likelihood of incontinence. Potential hazards (medicines, bleach, open fires, trailing wires, access to gas, boiling water, and so forth) may have to be eliminated or made safe.
- To reduce disorientation, a clock with large numbers and a calendar may be of value. In addition, individuals can be reminded daily of the date, corrected when they appear disorientated in time or place, and informed in simple terms of important family and world events.
- Display by the door a list of things to check and make safe (doors, windows, lights, electrical and gas appliances) or to pick up (money, umbrella, coat) before leaving the house. Choosing prominent and set places for frequently used items such as spectacles and keys can minimise the disruptive effects of impaired memory.
- Communication is best kept simple, using short sentences, spoken slowly and clearly. Eye contact, touching and physical guidance may also enhance communication.
- There are strategies that can be used to prevent or reduce wandering, agitation and aggression, including structuring the person's daily routine so as to maintain a sense of familiarity and avoid confusion, allowing him or her to engage in enjoyable activities, arranging visits to shops or pubs or drives in the country, ensuring that he or she gets regular exercise but avoiding fatigue, and reducing stress; at the first signs of disruptive behaviour, distracting or talking to the individual in a soothing voice, and using physical contact, should alleviate the situation.
- Looking after the emotional and physical health and the needs of the carer is also very important. Taking frequent breaks from caring, maintaining social ties and outside interests can prevent the strain of caring from becoming a burden.

8

Young-onset Parkinson's Disease

THE NATURE OF YOUNG-ONSET PARKINSON'S DISEASE

Since people with young-onset Parkinson's disease constitute a minority of those with the illness, they have not been widely investigated as a separate subgroup. Most of the medical research on young-onset Parkinson's has concentrated on certain specific issues:

- the family history of Parkinsonism or essential tremor among the relatives of patients, the subject of interest here being the degree of genetic contribution
- the association of the illness with other disorders such as hypertension, diabetes, thyroid disorder and pernicious anaemia
- the natural history of the disorder, or the way the symptoms of the disease develop and change over time
- the short- and long-term effectiveness of levodopa therapy.

The main question underlying this research has been whether young-onset Parkinson's is Parkinson's disease manifested at an earlier age or a separate disease altogether. Whether the incidence of Parkinsonism or essential tremor among the relatives of people with young-onset Parkinson's is higher than in the general population has not been firmly established, but more recent research suggests that it is not. More recent data also show no association between the young-onset illness and metabolic or systemic disorders. People with young-onset Parkinson's show the classic features of the illness, particularly resting tremor. Levodopa is clearly of benefit in most cases. Levodopa-induced dyskinesias and on–off fluctuations occur early and frequently in this subgroup. The incidence of dementia is very low.

In summary, the general medical consensus is that young-onset Parkinson's disease is Parkinson's disease occurring at a younger age, rather than a different disease.

What has remained relatively unexplored is the effect of the illness on the patients themselves, and on their spouses or partners and their families. The small amount of research evidence that exists suggests that people who develop Parkinson's at an earlier age show a high rate of depression despite the slow progression of the illness—in contrast to those with late-onset Parkinson's who have a lower rate of depression, even though the disease progresses more quickly. Furthermore, while in those with late-onset Parkinson's disease depression is directly related to the degree of functional disability, no such association is found in people with the early-onset illness. This suggests that other factors may contribute to depression in young-onset Parkinson's disease. When people develop a chronic illness at an early age, it can be emotionally more devastating for them and for their families. We don't expect to fall ill in our youth or middle years, and the early onset of a chronic disorder brings with it the modification of our aspirations and expectations for the future, as well as the prospect of living and coping with disability for the rest of our lives.

THE SPECIAL NEEDS OF PEOPLE WITH YOUNG-ONSET PARKINSON'S AND THEIR FAMILIES

Here we consider some of the special challenges faced by people with young-onset Parkinson's disease, and make some suggestions about ways of coping.

The Shock of the Diagnosis

To be told that you have Parkinson's disease, a disorder associated with old age, when you are in the prime of life, can be truly shocking. Recording his thoughts shortly after being given the diagnosis, Ivan Vaughan, a psychologist, wrote:

> How could it be true? I didn't get ill. Anyway, I was young and fit and only old people got Parkinson's. It was cold comfort that it was pretty extraordinary to get the disease at my age and that at least it supported my desire to be different and unique.

In his book *A Shadow over My Brain* psychiatrist Dr Cecil Todes, another person who contracted the illness early on, wrote about his inability to apply the image of the elderly person with Parkinson's disease to himself:

> For me, Parkinson's disease recalled the shuffling, drooling and speech-affected old men and women in the outpatients' departments at hospitals where I had worked. I couldn't imagine myself in this role. From the viewpoint of a healthy thirty-nine-year-old there remained a vast distance to cover.

The diagnosis of young-onset Parkinson's disease may produce almost as great an impact on the lives of the family members, and particularly on young children, as on the patient. The widely differing reactions of her two children to the diagnosis were described by Margaret, an optician, who had gradually developed symptoms since the age of 39:

> My daughter, aged 17 at the time of diagnosis, was very upset shortly after, but she soon returned to her usual self (a typically selfish teenager) when after two weeks she realised that I was not going to die tomorrow. My son, aged 15, said very little, despite my gently and slowly providing him with basic information about Parkinson's disease. Early on he asked, very reluctantly, if he was likely to suffer from Parkinson's disease in later life. However, the shock might have exacerbated his already worsening adolescent 'blues' that four years on have manifested themselves as depression, which raises its ugly head every 10–12 months.

Medication

Levodopa therapy produces a clear benefit for most people with young-onset Parkinson's disease. However, a large proportion of patients tend to develop levodopa-induced dyskinesias and on–off fluctuations relatively early in the course of treatment. As with those who develop Parkinson's at a later age, the first appearance of these drug complications is related to the rate of the illness's progression as well as to the duration of the levodopa therapy. (Levodopa-induced complications and their management have been described in detail in Chapter 3.) The complications are probably distressing for all who experience them, but their implications may be more drastic for someone who is in the prime of his or her personal and professional life. The dyskinesias and on–off fluctuations may disrupt daily activities, force him or her to stop work, and make socialising difficult. In Chapter 3, we noted that medical opinion is divided about whether levodopa therapy should be started early on or later. As may be imagined, the decision about when to start therapy is even more significant in the case of young people, who will have to live and cope with the illness for a longer period of time. Such decisions are usually taken after considering the life situations and needs of individual patients, and discussing the pros and cons with them and their families.

Work

In most modern societies, work serves many purposes other than enabling a person to earn a living. A considerable portion of our lives may be spent training for a particular profession or job. Subsequently, for most people work takes up a large part of the day, and many constitute a major aspect of an individual's identity and self-esteem. Work contributes to a person's self-esteem partly because it is through work that he or she takes on particular responsibilities, plays an active role in society, and achieves financial independence. In addition, the workplace is a social environment that provides the opportunity for interaction and friendship with colleagues both during and outside working hours. Active participation in the workplace has become such a fundamental feature of most people's everyday life that those who cannot fulfil such a role may sometimes feel like outcasts. Redundancy and unemployment can be associated with feelings of depression. The inability to work because of physical disability may be equally distressing.

If they are employed, people with Parkinson's disease should try to continue working for as long as possible, until the disability makes it impossible.

One of the immediate concerns associated with the diagnosis may be the fear of being seen as incapacitated and, as a result, losing one's job. For this reason, as with later-onset patients, mentioned earlier, some attempt to keep the illness a secret. In recounting his experiences, Ivan Vaughan commented:

I was absolutely determined to conceal from friends and colleagues that I was ill and, when I could no longer keep it secret, to minimise the seriousness of the illness ... During the first few months, keeping the illness secret from other people was fairly easy. I could not stand the thought of having to put up with people feeling sorry for me. The last thing I wanted was to be regarded as 'invalid': I wanted to go on being seen as a person to be reckoned with. I did not want to fall into the position where allowances or excuses had to be made because of difficulties of one kind or another.

Besides personal preference, and the unwillingness to be considered less able, the need for secrecy may also be generated by the problem of convincing employers that, at least in the initial phases when the disorder is mild, Parkinson's does not affect the individual's ability to perform his or her duties efficiently. In *A Shadow over My Brain*, Dr Cecil Todes describes the pressures on him to resign when he developed the illness:

> Demands for leadership in the clinic were coming to a head, as there was repeated talk of closure and, or, merging of the clinic with a neighbouring one. Unfilled sessions were left unfilled and voluntary redundancies were being sought. I appeared a vulner- able candidate and the pressure on me from my colleagues to resign, on the grounds of ill-health, was mounting. A meeting was convened by the fellow consultants in my clinic, to which they summoned me and told me that my presence at the Pad- dington Centre was negatively affecting the clinic in its struggle for survival, and that therefore I should resign or submit myself to the scrutiny of the Three Wise Men. This is a body of doctors drawn from a pool of consultants who would make an objective assessment of a doctor's fitness to work.

Depending on the nature of the job, in the early stages when the symptoms are mild, it is reasonable to expect colleagues and employers to make allowances for slowness and for the need to pace activities because of fatigue, and to accommodate the soft voice and the difficulty with and illegibility of handwriting. Such a degree of understanding and tolerance is to be justifiably expected if the individual has informed them about the nature of Parkinson's disease and the ways in which the symptoms may alter performance, and pointed out the areas of functioning that remain unaffected.

As the concerns and the degree of understanding and sympathy shown by employers are likely to vary considerably, it is difficult to recommend a standard way of approaching them or of breaking the news. But since the anxiety associated with secrecy can be as harrowing as the threat of losing one's job, it is generally best to inform employers about the diagnosis. In most Western countries, there are laws that protect the individual against unfair dismissal—in cases, for instance, where the presence of physical disability does not affect his or her work performance. But it is also important to remember that, besides having rights, each employee also has particular responsibilities towards the employer and in the workplace generally, foremost amongst which is the optimal performance of his or her duties. To give an extreme example, none of us would like to be operated on by an eye or brain surgeon who has the tremor and slowness of movement associated with Parkinson's disease! And the performance of many other skilled professionals would be hampered if they had the symptoms of the disease: actors, teachers, architects, draughtsmen, typists, hairdressers.

So the interests of the individual with Parkinson's disease should be balanced against those of clients and employers. When the point is reached where the symptoms interfere with the performance of an individual's duties or threaten clients' confidence in his or her abilities, then retirement may be the best course of action for all involved.

It is hardly surprising, since work allows financial independence, the fulfilment of professional roles, social interaction and a sense of positive self-esteem, that stopping work is often associated with a sense of withdrawal from society. And this is particularly true for those with young-onset Parkinson's disease; young people who are unable to work because of physical disability and are made redundant or forced to take early retirement often have a sense of premature social ageing.

Fortunately, much can be done to prevent such a reaction. Even if no longer able to hold an outside job, the person with young-onset Parkinson's may be able to work from home. And the development of new interests may prevent the mental and physical decline that is sometimes associated with early retirement and spending time alone at home during the day. Another option is to engage in a new hobby for which previously there may not have been time. Learning to play bridge, photography, a course with the Open University, adult education classes in modern languages—these are just some of the possibilities. In her book *An Old Age Pensioner at Eighteen: My Life with Parkinson's Disease*, Helen Rose describes how, despite never having been very academically minded, she decided to learn how to use a computer.

> The computer entered my life at a crucial time and has, I believe, kept me sane. It did most definitely change my life.

Alternatively, playing an active role in running the home can help the individual, man or woman, to maintain a relatively structured daily routine similar to that provided by most workplaces. As any full-time housewife can attest, running a household is an enterprising, demanding and time-consuming affair. Freedom from outside work can allow an individual to concentrate on being a parent or a wife or husband. Within the restrictions imposed by Parkinson's disease, it can still be satisfying to run a family. Given the sex-role stereotypes inherent in most people's upbringing, older men with Parkinson's disease, as noted earlier, may be resistant to the role reversal involved in switching from being the breadwinner to running the household. But if the concept of the 'new man' means anything, then younger men with Parkinson's disease should have no problem adapting.

Sidney Dorros, who recounted his experiences of young-onset Parkinson's in his book *Parkinson's Disease: A Patient's View*, wrote about the need to adjust to retirement by focusing on its benefits:

> Accepting retirement at age forty-eight was as difficult as accepting the diagnosis eleven years earlier that I had Parkinsonism. It took Debbie [his wife] and me quite a while to acknowledge 'permanent disability' as really permanent, but eventually we did . . . As we learned to adjust to retirement we found some advantages in my relief from the pressures of time and responsibility. Retirement enabled us to enjoy our lives more, to cope more effectively with any ailment, to improve our relationships with our children, and to render increased service to others.

See 'Work and Leisure' in Chapter 5 (p. 120), for a discussion of work and leisure activities that includes aspects of equal relevance to the younger Parkinson's patient.

Finance

People with young-onset Parkinson's disease are still in the productive phase of their lives when the illness strikes. The financial burden of the illness is therefore likely to be higher than for those with late-onset Parkinson's. Besides meeting the costs of daily living, keeping up mortgage repayments and running a car, many have to accommodate the financial needs of children, including the cost of clothing, leisure activities and, sometimes, school fees. These may pose less of a problem in the initial stages, when the individual is still in employment, but when he or she has to stop work, financial hardship may be experienced. Financial problems are likely to be less acute in families where the person with the illness is a woman who has never worked or has made a smaller contribution to the family income. Conversely, when a man who was the main or sole breadwinner develops Parkinson's, it may become necessary for his partner to seek outside employment if she does not already work. The unmarried person with young-onset Parkinson's is usually in a less favourable financial situation. Contact with a social worker who can provide advice on benefits may prove useful (we discuss the various benefits available in Chapter 9). In addition, shortly after the diagnosis, a financial adviser may be able to suggest ways of maximising income through investment of any savings that the couple may have.

The Spouse or Partner, and the Marital Relationship

Coming to terms and living with the chronic illness of a husband or wife, particularly when it develops early in life, affects the other person in as many ways as it affects the patient. Besides the emotional impact of the diagnosis, the spouse or partner has to cope with the prospect of being less able to rely on the ill person to share life's burdens with. The disruption of future aspirations and expectations, the possibility of loss of social life and outside activities, and the likelihood of financial insecurity may all provoke anxiety in the partner. We all have conscious and unconscious images of how we hope our futures will turn out. Like the person with Parkinson's disease, his or her partner has to come to terms with the disruption of their future plans. The daily routines of both may be drastically altered by the illness. And when the ill spouse has retired, if the partner does not go out to work there may be concern about the likely effects of being 'thrown together all day long'. Sidney Dorros, who retired at the age of 48 after developing young-onset Parkinson's when he was 37, wrote:

Like many other couples, Debbie and I had feared that too much togetherness might break our already strained marital relationship. However, within a year after retirement our love and respect for each other began to increase. After more than twenty-five years of frustration over differing attitudes and habits on a few crucial matters, we began to accommodate to each other.

A range of mixed feelings often accompanies the news that a loved one has Parkinson's disease. These may include sadness, helplessness and hopelessness. No matter how willingly a partner or spouse or other relative takes on the role of carer, there are likely to be periods of frustration, resentment and anger, now and later, about the additional responsibilities, the practical demands, and the restrictions that the illness imposes on the lives of everyone concerned.

Such feelings may also be experienced by the ill person. Loss of independence and the need for role reversal can bring on feelings of helplessness and frustration. Right from the start, it is important to allow him or her to do as much as possible within the limitations imposed by the symptoms and the associated disability. The carer needs to bear in mind that being unrealistically demanding can be as harmful as being overprotective. And it is equally important that the ill person acknowledge the major impact that his or her disorder will inevitably have on the lives of spouse and family. Ivan Vaughan talks about his initial resistance to taking medication, and the implications of this and other unilateral decisions for his wife Jan:

> The trouble was that Jan was highly implicated in the consequences of any decision I made concerning the illness. I decided this to myself for a long time and exaggerated the degree to which I was succeeding in maintaining my independence for coping from day-to-day ... In truth, I couldn't hope to have a more sustaining companion. I wanted her to support my desire to be self-determining and independent. What an impossible paradox! And what an uncomfortable role for Jan.

In *The Spaces in Between*, the graphic artist John Harris writes about the effect of his illness on his wife Caryl:

> The other type of side-effect, and one that should not be underestimated, is the effect that my illness had on the family, and especially Caryl. First, there was the worry, for it is far worse to worry about someone other than oneself. Then there was Caryl's feeling of added responsibility and her extra work: taking on more of the domestic chores (Caryl would say she did these anyway). However, even one or two more are an added burden. Most of all there was the difficulty of knowing how to act towards me and my symptoms. Finally, there was the unease of not knowing how I would deteriorate in the future.

Love, understanding, communication, mutual respect, and above all give and take and compromise—the usual essentials of a happy marital relationship—are even more important when one partner suffers from Parkinson's disease. In his book *Heading for Goal*, Paul Baynes, who developed young-onset Parkinsonism following a football injury, says:

> This story is dedicated ... mainly to someone who has stood by me through it all. Through thick and thin, she has always been there when I most needed her and has also brought up two tremendous young boys through the difficult years. Through it all she has shown me the most love and affection that anyone could expect. That person is my wife, Margaret.

In the epilogue to the book, Margaret writes:

As Paul's wife I have shared the trauma of this period of his life. My role has been primarily to keep as normal a life as possible for our two children ... I could not have done this without the support of our families and friends ... There have been some very difficult periods for both of us. These have, however, made me appreciate better those things which I may have taken for granted, and it has made me stronger and more self-sufficient.

To an extent, the onset of a chronic illness such as Parkinson's can make or break a marital relationship. As discussed in Chapters 5 and 6, the quality of the relationship before the onset often determines how well the couple cope. But there are also a few basics that both patient and partner can do—or avoid doing—to guard their relationship against the stresses of the illness.

- Try to strike the right balance—give the individual the necessary help, but don't take away his or her autonomy and independence by doing everything for him or her.
- When there is a problem, discuss it openly.
- Allow each other space.
- Don't nag or criticise. Instead, make positive comments that motivate and help the other person to change.

Sex

Until recently, the topic of sex in relation to people with disabling disorders has been relatively taboo, avoided by those with chronic illness and by medical professionals alike. To overcome this, we recently conducted a study of sexual function in a group of people with young-onset Parkinson's disease. Their spouses or sexual partners also participated in the study. The majority—about 57 per cent of those who took part—were satisfied with their sexual relationship. So we concluded that having Parkinson's disease does not mean that sexual problems are inevitable. A 41-year-old man whose wife of 12 years had had Parkinson's since the age of 32 wrote:

> The only slight problem we have had is adapting to the various physical handicaps that PD presents—i.e. involuntary movements, tremor, rigidity, etc.—but these have been overcome by varying slightly our techniques of love-making. Neither of us is sexually inhibited, so we have great fun experimenting—patience is a virtue!

Partners tended to agree as to whether or not their sexual relationship was satisfactory. About one-third of those who took part reported that it was *un*satisfactory. More problems were reported by couples when it was the man who had Parkinson's disease. As described in Chapter 5, when a sexual problem exists, it isn't any different from the corresponding sexual problem reported by other people. Other factors that can contribute to the development of sexual problems, besides slowness, rigidity and tremor, increased fatigue, and difficulty in non-verbal communication, need to be mentioned here too. Paramount among these are the stress of coping with the illness, worry about physical health, anxiety over job redundancy, financial concerns; and the possible need fundamentally to restructure family life, with individuals taking on new roles as provider or housekeeper or carer.

Lack of communication, or the inability to talk about it, was often mentioned as a stumbling-block by couples who were dissatisfied with their sexual relationship. Acknowledging that a sexual problem or dissatisfaction exists is the first step towards addressing it. There are many ways in which people with Parkinson's disease and their sexual partner can avoid or overcome sexual difficulties:

- Finding out more about the sexual response, and understanding it, can help promote better adaptation. (Most people have a relatively rudimentary knowledge of sexuality and the human sexual response, often based on very elementary teaching at school combined with what they have picked up from friends in their youth.)
- Examining attitudes to sex may reveal where any inflexibility or anxiety stems from.
- Being relaxed, seeking to give as well as to receive pleasure, being considerate of the needs of your sexual partner—all of these are associated with good sex.
- Communicating what you like and don't like, what gives you pleasure and what does not, is the only means of obtaining pleasure.
- Being open to experimentation and trying new positions and techniques can add a spark of novelty and excitement. Altering positions and adopting different sexual roles may improve your sexual satisfaction. As described later, such adaptation is necessary anyway to accommodate the symptoms of Parkinson's disease.
- Adequate contraceptive protection reduces the anxiety that may be associated with the risk of catching AIDS and other sexually transmitted disorders or the problem of unwanted pregnancy. See p. 194 for details on suitable contraceptive methods.

A word about physical attraction is relevant here. Through the media and advertising, we are all exposed to idealised images of the male and female body. Although very few of us in fact possess bodies that match such images, years of exposure result in 'internalisation' of these images as norms: we adopt them as a sort of reference against which to measure ourselves and others. Feminists such as Naomi Woolfe have made us aware of the pitfalls and psychological costs of 'the beauty myth'. If we don't measure up against the image, the feeling is, there must be something wrong with us.

The damage that these fantasies do to a person's self-esteem and sexuality can be even greater for someone with a physical disability than for the rest of us. The person with Parkinson's may well feel less physically attractive and fear rejection by his or her partner. This negative body image was reflected in the accounts of some of the people in our study. There is no doubt that symptoms such as increased salivation and dribbling, oiliness of the skin and hair, and involuntary movements, may make the individual appear less attractive to his or her partner. Physical attraction is undoubtedly important for sexual arousal, performance and satisfaction. However, in any long-term relationship people learn to love and appreciate different aspects of the person who is their spouse or partner. For many, particularly those with decades of marriage or companionship behind them, it is the 'person within' rather than the 'physical appearance' that matters most.

If the problem is not merely one of diminished contact or general dissatisfaction, but something specific, it needs to be addressed. Some difficulties can be dealt with relatively easily:

- It may be possible to partly overcome problems of arousal through longer periods of foreplay.
- It the man has problems obtaining a full erection, or if it is lost before intercourse begins, rhythmic stimulation may help maintain it. A relatively limp penis may still be stimulating when rubbed against the clitoris.
- Premature ejaculation can be prevented or delayed by gripping the area close to the tip of the penis and gently pressing it between the thumb and forefinger.
- In the woman, insufficient lubrication may result in discomfort or even pain. Lubricants such as KY Jelly bought over the counter can help to overcome this.
- Most people are unwilling to use sexual aids, because they tend to be seen as kinky. But none of us has any reservations about using aids where other functions such as seeing or hearing are concerned— we willingly correct them with glasses and hearing aids. Sexual function is no different. Aids such as the energising ring, which can

help to overcome incomplete erections, or a vibrator that can substitute for a penis if erections are impossible, can enhance sexual performance and pleasure. Details of these can be obtained from Sexual and Personal Relationships of the Disabled (SPOD), a charity concerned with the sexual needs of the disabled.

Specific sexual problems such as premature ejaculation may require professional treatment, if they are severe or disruptive. But the main challenge faced by a couple one of whom has Parkinson's disease is to compensate for any problems produced by the symptoms of the illness, and there are a number of strategies that may prove useful:

- With diminishing physical capacity, a change in sexual roles may become necessary in which the partner with Parkinson's, whether it's the man or the woman, plays a more passive role.
- A shift in the timing of sexual activity may be called for, so as to take advantage of the period when the motor status of the individual is at its best. So the time of taking medication may need to be altered.
- Since the person with the illness is more prone to fatigue, it may become necessary to take brief breaks in the course of sexual activity. Or the well partner could adopt a more active role from time to time.
- Instead of the standard man-on-top, or missionary, position, other positions may reduce the pressure on the joints of whichever partner has Parkinson's.

A sexual relationship is not just about sexual intercourse, and orgasm is not the only goal. Besides obtaining and giving pleasure, the aim of the relationship is to create intimacy between two individuals. The sense of intimacy can also be created by embracing, kissing, caressing and fondling. The need for human warmth is a primary one. For most people, expressing warmth is embodied in the sense of touch: holding hands, touching and caressing, giving a hug, having a cuddle, holding someone in an embrace. Even if there are problems with full sexual intercourse, or if there is anxiety associated with having to 'sexually perform', all these other means of communicating warmth can be rewarding.

Family Planning

A concern of many young couples where one partner has Parkinson's disease is whether they should have children, if they do not already have any. Or they may be hesitant about whether they should have any *more* children. The central worry here is the question of whether children will inherit a predisposition to Parkinson's. Obviously, this risk will differ according to the particular circumstances. In the very unlikely event that both parents have Parkinson's, the risk is relatively high. And there may be some risk if, besides the partner with Parkinson's disease, a primary or secondary relative has the illness or a related disorder. Conversely, there is no risk if the person has secondary Parkinson's disease (see p. 18), which has developed after injury. Both partners need to be reassured that, in the majority of cases, Parkinson's is not an inherited disorder and that their present or future offspring are not at any greater risk of developing it than is the general population (see p. 24).

A more important consideration for the young couple may be whether the individual with Parkinson's will be able to give his or her best to the parental role—and this should be evaluated in the long term as well as the short term. As discussed earlier, it is difficult to predict the likely course of Parkinson's disease. People have to consider five, ten, fifteen years hence. Providing for children's emotional and financial needs can be demanding not only during infancy and pre-school years but also later, in adolescence and even into adulthood. So the joys of parenthood have to be weighed against the responsibilities, burdens, financial strains and daily practicalities that go with the role of parent.

Parkinson's disease does not affect fertility, either in men or in women. If the couple do not wish to have children, or wish to have no more, safe methods of contraception have to be considered. Besides the more permanent and irreversible options of vasectomy and hysterectomy, other safe methods of contraception are available such as taking the contraceptive pill or having an intra-uterine device (IUD) or a cap inserted. Each couple should select an appropriate method by first discussing their particular needs with a doctor. The effects of the contraceptive pill on Parkinson's disease are unknown. The IUD may not be appropriate for some. For others, tremor and rigidity may make it difficult to insert caps.

For men and women of child-bearing age who are planning to have a family, another concern is the possible effects of anti-Parkinsonian medication on the unborn child and during breast-feeding. The medications commonly used in the treatment of Parkinson's are not considered to damage the unborn child. If it is the woman who has Parkinson's disease, it is usually best not to discontinue the medication during pregnancy, because this may result in increased muscle stiffness, with a risk of premature delivery or problems with labour and natural birth. Possible difficulties are best discussed with the doctors concerned—that is, the neurologist treating the illness and the obstetrician involved in the care of the woman during pregnancy. When it is the man who has Parkinson's, neither the illness nor the medication should have any effect on the sperm or hence on the unborn child. A further concern for a woman with young-onset Parkinson's disease may be to do with the likely effects of pregnancy on the symptoms and course of the illness. At the moment, there is no systematic information available about the possible influence of the hormonal changes associated with pregnancy on the symptoms of Parkinson's.

The onset of the *menopause*, which can sometimes be accompanied by symptoms such as hot flushes and mood changes, can place an additional burden on the woman with Parkinson's disease. Hormone replacement therapy (HRT) is an option available to menopausal women that can help alleviate some of the symptoms and reduce the risk of others such as osteoporosis, a condition in which the bones become porous and brittle and less dense. An informal survey of female members of YAPP&Rs (Young Alert Parkinson's Partners and Relatives, see p. 201) in the winter 1992 issue of *YAPmag* reported that about half of those who participated were on HRT while on levodopa therapy, with only one person complaining that HRT worsened her Parkinson's disease.

Children and Their Reactions to Parental Illness

An often difficult issue after the diagnosis, for people with young-onset Parkinson's disease, is the question of telling the children. Parents can be uncertain about whether or not to tell young children about the illness and, if they decide to, how much to tell. As noted in Chapter 5, as a general rule it is best not to try to keep it a secret. The more dramatic conclusions that a child may draw from silence on the subject can have shattering effects on his or her emotional well-being, general behaviour and academic performance. Remember that the responsibility lies with you, the parent, and not with your child to open the topic for family discussion. Choosing a suitable time to be alone with the child or children to explain in simple terms and in ways that are appropriate to their age and maturity what Parkinson's disease is, will alleviate fears and prevent unfounded speculation. Upsetting news may not be registered easily, so to avoid overloading the child, offer information gradually, maybe over several occasions. It may also help to describe the ways in which you or your partner may no longer be able to contribute to your child's upbringing as you have hitherto—all the time reassuring him or her, of course, that you would love to be able to. You might consider something along these lines:

Dad/Mum has Parkinson's disease. Parkinson's is an illness that affects a small part of the brain that controls movements. Because of this, Dad/Mum has difficulty moving, can only walk very slowly, talks in a soft voice, and his/her hand shakes. You may notice other things, such as that he/she can't swallow his/her saliva or do up buttons. These are all caused by the illness. It doesn't affect the mind, so he/she can think and feel normally. Doctors don't know why people get Parkinson's, but it's nobody's fault that Dad/Mum has got it. He/she is not going to die, but the disease is likely to get worse over the years, so that he/she will need more and more help in doing things. The fact that Dad/Mum has Parkinson's doesn't mean that you or the rest of the family are going to get it as well. It isn't an infectious illness like flu. You can't catch it from other people. Because of Parkinson's disease Dad/Mum can no longer spend as much time playing with you, or may not be able to play football or race with you. There will be times when he/she will be upset or irritated and snap at you, but this doesn't mean that he/she loves you any less.

Children should be encouraged to ask questions and to express their feelings and reactions to the news. They should also be given lots of reassurance. It is important to paint a realistic picture—not to be too dramatic, but not to minimise the meaning and implications of the illness, either. The aim is not to frighten them, but to inform them. Such explanations can also help children to provide explanations to their friends about the ill parent's reduced participation in their upbringing or social life.

Besides the question of whether to tell the children about the illness and how much to tell them, parents with Parkinson's disease often have other, related, concerns. The ill parent may be worried about his or her inability to spend more time with the children or to interact with them. Because of the physical restrictions imposed by the illness, there may be feelings of missing out on the children's childhood. The on–off fluctuations, the increased susceptibility to fatigue, and the need to take more frequent rests may make the ill parent less able to participate in play, more irritable and less tolerant of noise or misbehaviour. On occasion, the well parent may become the 'mediator', preventing the needs and demands of the children from impinging on the other parent, or, on the other hand, shielding the children from the negative impact of parental illness by means of compensatory strategies, such as trying to be both mother and father. In some cases, so as to allow the well parent to go out to work, the children may take on a greater proportion of the household chores. This may interfere with their homework or limit the time spent with friends.

When confronted with a parent's illness, children may experience a wide spectrum of feelings. They may have a sense of grief, brought on by the evident changes in their ill parent and the fact that, compared to their peers, they are missing out on input from and interaction with this one parent. Fear may be associated with thoughts that the illness may cause the family to split up. They may feel rejected, in the sense that they are no longer the centre of attention in the family. Embarrassment may result from the fact that, despite being an adult, the ill parent is no longer able, in the more advanced stages of the illness, to do basic activities or look after his or her own needs. Older children may become particularly embarrassed by the parent's more evident symptoms such as tremor or rigidity, and ask them not to come to parent–teacher meetings or accompany them on shopping trips; or they may refuse to bring friends home. This can be upsetting for the parent, but the first rule of tolerant parenting is to make every effort to bridge the generation gap and view life from the adolescent's perspective. Making time to discuss the embarrassment openly, and finding ways of overcoming it, may well prove helpful for all concerned.

Children show diverse reactions to the changes that living with an ill parent may entail. Some become very upset and weepy. Others become stubborn, lazy and self-centred. Yet others withdraw from family life and spend more time in their room or away from home.

Besides practical help, children, particularly older ones, sometimes provide emotional support for the carer-parent as well as for the ill one. Parents tend to worry and feel guilty about this burden of care falling on their children's shoulders. Certainly, even if they are willing and although circumstances may seem to necessitate it, children should not be expected to take on major responsibilities or to perform the role of sole carer. This would be unfair—they would miss out on their childhood and the responsibility might be too great for them. On the other hand, many children willingly take on new duties to help the ill parent. In her book, Helen Rose expresses her appreciation of the help given to her by her son Stuart:

Now that I have to use the wheelchair every time I want to go out, I quite often feel that I am more of a nuisance than a wife or a mother to my family. Ashleigh [her older daughter] no longer lives at home, so poor Stuart has it all to do, along with his Dad. Stuart is thirteen and does a lot more than Ashleigh did at thirteen. Of course I was much more able then than I am now. Apart from the weekly shopping trips in the car with Peter [her husband], Stuart pushes me in the wheelchair to the village and quite often he will take me and the wheelchair on the bus to the shopping centre ten miles away. The first time he did this an old man was so pleased to see someone his age taking his mum on a shopping spree that he patted him on the back and gave him fifty pence.

Helen Rose's book helps to illustrate other problems that may have to be faced by children when one parent has Parkinson's disease. In their search for fun or a good laugh, children can sometimes be incredibly insensitive and cruel. Lack of understanding and misinterpretation of symptoms such as tremor, slowness and involuntary movements can result in classmates making fun of the ill parent, maybe calling him or her 'drunk', 'mad' or 'bizarre'. Others may not understand why it is necessary for the particular boy or girl to spend more time at home with the ill parent, and make fun for this reason. This was the case with Helen's son:

[Stuart] arrived home from school one afternoon in tears. I comforted him and we had a heart-to-heart. It appeared that two boys taunted him by calling him a cissy because he chose to come home after school to help his mum.

On this occasion Helen intervened and talked to the headmistress, who spoke to the boys concerned, who then apologised to Stuart and to her.

With experience and maturity, children can learn not only to cope with the day-to-day needs of the ill parent, but also to attain a better understanding of the challenges faced by him or her and the sacrifices made by the well parent. Ashleigh, Helen Rose's daughter, writes:

I suppose after fifteen years you just get used to the fact that you have a disabled parent. I could not imagine my Mum any other way than the way she is now. I do know she gradually becomes worse, but I have watched this since I was about two years old when she had her first symptoms . . . But no matter how bad she gets, I will always love her and she will always be *my mum* . . . Now that I am older and understand more of what Parkinson's disease is, I realise how much my Dad has gone through. It is not only the disabled person who suffers, and it has made me love and respect him even more. There are a lot of men who wouldn't stay with their wives and children with such responsibility, as he has. Only a few years after they married he had to dress her, bath her and sometimes toilet her at bad times, and knowing her pride has all gone, you can see in his face at times the pain he is feeling.

As mentioned earlier, children's expectations for their own future may be tainted by the parental illness and by the burden of increasing dependency. Older children may feel responsible, and may be concerned about what will happen to the ill parent or how the other parent would cope alone if they were to marry or simply move out of the family home. These concerns shape children's decisions about their future, and should be openly discussed.

Within the framework of the new *holistic approach* to health and illness, the family is considered as a *system*. Within this system, the interaction of individual members has implications for their collective functioning and well-being. When one person falls ill, the functioning of the whole system is affected and its previously well balanced working may be disturbed. To compensate for this imbalance, individual members such as the spouse or partner and children, and even members of the extended family such as grandparents, aunts and uncles, may take on new roles. Such attempts may not always be successful, and friction and tension may develop. When this happens, family get-togethers to enhance communication, allow the airing of discontent, and to clarify roles, joint aims and means of achieving them, can prove helpful. Such informal 'lay therapy' can often nip a problem in the bud.

However, if difficulties are not resolved by such informal *family therapy*, it may be appropriate to seek outside help so as to promote the necessary adjustments. Formal family therapy from a trained *counsellor* or *therapist* need not be very lengthy. Depending on the precise nature of the problems, six to twelve sessions, or even as few as three or four can prove useful. When problems with communicating and relating to each other develop, family therapy may help re-establish communication, unmask hitherto unvoiced or unrecognised feelings or problems, and help individuals to develop insight into the ways in which difficulties have developed in the past, or escalated from minor to major. The therapist can also help the family create alternative ways of behaving or relating to each other that may stop difficulties developing, and explore realistic ways in which individuals may adopt new roles or help each other. In this way, the family system as a whole can cope better with the daily strains and stresses posed by the challenges of Parkinson's disease.

In a study conducted by the National Children's Bureau to assess the impact of Parkinson's disease on children, some of the families interviewed expressed a need for specific help in relation to children. They said that an exploratory booklet or contact with other children in the same situation would have been valuable. As far as we know, no such booklet is available and no kind of formal network between children whose parents have Parkinson's disease has been organised. But, where there's a will—and a need—there's usually a way! Such a network could be instigated by two sets of concerned parents—that's all it would take.

Unattached People with Young-onset Parkinson's

Much of the above is written on the assumption that the young person with Parkinson's disease has already formed a long-term intimate relationship, whether inside or outside marriage. However, this is likely to be a gross stereotype, particularly since the available statistics suggest that during the last two decades there has been a tendency for women to concentrate on their careers in their twenties and thirties, waiting until later to form lasting relationships or family units. So the onset of Parkinson's disease before the age of forty is likely to strike a proportion of women and men before they have had the opportunity to 'settle down'.

The sexual and relationship problems that may be experienced by those with young-onset Parkinson's disease who are not married or in a stable relationship need to be considered. Those who have already left home may have to cope with the isolating effects of the illness. Those still living at home may be very aware of the burden of care falling on their elderly parents. Single people with Parkinson's may find it harder to cope than the 'attached', as they may feel that their illness has deprived them of the possibility of lasting human contact and warmth, or that it cannot fail to limit their experience.

It is true that people with disability may have additional difficulty in finding and attracting a partner. First impressions do count, but appearance and physical attraction are not the only factors when it comes to establishing relationships. Certainly, staying at home and blaming the illness and disability is unlikely to be helpful. And there are in fact many people with Parkinson's or other kinds of physical disability who have no problem in establishing and maintaining relationships. Everything in life is relative, even misfortune. In comparison with some illnesses and disabilities, Parkinson's disease may appear benign! Instead of withdrawal and giving up without a fight, the first step may be *self-acceptance*. If you have got to know and to accept your strengths and weaknesses as a person, understood what you can give and what you can expect from a relationship, you will be much more able to convey these important things about yourself to another person when the occasion presents itself. One complaint may be lack of opportunity. The answer is, make your own opportunities. Instead of social isolation, choose social networking. Anyway, even among those not hampered by a chronic illness, not everyone develops a long-term relationship or gets married. Not every marriage is happy, or lasts—statistics tell us that one in four ends in divorce. So, if it's any consolation, it's worth remembering that as far as ability to establish and maintain satisfying relationships is concerned, even people who are not disabled by illness have problems in this department!

YAPP&Rs

The Young Alert Parkinson's Partners and Relatives (YAPP&Rs) group was born in 1988 in Lancaster in the course of a 'young think-tank' weekend organised by the Parkinson's Disease Society. The acronym was coined by Paul Lewin, a computer specialist with the illness. Although YAPP&Rs is strongly affiliated with the PDS, it operates relatively independently and is mainly run by people with the illness and their spouses, partners and relatives. YAPP&Rs now have their own newsletter, *YAPmag*, and hold regional and national meetings. The first European meeting of young Parkinsonians, Euro YapMeet, was held in May 1994 in Peterborough. As the members of YAPP&Rs are particularly interested in looking after the interests of people with young-onset Parkinson's, joining them may be a useful way of making contact with people in a similar situation, with similar problems and challenges at a similar stage in their life.

KEY FACTS 8

What is young-onset Parkinson's disease?
A person is said to have young-onset Parkinson's when the symptoms develop before the age of forty. Although Parkinson's is usually a disorder of old age, about 20 per cent of people develop it at this earlier age in their lives. From available evidence, most doctors are of the opinion that the young-onset illness is Parkinson's occurring at a younger age rather than a different disease.

What are the considerations in the medical treatment of people with young-onset Parkinson's?
Levodopa therapy produces symptomatic relief, but for those with young-onset Parkinson's disease it is associated with on–off fluctuations and dyskinesias relatively early on in the course of treatment. As discussed in Chapter 3, for the individual who will have to live with the disease for 30 to 40 years, the decision about when to start medication is best taken after considering his or her present disability and quality of life as well as longer-term needs. Decisions like this must take into account the particular circumstances and needs of each person.

What are their special needs?
As the illness strikes at an early stage in life, its disruptive effects are likely to be felt more acutely and for longer. The need to give up work sooner or later and the ensuing financial problems are a major concern. If the individual is married or in any other kind of stable long-term relationship, the marital/sexual relationship may be adversely affected by the stresses of the illness. Parkinson's disease affects the whole family, and not just the ill person. The illness has major implications for the present and future life of the spouse or partner. Children react in diverse ways to parental illness: for example, by showing greater co-operation and taking on new responsibilities, or by withdrawal from family life and spending more time outside the home, or by becoming lazy, stubborn or self-centred. Fear, sorrow and embarrassment are

commonly experienced by children of whatever age. If a couple are planning to have a family, they may be concerned about the effect of anti-Parkinsonian medication on the unborn child or the effect of the pregnancy on the symptoms of Parkinson's (see below).

What strategies promote better coping?

Many of the recommendations in Chapters 9 to 12 also apply to those with young-onset Parkinson's disease. The strategies that follow may help you to deal with the specific challenges that you face:

- Continue working for as long as physically possible. But when it becomes a major burden and source of stress, or when duties can no longer be reliably performed, it's best to stop.
- Stopping work does not mean becoming idle. Explore possible ways of working from home. Alternatively, whether you are a man or a woman, running a house and looking after the needs of one's family can be challenging and rewarding.
- Secrecy is often motivated by fear—fear which in this instance may relate to losing your job or being considered different or incapable by others. As the symptoms of the illness will become noticeable sooner or later, secrecy only deprives you of the understanding and help that others would probably offer, if you let them know the situation. By far the best strategy is to tell family, friends and colleagues about Parkinson's disease and how it affects you. Only then will they be in a position to help.
- If you are married or have a partner, remind yourself from time to time that your spouse or partner is also affected by your illness and that it is a burden that you need to share and cope with together. Making time to talk, to share concerns and to vent emotions will prevent the build-up of frustration, discord and emotional outbursts.
- The symptoms of Parkinson's and the stress associated with the illness can adversely affect sexuality. Communicating with your sexual partner, being open to experimentation and exploring new ways of coping with the problems created by the illness can be productive strategies. When marital or sexual problems develop that you cannot deal with, it's time to seek outside help. A short course of marital and/or sexual therapy may resolve the problems.
- Parkinson's disease does not affect fertility, and there is no reason why you should not have children if you wish. No clear scientific evidence yet exists about the effect of anti-Parkinsonian medication on the unborn child, or about the way in which pregnancy affects the symptoms of the illness. Both you and your spouse or partner

need to weigh up the joys of parenthood against your ability to perform the parental role adequately in the long term, and the likely effects of the additional burden of child-rearing on your symptoms.

- The fact of the illness should not be hidden from children—otherwise, they may reach more worrying conclusions about the changes they observe in the ill parent. It is parents' responsibility to adequately inform their children about the illness, and the explanation should be simple and appropriate to their ages. Children need to be reassured that they will not develop the illness, and that the family will not split up as a result of it.
- Joining self-help groups such as YAPP&Rs will bring you and your family into contact with others who are facing and coping with similar life challenges.

Part III

Coping with Parkinson's Disease

9

Getting Help from Others

The Parkinson's Disease Society recommends that all 'health purchasers' should ensure that patients with Parkinson's disease living within their health authority have access to the following services: a GP, a consultant neurologist with a specialist interest in the illness, a specialist nurse, a physiotherapist, an occupational therapist, a speech and language therapist, a dietitian, a social worker, a psychologist, a counsellor, a chiropodist, a community nurse, a community psychiatric nurse, a continence adviser and a wheelchair service. In addition, facilities for day care, respite care and institutional care are considered necessary.

This chapter considers the various sources of help available to the person with Parkinson's disease and his or her carer, and the exact ways in which each resource can help them cope better with the illness. These other resources—referred to as *adjunct therapies*—can help to alleviate symptoms and delay the onset of disability and handicap; they are adjunct, or additional, to the standard treatments such as medication and surgery. Adjunct therapies and other sources of help fall into several broad categories:

- The main types that are aimed at alleviating the symptoms of Parkinson's are speech therapy, physiotherapy and conductive education.
- Other kinds of adjunct therapy, that can help prevent or reduce disability and handicap, or promote ways of coping better with emotional reactions to illness or with the psychological burden of caring, are provided by the occupational therapist, the social worker, the nurse practitioner, the dietitian and the psychotherapist or counsellor.
- Day care, respite care and residential care are other sources of help,

that may be necessary to relieve the burden on the primary carer.

- Holiday breaks, essential means of relaxation and relief from daily duties, can be arranged for people with special needs.
- The various procedures under the label *alternative medicine* constitute another option aimed at promoting health and combating disease.
- Voluntary organisations such as the Parkinson's Disease Society and the Carers' National Association can also be of value.

When considering the range of services available, there are a few points that are worth remembering:

- Don't be too proud to ask for and to use these services—they exist in order to offer help to people in your situation.
- On the other hand, when asking for the various services, don't assume that you will necessarily be provided with everything that you have asked for. In most areas, resources are limited and there may be others whose needs are as great as or greater than yours.
- As we have already noted, the needs of the person with Parkinson's disease and his or her carer vary at different stages of the illness; so the resources required and the frequency of contact with each source of help will vary similarly. Even though you may be able now to shop, clean, cook and look after yourself or your relative with Parkinson's, a time may come when you will appreciate even a few hours of outside help.
- Some of the services are free to anyone who is entitled to free health care under the National Health Service. You can contact the local Social Services, who may send a Social Security officer to assess your needs for care and support. He or she will also be able to give you information about, and arrange access to, equipment or resources such as home help, sitting services, laundry services, nursing and residential homes. *Health services* such as physiotherapy, occupational therapy, speech therapy, chiropody and nursing are free when provided through the NHS. *Social services* such as home help, attendance at a day centre and meals-on-wheels have to be paid for. If your financial resources allow it, you will be able to obtain some of these services privately.
- Some of the adjunct services are home-based and require you to welcome a stranger into your home so that he or she can attend to your more private functions. Initially you may find this intrusive, but as you get used to it you will find it more acceptable and worthwhile.

ADJUNCT THERAPY: IMPROVING THE SYMPTOMS

A survey conducted by Dr Marie Oxtoby in 1978 for the Parkinson's Disease Society found that of the people with Parkinson's who were members of the society, 17 per cent had seen a physiotherapist, 13 per cent had seen an occupational therapist, only 3 per cent had been referred to a speech therapist; and, in addition, many were found not to have the necessary aids. The low level of referral was confirmed in a survey carried out in Aberdeen. The conclusion to be drawn is that doctors do not automatically refer people with Parkinson's disease for these kinds of adjunct therapy. If you think you will benefit from any of these services, ask your GP or neurologist for a referral.

Speech and Language Therapy

About two-thirds of people with Parkinson's complain of some sort of speech problem. In addition, about 40 per cent suffer from dribbling and about a quarter have difficulty swallowing. The speech and language therapist can help improve all aspects of communication, which include the following problems:

- weak and monotonous voice, delay in speech initiation, slow speech, speech that starts off at a normal rate and then speeds up
- blank and mask-like facial expression, infrequent blinking, lack of gestures
- handwriting that gets gradually smaller, or that is spidery and diffi-cult to read
- difficulty in swallowing, choking, dribbling.

A speech and language therapist will start off by doing an assessment to determine the precise nature of the speech and related problems in each individual case. Then, advice will be given and particular exercises will be demonstrated and practised, as appropriate:

- Exercises that can be practised in front of a mirror, for achieving general relaxation or for reducing the rigidity of the facial muscles.
- Optimal methods of breathing using the diaphragm (the muscle sepa-rating the upper and lower parts of the chest) and ways of moving the mouth and tongue, to prevent the individual from 'running out of air' when speaking and to enable him or her to pronounce all sounds clearly.
- Intonational exercises using equipment such as Vocalite, which

records and then plays back speech so as to provide feedback. This allows the individual to monitor the volume, rate and changes in pitch and rhythm of his or her own speech. A metronome may be used for teaching rhythm and timing of speech, and a tape-recorder for providing auditory feedback.

In addition:

- The individual is taught to overcome the delay in initiating speech by mentally counting 1–2–3 and then starting to speak. To make it easier for others to comprehend the individual's speech, the patient is encouraged to utter each word slowly by opening the mouth widely, using short and precise sentences, and varying the way a request is expressed when repeating it. To help increase volume, the individual with the illness will be reminded to speak loudly at all times, as if addressing an audience in a large room.
- The speech therapist is the best source of advice about mechanical aids such as portable microphones and amplifiers that can be worn around the neck. Remember that voice amplification will be of value only if the speech is intelligible. Other equipment that may improve communication are telephones with microphones and amplifiers, and small typewriters with specially adapted visual displays for giving easily recognised messages, thus bypassing altogether the need to talk.
- The speech therapist will recommend various strategies for combating swallowing difficulties. Maintaining a good posture when eating and drinking can reduce both swallowing problems and the risk of fluid entering the lungs. Never swallow with the head tilted backwards. Instead, take a mouthful, lower the chin towards the chest, and then swallow. Yawning a few times before the start of each meal and drinking very cold fluids can help, too.
- Writing on lined paper can help maintain a constant size of script, and illegibility can be overcome by typing your messages.
- The speech therapist may advise the carer to be patient and not to rush the ill person when he or she is speaking or eating, as this can only complicate matters and result in mounting frustration.

Because of the need for special equipment, speech and language therapy is usually provided in hospital departments. Occasionally the speech therapist can see people in their own homes. Referral to a speech therapist can be organised by your GP or by the consultant neurologist. A tape entitled *Speech Exercises for People with Parkinson's Disease*, which includes relaxation, breathing, volume, speed, stress, pattern, pitch and articulation exercises, can be obtained from the PDS.

Physiotherapy

The aim of physiotherapy in Parkinson's disease is to use specific exercises to prevent or relieve musculoskeletal problems. Although most patients are referred to physiotherapy when moderate to severe disability has already developed, it may be more useful to have physiotherapy at an earlier stage, to prevent problems becoming severe in the first place. The aims of physiotherapy exercises are:

- to reduce joint stiffness
- to increase the range of joint movements
- to prevent muscle weakness
- to improve posture and balance
- to retrain gait with a view to preventing falls
- to teach methods of counteracting 'freezing'
- to promote relaxation
- to teach techniques for getting up from a chair or out of bed
- to teach strategies for rolling over in bed.

Physiotherapy focuses on some of the symptoms and associated problems of the illness. The course usually starts with an assessment of what the patient can and cannot do—how posture, balance and walking are affected, to what extent rigidity and slowness affect movements, and whether pain or discomfort are present and if so, where. Then an individualised treatment plan will be drawn up. This may include passive movements of body parts carried out by the physiotherapist, as well as active exercises performed by the patient. Hydrotherapy—exercises in a swimming-pool—may also be used to overcome some of the musculoskeletal problems.

Posture

The physiotherapist advises on ways to improve posture while sitting or standing or walking. Practice in front of a mirror will provide visual feedback and allow you to make adjustments and corrections where necessary. You can practise standing straight by standing against a wall with your heels, shoulder blades and back of the head actually touching it. Sitting on a high-backed upright chair with a cushion to support your back can prevent stooped posture while you are sitting.

Walking

Because movements such as walking that are usually performed auto-matically—that is, without much effort or conscious planning—are affected most in Parkinson's disease, physiotherapy concentrates on breaking movements into smaller component parts and teaching the patient to consciously control each part in turn. To improve walking, the physiotherapist can teach you to strike the heel down and to reinforce the action by thinking to yourself, 'Heel first' with every step. A military-style heel strike, in particular, will improve gait. In addition, you will be asked to counteract the forward-leaning, or flexed, pos-ture—which results in the displacement of the centre of gravity, shuf-fling, speeding up and freezing—by trying to stand straight or by holding the shoulders slightly back. And keeping the feet a few inches apart can improve the stability of walking.

Falls

If falls have become a major problem, the GP or neurologist may be asked to check your blood pressure in order to exclude postural hypotension—a sudden drop in blood pressure when standing up from sitting—as a cause. If most falls occur when you get up first thing in the morning or after an afternoon nap, postural hypotension is likely to be the main cause. For falls that have other causes, the physiotherapist can give advice: equipping yourself with sensible shoes and a walking-stick, for instance, may help. Soft slippers can result in falls, and should be avoided, even at home.

Turning

Those who have difficulties with balance and turning will be taught to turn slowly in a large semicircle, and to consciously lift their feet higher than their natural tendency and to lengthen their pace at every step.

Freezing

The physiotherapist may suggest a number of steps for unfreezing. First, learning to put the heel down first. Second, straightening up to correct the flexed posture. Third, using 'trick' movements such as walking over imaginary lines or marching on the spot, which can get you going from the stationary position.

Getting up from a chair

A suitable chair for a person with Parkinson's is a high one with arms that make it easier to rise, and a high back that provides back support when sitting. To get up from a chair, patients are taught to move to the edge of it, tuck the feet back, then throw their body weight forward—for example, by rocking themselves forward and then pushing up with their hands on the arms.

Rolling over in bed

This can be made easier by teaching the patient a number of steps. First, with the feet flat on the bed, bend your knees. Second, clasp your hands together and raise your arms into the air with the elbows straight. Third, turn your head and arms to one side—this can flex the hips sufficiently to allow you to roll on to your side. Fourth, use your arms and upper trunk to complete the movement. Rotational exercises such as twisting the trunk alternately to the left and right while sitting or standing, or rotating your legs from side to side while lying on your back, can make rolling over in bed easier.

Home exercises

The ultimate goal of physiotherapy is to achieve functional improvement in the patient's everyday life. To this end, in addition to the exercises carried out in the clinic, you are taught a range of exercises to practise regularly at home. These include breathing and relaxation exercises, and exercises for the neck and head, the facial muscles, the shoulders and arms, hands, legs and back; and exercises to help with rolling over. They should be practised for between 10 and 20 minutes once or twice a day, to prevent muscle weakness and to maintain a good range of movement in the joints.

Advice about remaining active

Because of fatigue, reported by about half of all those with Parkinson's disease, there is a tendency to be inactive. The fear that tiredness caused by exercise can cause setbacks is unfounded. Despite disability, you should remain as active as possible. It's a good idea to go for a walk every day, even though this may be only for a short distance in the later stages of the illness. Sports such as golf, swimming and boules should be continued for as long as possible.

Advice to the carer

The physiotherapist can teach the carer the best methods for lifting the patient and for helping him or her to get up from a chair or out of bed, and how to support him or her while walking. These methods involve strategies that produce no damage to either the back muscles or the spine, and are safe for both parties. Carers need to be encouraged to take regular exercise, and to look after their general physical health and fitness.

The majority of physiotherapists work in hospital departments, and some work privately. Although physiotherapy is usually offered in a hospital or clinic, some physiotherapists also make home visits. A referral can be arranged by your GP or neurologist. Specific physiotherapy exercises to increase mobility and combat other musculoskeletal problems in Parkinson's disease are described in the booklet *Living with Parkinson's Disease*, which can be obtained from the Parkinson's Disease Society. In an accompanying audio-cassette, also available from the PDS, the exercises are set to music.

Conductive Education

Conductive education is a technique developed in Hungary after the Second World War by Dr Andras Peto, a doctor with a special interest in rehabilitation, and was originally developed for children with motor disabilities. It is used in the rehabilitation of children with cerebral palsy, and adults with stroke, multiple sclerosis or Parkinson's disease. The technique involves teaching people with motor disability how to control their movements, and is modified to fit the symptoms and meet the needs of each disorder. The courses are intensive and are often carried out in groups of up to 12, led by teachers or 'conductors' who lead their pupils through the process of learning.

There is firm emphasis on four principles:

1 The active participation, but independence, of the patient.
2 The breaking-down of motor tasks into small steps, to make them more manageable.
3 The use of rhythm, music and harmonic chanting—called *rhythmic intention*—to help the patient regulate his or her motor skills.
4 The use of speech to control motor tasks. When a sequence of actions is being learned, the conductor verbalises the action as it is happening and the student repeats it out loud. As the action becomes automatic, the student can reduce the use of audible verbal regulation.

In addition, the conductor recommends daily practice of the exercises and inspires the student to strive to surpass yesterday's achievement. The conductor facilitates this process by fostering a positive attitude, encouraging effort, reinforcing progress and structuring tasks so that failure is prevented or minimised.

Conductive education exercises target the types of motor activity that are particularly impaired by Parkinson's disease, such as doing two things at once, controlling posture and performing sequential or repetitive movements. The aim is to facilitate everyday activities such as getting up from a chair or from the floor and rolling over in bed, as well as to alleviate writing and speech difficulties. The exercises are performed in different positions, such as while lying on the back or stomach or while standing or sitting. In the course of a session most muscles of the body are stretched and relaxed to some extent. During each exercise, the patient is encouraged to repeat the instruction given by the conductor—'I raise my left arm', 'I lower my right leg', and so on. The verbal instruction is considered to create the intention of performing whatever action it may be. Rhythmic counting aloud—for example, 1–2, 1–2— is also used frequently when actions are being performed.

The Birmingham Institute for Conductive Education was set up in 1987 to provide and evaluate conductive education for children with cerebral palsy. Some of its conductors were trained at the Peto Institute. Other conductors who trained there work in London and other parts of the country. Some of them hold weekly group training sessions for people with Parkinson's. The PDS can provide the names of conductors specialising in the illness.

ADJUNCT THERAPY: PREVENTING OR REDUCING DISABILITY AND HANDICAP

The services of the occupational therapist, the social worker, the nurse practitioner, the dietitian and the psychotherapist or counsellor are all geared to reducing disability and handicap.

The Occupational Therapist

The community- or hospital-based occupational therapist (OT) aims to improve an individual's motor skills and mobility, as well as his or her ability to carry out the activities of daily living, including work. First, the OT assesses the patient's daily activities so as to find out what he or she can still do efficiently as well as which activities are adversely affected and in what ways. In light of this assessment, the OT will recommend the use of particular aids and equipment, or alterations to the home. When necessary, training is provided to modify the way in which the patient does things or to teach alternative skills. The activities of daily living are usually assessed during a home visit, to determine the special needs of the individual within the context of his or her environment. This also enables the OT to appraise the practical and physical demands made on the primary carer.

The degree of disability experienced by the patient in the course of daily living is only one factor considered in the choice of aids and equipment. The lifestyle of the individual and his or her family, the home setting, and the ability of both patient and carer to cope with the equipment as well as the effects of that equipment on them are other important considerations, as are safety, comfort and convenience.

The range of daily-living aids and equipment is very wide, covering the requirements of eating and drinking; kitchen, bath and toilet activities and dressing; walking and mobility generally; sitting, getting up from a sitting or lying position, getting in and out of bed, using the phone and television; reading and other leisure activities. Other aids and equipment may be provided to meet employment demands. Some kinds may require structural change to the home, such as the installation of stairlifts and through-floor lifts; overhead hoists, showers, extra baths, toilets or bedrooms; kitchen extensions, ramps and rails; changes to gates, garden paving, paths, garage and car ports; door-locking and -opening, and alarm systems. The OT may also suggest changing the arrangement of furniture and other objects in the home so as to improve safety and access and generally facilitate getting around the house.

The various types of aids and modifications that people with Parkinson's find valuable are listed in Table 4 and briefly described below. But don't rush off to get them all! To be of value, aids must match the individual's disability and the activities that he or she has trouble with, and be introduced at the correct time. If they are acquired before disability indicates, they are likely to be left unused or lead to loss of self-confidence and of skills. If supplied too long after disability sets in, it may become difficult for the individual to incorporate them into his or her routine activity. The importance of the correct timing is illustrated by the following passage from John Williams' pamphlet, *Parkinson's Disease: Doctors as Patients: Eleven Autobiographical Accounts*, in which Dr A., a psychiatrist, says:

The occupational therapist at the centre for old people was most helpful. She visited our home and swathed the tops of corner posts of the banisters with soft material, fearing that I might fall. In fact I can manage stairs without too much trouble: we have a stair-lift, but we seldom use it. Likewise, the OT supplied me with a plank and steps for getting into the bath, but since having a bar fixed to the wall at the side of the bath I do not use them. The OT also fitted Velcro to one of my shirts, but I can still manage the buttons. However, a built-up spoon for the left hand is particularly valuable to me, and as my left side is still relatively good I can eat soup and other soft food with this spoon.

Table 4   Equipment found useful by people with Parkinson's
disease

Bath and toilet aids	Eating aids
Bath step	Cup with lid and handles
Bath seat/board	Dycem mat
Bath mat	Melamine (or other tough
Shower	plastic) plate with rim
Stool	Cutlery with large angled
Handrail	handles
Toilet seat raiser	
Commode	Bedroom aids
Electric shaver	Electric bed
Electric toothbrush	Monkey-pull
	Rope for pulling up on
Dressing aids	Bed-raiser
Velcro fastening	Satin sheets and night-clothes
Large-tabbed zippers	
Long shoehorn	Walking and mobility aids
Slip-on shoes	Walking-stick
Easy-to-change and washable	Wheeled walker
clothes	Wheelchair and ramp
Footstool	
	Other aids
Kitchen aids	High-backed chair with arms
Cooker safety-guard	Chair-raiser
Electric can- and jar-opener	Chair with ejector seat
Trolley	Telephone-amplifier
Tap-turners	Telephone with large
Dycem mats	button-press numbers
	Hands-free telephone
	Typewriter/word-processor
	Ruled paper

Once the appropriate aids and equipment are obtained, it may be
necessary for the OT to come and demonstrate their use. Similarly, as
the degree of disability progresses, the OT will need to pay follow-up
visits to reassess the individual's needs and abilities, on the basis of
which he or she will be able to recommend new aids or suggest the
modification of those already in use.

Mobility aids

The disturbance of balance and the walking problems associated with
Parkinson's disease, particularly in the later phases of the illness, mean
that the provision of walking aids is a major focus. Wheeled walkers,

crutches and canes make the gait more efficient by transferring weight-bearing to the arms, thereby reducing the need for support. To use these devices safely, arm-strengthening and gait training may be required. Wheeled walking-frames such as Delta-aid and Rollator, particularly if fitted with hand-operated breaks, are best suited to the walking problems of Parkinson's patients. These are more useful than Zimmer frames, which require stopping and starting too frequently—something that patients do not find easy because of the hesitancy in starting that Parkinson's often brings. Shoes should be appropriate for walking and loose-fitting slippers that might cause tripping and falling should be avoided.

For most people, using a wheelchair signals loss of independence, or is somehow akin to being officially declared disabled. For this reason, many try to postpone using one for as long as possible. There is no denying that there is some stigma attached to using a wheelchair, especially in public places, most of which still do not allow easy access. However, a wheelchair is a walking-substitute—it allows the individual to move around, thereby permitting mobility and independence to someone who may otherwise be confined to sitting in one spot. Before you buy a wheelchair, it is essential to have it assessed by your OT, who will be able to take into account your particular circumstances. The relevant factors are whether it needs to be used inside as well as outside the home, whether modifications to doors or paths are necessary, whether it needs to be foldable to fit in a car boot, or lightweight to be handled by an elderly carer, and whether it will be self-operated or operated by others.

Washing and toileting aids

A shower cubicle is easier to get in and out of, and can reduce the risk of slipping and falling. The danger of falls while bathing can also be reduced by installing handles or rails on the wall near the bath or shower, as well as by using bath seats and a bath mat; a bath step can help you to get in and out. A toilet seat raiser and an adjacent handrail can help with getting up from the toilet. A stool of medium height in the bathroom allows you to rest while washing or shaving or putting on make-up. If tremor makes shaving with a razor hazardous, substitute an electric shaver. Similarly, an electric toothbrush may prove useful.

Dressing aids

Clothing and footwear should be selected for ease of dressing and undressing as well as for washability. As already mentioned, dressing can be made easier by using Velcro or large-tabbed zip-fasteners instead of buttons, which Parkinson's patients have difficulty doing up and undoing. Wearing looser-fitting clothes—skirts and trousers with elasticated waistbands, cardigans instead of jumpers—can also make dressing and undressing easier, as can front-fastening bras and front-buttoning dresses. Hems can be adjusted to counteract the effects of stooping, and drooping shoulders can be boosted with shoulder pads. Slip-on shoes eliminate the need for tying shoe-laces, and leather soles are less likely than rubber ones to catch on the ground. A foot-stool can make it easier to put on socks, tights and shoes, and a long shoehorn can also be useful. Suggestions for other adjustments to clothing and a list of manufacturers and suppliers of appropriate clothing can be obtained from Disability Scotland.

Cooking and kitchen aids
Judicious reorganisation of utensils and working surfaces in the kitchen will improve access and reduce fatigue. Safety can be improved by the use of electric appliances such as an electric cooker and kettle, and a cooker safety-guard. Special peelers and electric jar- and can-openers are available. A tap-turner can be fitted on to kitchen taps to make them easier to turn on and off. A stool in the kitchen can provide support while cooking or washing up, or for periods of rest, and a small trolley or a basket attached to a wheeled walking-frame can be handy for carrying objects between rooms.

Eating and drinking aids
Eating can be made easier with the help of cutlery with large handles and curved at angles; cups with special handles, a lid and a spout which provide a firm grip and prevent spilling; plates made of unbreakable Melamine or other tough plastic and with a rim to prevent food escaping; Dycem mats to ensure that dishes remain stationary on trays or tables. A straw can make drinking from a glass or cup easier and prevent spilling.

Getting in and out of chairs and beds
To facilitate these procedures, metal leg raisers can be fitted to increase the height of chairs and beds to a level that suits you. An ejector seat can help with getting up and out of a chair, and you can make getting out of bed easier by having a rope attached to the bed frame, to pull yourself up with. Satin sheets and bedclothes can help with turning over in bed—and they feel nice too. Alternatives are an electric bed and an overhead triangle, as Cecil Todes found:

Mobility in bed was much less of a problem since a friend gave me an electric bed which jacked me up from a horizontal to a sitting position and, combined with an overhead monkeyhold, helped me in turning from side to side and getting out of bed. I feel I know every corner of my bed and how to get to it.

Communication aids

As mentioned earlier, telephones with voice amplifiers may improve communication over the phone; large push-buttons for dialling and hands-free telephones can also be useful; speech amplifiers may overcome the low-volume voice. Writing problems can be dealt with by using a typewriter or word-processor. For more information, see under 'Speech and Language Therapy', p. 209.

Besides the OT and the physiotherapist, the *community nurse* attached to a general practice and the *health visitor* can also provide information about such aids. Some kinds of equipment are occasionally loaned by occupational therapy or physiotherapy departments and by some voluntary organisations. Other kinds may have to be purchased. The occupational therapy department of your local hospital, the local DSS office, and some of the voluntary organisations listed in the Appendix can provide information about obtaining equipment. Many of the aids listed in Table 4 are available through Boots the chemists, who can supply a catalogue with photos and details of each item. This kind of equipment is also sold by mail order companies (catalogues can be sent for) and by a number of specialist high-street shops. In the UK there are over 30 Disabled Living Centres (DLCs), which demonstrate equipment and assess special needs (for details contact the Disabled Living Foundation, or see pp. 548–50 of the booklet *How to Get Equipment for Disability*. In Scotland there is a mobile DLC which gives demonstrations at hospitals, health centres, schools and shopping centres in the region. The DLC can also lend equipment for trial periods, and provide the names and addresses of suppliers and manufacturers. Where structural adaptations to the home are necessary—such as installing a lift, a shower or an extra toilet—it may be possible to obtain a grant from the local housing authority; an environmental health officer or other housing authority personnel may visit to assess eligibility and technical feasibility.

The Social Worker

Social workers offer a variety of help and advice:

- They are often the best source of information about welfare and benefit entitlements. If necessary, the social worker can help you to make applications for benefits. For example, because of the changes in mobility associated with on–off syndrome in Parkinson's disease, the social worker may advise keeping a diary of such changes to support an application for the Disabled Parking Badge or Mobility and Attendance Allowances.
- They can offer practical advice about ways of reducing some of the pressures of the illness on the family or the carer. They do this partly by acting as *key-workers* and arranging referral to other services. For example, by arranging for a home help, a community nurse or a sitter, or organising attendance at a day centre or club for the patient, some of the burden of caring can be lightened. A social worker can also arrange for meals-on-wheels, a service run jointly by the Women's Royal Voluntary Service and local authorities that provides the patient with a hot meal every day or several times a week. In some areas, a laundry service may be available for incontinent people, which collects and launders soiled clothes and sheets—the social worker can arrange access to this service too.
- Social workers can offer advice about local residential care and nursing homes and arrange short- or long-term admission where appropriate.
- As part of their training, social workers develop listening and counselling skills, so both patients and carers can discuss their worries with them.
- They can also give advice on leisure activities and holidays.

If you do not have a social worker, and think that contact with one may be beneficial, ring your local Social Services department, describe your circumstances and arrange an appointment for a home visit. The clinical team that you consult at your hospital may have a social worker attached who has particular expertise in dealing with Parkinson's disease. Ask the consultant neurologist or the doctor you see at the clinic for a referral.

The Nursing Services

Most people associate nursing care with hospitalisation, but there is quite a variety of other nursing services. In recent years, there has been a trend towards providing community-based nursing care. The several types of service are provided by community or district nurses, health visitors, nurse practitioners and community psychiatric nurses (the latter are rarely involved in the management of Parkinson's disease, except when severe dementia is present).

Community or *district nurses* provide home-based care. The range of help and advice that they offer includes:

- practical help with bathing, dressing, eating, changing dressings on pressure sores
- advice on the best ways of eating, such as ensuring good posture to prevent choking or the aspiration of liquid
- advice for the carer on the best ways of lifting and turning the ill person in bed
- advice on the management of incontinence, when present—the nurse may first recommend charting the pattern of the incontinence.

Health visitors are state-registered nurses with some additional training. Their aim is to advise people about their physical and mental health, in the community, and to prevent the need for hospital admission. Health visitors are usually attached to local clinics or GP practices, and they mainly visit people in their homes. They can advise on other services that are available locally, and how to obtain access to them.

The involvement of *nurse practitioners* in the management of chronic neurological illnesses such as Parkinson's disease is a relatively new idea. A nurse practitioner has background training in nursing and a specialist expertise in dealing with Parkinson's patients and their carers. You may meet the specialist nurse practitioner at the out-patient clinic or during a home visit, or he or she may contact you in follow-ups over the phone. The nurse practitioner can play several important roles in the management of Parkinson's disease:

- Immediately after diagnosis, he or she can provide the patient, the carer and the family with support, and help them come to terms with the diagnosis.
- Supply information about the illness and the various medications used in its treatment; help the patient to monitor changes in his or

her drug regimen and to cope better with the difficult side-effects that can sometimes accompany drug therapy.

- Act as a key-worker, assessing the needs of the patient and asking the GP for appropriate referrals for adjunct therapy such as physiotherapy, speech therapy and occupational therapy; arrange consultation with a dietitian, a chiropodist or a dentist.
- Be easily accessible to both patient and carer so as to offer them practical as well as emotional support. By being there and listening to their worries, the nurse practitioner can help them to vent their emotions and reduce stress.

In a study conducted with the Parkinson's Disease Society and the Dystonia Society, we evaluated the effects of even minimal contact— two home visits and four phone calls during a six-month period—with a specialist nurse practitioner. The service turned out to be highly valued by the patients and their carers, and led to new referrals to other health care agencies and to a take-up of state-provided benefits. The patients and their families particularly appreciated the 'opportunity to talk to someone about the illness and the problems caused by it' and 'knowing that the nurse practitioner could be contacted if problems arose'.

These responses reflect the patients' perceptions of the services normally available to them. All were under the care of a specialist neurologist and all had access to their GP, but it would seem that few patients, or their carers, felt able to pick up the telephone and call their neurologist for help or advice. And even GPs are rarely available, except through appointment. The attraction of the specialist nurse practitioner to people with Parkinson's disease and their carers, therefore, may be in his or her accessibility, specialist knowledge of their condition, and possession of a network of contacts in the other health professions. While awareness of such accessibility would be a comfort to patients on a day-to-day basis, its real value would be felt when major problems occurred. Nurse practitioners are ideally placed for crisis management, particularly if patients feel that they can call them at such times. The PDS has a team of specialist nurse practitioners who are associated with particular movement-disorder clinics around the UK.

Counselling and Psychotherapy

Even today, in most Western societies there is still some stigma attached to seeing a psychotherapist or counsellor. The stigma derives partly from the assumption that everyone should be able to cope effectively with all the hardships that life throws their way, and if they can't then there's something wrong with them. This is a false assumption. No one can be expected to cope all the time with hardship, particularly of the long-term and changing kind typical of chronic illness, without any help or support. Counselling or therapy is usually used for crisis intervention—that is, the help of a therapist or counsellor is sought when problems have persisted for a long time or when they build up to crisis point. But instead of waiting for a crisis to build up, consulting a therapist shortly after the problem is first experienced could actually prevent that crisis from developing.

Regardless of the nature of the therapy or counselling provided, a counsellor or therapist is not there to judge, to provide a personal opinion, or to give direct advice or practical help. Rather, the aim of most types of therapy or counselling is to establish a therapeutic relationship based on understanding, warmth, genuine concern and respect. This allows the individual to vent his or her emotions, voice concerns and sort out thoughts and feelings about specific matters. Clarifying the exact nature of the problem and gaining some insight into its source and the factors that contribute to it make it easier to work out ways of dealing with it within the context of the individual's special circumstances and abilities, and allows him or her to set him- or herself both short- and long-term goals for change. The British Association for Counselling defines counselling as 'an interaction in which one person offers another person time, attention and respect, with the intention of helping that person explore, discover and clarify ways of living more successfully and toward greater well-being.'

The particular type of therapy or counselling selected depends on the nature of the problem.

Individual therapy

The onset of Parkinson's disease requires a major change in the individual's view of what he or she can and cannot do and in his or her expectations. Some find it difficult to accept the reality of the illness, even after years of living with it, and experience depression or anxiety. As noted earlier, feelings of helplessness and hopelessness may also be experienced by the carer, whose life is affected by the illness in fundamental ways. Contact with a psychotherapist or counsellor on a one-to-one basis may help both the patient and the carer to examine their worries and fears and the roots of their depression by exploring their thoughts and feelings about the illness and its implications for their lives.

Family therapy

When someone in the family falls ill, the previously balanced functioning of the family system may be disturbed. And when communication problems develop, family therapy may help re-establish positive rapport, provide insight into why the difficulties have occurred, and explore ways in which the family members can help each other. This can enable all concerned to cope better with the daily strains and stresses posed by the challenges of Parkinson's disease. Family counselling can help children caught in the web of the family living through stress to come to terms with the implications of the illness both for their ill parent and for themselves.

Marital therapy

This form of therapy can help couples to live through a problematic period in their relationship. The therapist is there as an impartial mediator to help them to learn to listen and talk to each other more effectively, sort out their feelings about each other, objectively examine what is happening in their relationship, establish a more realistic view of their expectations, and develop more productive ways of relating to and interacting with each other. As with most problems, it is best to seek help when they first arise, rather than leaving them to fester.

Sex therapy

We discussed sexual problems and strategies for overcoming them in some detail in Chapter 8. During the initial assessment sessions of therapy, the nature of the sexual problem and the circumstances under which it occurs, will be discussed. Once the problem itself and the factors that may contribute to it have been clarified, methods for dealing with it will be discussed, and simple 'homework' tasks set to be carried out by the couple in the privacy of their home. The aim is to improve sexual awareness and communication, induce sensitivity to the other partner's needs, and improve sexual performance within the context of a relaxed and pressure-free relationship. The 'home exercises' recommended by the therapist are tailored to the particular problem that the couple are experiencing. There are specific techniques for helping with impotence or premature ejaculation, and for orgasm problems in women.

A referral for any of these kinds of therapy can be arranged by your GP.

The Dietitian

Dietary factors are relevant to the management of Parkinson's disease, and a consultation with a dietitian may be helpful in many ways. Dietitians usually work in general hospitals—a referral can be arranged through your GP. The information and advice offered by a dietitian include the following:

- As mentioned on p. 65, a high-protein meal taken at about the same time as the levodopa dose has been found to interfere with the absorption of the drug. To optimise the absorption of levodopa, a *protein-redistribution diet* is recommended in Parkinson's disease. This involves postponing the meal with the highest protein content until the evening. This diet may be particularly useful in people who have developed a fluctuating response to levodopa; occasionally, the protein intake may be kept below the recommended daily allowance of 0.8g per kilogram of body weight,
- The body needs *vitamins* only in minute amounts. A balanced diet should meet all the vitamin requirements of most people except the elderly, and pregnant women. Normally, therefore, it is not necessary to take vitamin supplements. In Parkinson's disease, it may be best to avoid large doses of certain vitamins and advisable to take others. Although vitamin B6 is necessary for the operation of the enzyme that converts levodopa to dopamine, you should avoid large amounts of it because it causes a quick conversion of levodopa to dopamine before it gets to the brain, with a resultant loss of efficacy. The amount of vitamin B6 contained in ordinary foods—such as bran, brewer's yeast, wheatgerm, tomatoes, soyabeans and liver— is not so high as to make it necessary to avoid them. There has been some concern that too much vitamin C (ascorbic acid) may result in the need to increase the dosage of levodopa, so don't take large amounts of vitamin C. Evidence suggests that vitamin E (alpha-tocopherol) may slow down the progression of Parkinson's disease, when taken at bedtime in large doses such as 400 international units. Dosages larger than this may interfere with the absorption of vitamin A.
- The dietitian may also advise on the intake of certain dietary *minerals*. With age, the bones tend to lose their calcium, becoming brittle and thin and more likely to break if you fall. So taking calcium is recommended. Iron supplements are also recommended, especially to women, who lose a proportion of iron through the menstrual flow. Small amounts of these supplements are not harmful, but all the

same, consult your GP or neurologist before starting any vitamin or mineral supplements.

- As mentioned on p. 78, constipation is a common problem in Parkinson's disease. The long-term use of laxatives is not advisable, and the dietitian will be able to suggest other ways of dealing with it. Increase your intake of dietary fibre by eating more cereals, fruit and vegetables. Frequent physical activity and exercise, as well as drinking four to six glasses of water a day, can facilitate bowel movements. Going to the toilet at a regular time each day and when bowel movements are more likely, such as after a meal or exercise, may also be effective.

- Given the reduced mobility and reduced physical activity, it is easy for the patient to put on weight. Obesity can exacerbate the sense of imbalance and difficulty in walking, and make it more burdensome for the carer to help the patient to get up and move about in the later phases of the illness. Obesity can be combated by cutting down on starch and fatty foods and by taking regular exercise.

- Instead of gaining weight, some people with Parkinson's disease lose it. Weight loss may be partly caused by the fact that, because of their slowness, some individuals manage to eat only half of what was their normal amount in the course of a mealtime. If this is a problem for you, it can be overcome by allowing yourself longer to finish your meals and serving them in two portions on two plates, one of which you keep warm in the oven. In other cases, weight loss may be related to the excessive sweating or the physical effort associated with the dyskinesias. Here, dietary supplements such as Complan or Build-Up may be necessary to promote weight gain.

- Alcohol in moderate amounts does not interact with medication, and can be enjoyed at mealtimes. Although the tremor in Parkinson's is not particularly responsive to alcohol, by creating general relaxation it may to some extent alleviate tremor and rigidity.

- If problems with continence develop, advice about what to eat and drink may be crucial to preserve the individual's dignity and to allow him or her to continue living at home.

WELFARE RIGHTS AND BENEFITS

As a result of disability your capacity to work full-time may be reduced, as may that of your carer. Consequently, your household income may be much reduced too. And disability does entail extra costs, as you may already have discovered. Besides aids and equipment, and possible modifications to your house or flat and to your car, the extra costs of transport, and of obtaining extra help with caring, household work, laundry or gardening, all add up. Most people are not able to meet these extra costs solely from their income. But many with disability who may be entitled to benefits that will help meet the extra costs are often unaware of the range of benefits available and so fail to apply for them.

These are some of the benefits that you or your primary carer may be entitled to:

Disability Living Allowance
A tax-free benefit, payable after three months' disability, for people from birth to 65 years who need care and/or have problems with mobility. It is not means-tested, and should be claimed before you reach the age of 66, after which it can continue until any age. The care component of this benefit is paid at one of three rates, depending on the nature and degree of care that you require. Similarly, there are two rates for the mobility component, contingent on how difficult it is for you to walk.

Disability Working Allowance
Tops up the earnings of disabled people who work part-time or hold low-paid jobs. To be eligible for it, you have to work more than 16 hours a week and be aged over 16. The amount of the allowance varies, as it is means-tested.

Income Support
A benefit for people aged 18 or older, who do not have enough money to live on. It is therefore means-tested, and the income of both the ill person and his or her partner is taken into account. Income Support is not paid to those with savings in excess of £8,000. Even savings between £3,000 and £8,000 can affect the amount of Income Support allotted. Normally, to be eligible for this benefit, neither the ill person nor his or her partner should be working for more than 24 hours a week.

Attendance Allowance
A tax-free cash benefit for those aged 65 or over who require constant care. It is not means-tested and can be obtained in addition to other benefits. There are two rates—a lower rate for those who need care only during the day or only during the night, and a higher rate for those who need twenty-four-hour care (referred to as the Constant Attendance Allowance).

Invalid Care Allowance
An allowance for those of working age (16–65) who have earnings below a set limit and who spend a large proportion of their time (35 hours a week or more) looking after a person who is disabled and receives Attendance Allowance, Constant Attendance Allowance or Disability Living Allowance at one of the two highest rates. The Invalid Care Allowance is paid weekly and is a taxable cash benefit.

Incapacity Benefit
This benefit, which relates to inability to work, replaced the Sickness and Invalidity Benefits in 1995. Eligibility is based on a certificate issued by your GP giving, as well as the diagnosis, an assessment of your ability in relation to functions such as walking, standing, manual dexterity, speech, hearing and sight. For the first 28 weeks after the onset of the illness, the assessment will consider incapacity to mean inability to work in your own occupation; thereafter it will mean inability to do any type of work.

Council Rate Benefit and Housing Benefit
Council Rate Benefit reduces the Council Tax paid by the person who is disabled, while Housing Benefit is help with payment of rent. Both of these benefits are means-tested, and both include a Carer Premium, if the carer is entitled to Invalid Care Allowance.

Family Credit
A tax-free benefit paid weekly to families with children. One of the partners must be working at least 16 hours a week. It is means-tested and not payable to those who have savings of more than £8,000.

Social Fund Payments
Helps people of low income with expenses that cannot be met from their regular income. It includes Maternity, Funeral and Cold Weather Payments, and Crisis Loans. The payment is in the form of a grant or an interest-free loan, depending on the individual's earnings and savings.

Free Prescriptions
Available to all pensioners, pregnant women, women over the age of 60 and men over the age of 65, as well as to anyone who cannot leave home without assistance. Those who are not entitled to free prescriptions can still make savings if they need prescriptions frequently, by getting a four- or twelve-month prepayment certificate, obtainable from the post office or from chemists.

NHS Benefits

Free dental treatment, sight tests and help with hospital travel are available to anyone receiving either Income Support or Family Credit.

The Disabled Parking Badge

Also called the Orange Badge Scheme, this permit allows concessions such as parking in spaces reserved for disabled drivers and, under some circumstances, parking on a yellow line.

These benefits are extra to any retirement pension and the statutory Sick Pay that employers pay to employees for the first 28 weeks of sickness. It is important to claim all the benefits you are entitled to in order to prevent the financial hardship that may be associated with inability to work, reduction of earnings, and the additional costs of disability. In addition, help with travel costs can be obtained via various concessionary bus and rail schemes operated by British Rail and local bus companies, and local transport schemes such as Dial-a-Ride. Some London boroughs operate a special concession with taxi drivers for disabled users. The local DSS office can also provide top-up funds to help pay for residential care or nursing homes. Charitable trusts (listed in *Charities Digest*, which can be consulted in libraries) will sometimes help to cover the cost of holidays or residential care, or the cost of a piece of equipment or of carrying out modifications to the home.

You can get information about benefits and how to claim them from the following sources:

- Your social worker, health visitor or nurse practitioner (see p. 222).
- Your local Citizens' Advice Bureau.
- Your local Department of Social Security (DSS). You can either attend the DSS office in person or obtain the relevant information over the phone (freephone 0800 666555 in England, Scotland and Wales; 0800 616757 in Northern Ireland). Some offices will arrange for a Social Security officer to visit at home, to assess your needs.
- A Benefits Enquiry Line, set up by the Benefits Agency, which is an executive section of the DSS. Call freephone between 9 a.m. and 4.30 p.m. on weekdays, to obtain information about the available benefits and criteria for eligibility, and the procedure for claiming. Information given on the phone can be confirmed in writing. For some benefits, the agency even completes the claim form for you, and sends it to you to check, sign and send off.
- The welfare and benefits officer of the welfare department of the

Parkinson's Disease Society, who can be contacted for advice about welfare rights.

SERVICES FOR THE MIDDLE AND LATER PHASES

Day Care

In the UK, day care is usually provided through day hospitals or day centres that the individual can attend one or more times a week. Transport to and from day centres is usually provided, although the time of pick-up and drop-off may not be very reliable. Day centres usually provide meals, and various types of social activities and games may be scheduled; other services such as hairdressing, foot care and bathing may also be available. Appropriate and good-quality day care can be stimulating for the patient and provide a weekly outing to look forward to. It also provides the carer with a break, and may make it possible for him or her to continue in part- or full-time employment. Lily Warren, whose husband has Parkinson's disease, writes in her book *The Road Beyond*:

> As time went on and to give me a break, it was suggested my husband spend one day each week at a day centre. He quite enjoyed the change and I enjoyed the freedom. He was picked up by ambulance in the morning and returned about tea time.

Information about day centres can be obtained from local Social Services departments, and Age Concern, too, runs day centres for the elderly. In areas where there is more than one local day centre, patient and carer may want to visit each before choosing the one that is most likely to meet their needs.

Respite Care

Like day care, respite care aims to provide the carer with a break from caring. Respite care can be provided either away from, or in, the person's own home. Carers are sometimes unwilling to ask for or accept respite care, and this is usually because neither carer nor patient wants to be separated from the other. Occasionally negative past experiences, such as the patient having returned from respite care less mobile and more confused, are to blame for a carer's unwillingness to accept such help. A third reason may be the mixed feelings of the carer—feelings of guilt at what he or she wrongly perceives as his or her 'betrayal' of the patient if respite care is accepted. Lily Warren writes about her feelings of concern and relief when her husband spent a short while in hospital:

> Although I did not wish my husband to go away, I must admit it came as a great relief to know someone else would have the responsibility of looking after him. I travelled with him in the ambulance and I knew he was disturbed and upset to be taken from his natural surroundings, but I cannot explain how I felt that night when I returned home. It was wonderful to go to bed and know I could sleep through the night. The house seemed very strange and empty and I couldn't wait to visit the hospital as I knew he would miss me and be quite fretful.

Lily Warren's concern about her husband reflects the worries that can be brought on by the separation caused by respite care. Clearly, to some extent this defeats the purpose of the exercise, which is to give carers a physical and mental break from the duties of caring. Although it may be hard, carers should try to reassure themselves that their relative is being well cared for. They need to make the most of this period by going away to visit relatives or friends, engaging in social and leisure activities that they would otherwise not be able to enjoy.

Other respite care schemes such as Crossroads Care Attendant Scheme can offer this kind of relief at the individual's own home, thus avoiding separation from spouse or partner and family as well as the need to move to unfamiliar surroundings. Usually, the type and amount of respite care provided are flexible, and will be determined after an initial assessment aimed at accommodating the needs of the carer, the ill person and the rest of the family. Crossroads offer regular weekly support or occasional breaks from caring. They take over the caring duties normally performed by the carer, and timing—whether during the day or at night—is arranged to suit the carer. During the period of relief the carer may be at work, relaxing at home or attending to other duties, or taking time off for social and leisure activities. Although the service is free to the client, the care attendants are trained and paid; they are recruited locally, and work for Crossroads on an hourly basis. Referrals can be arranged by GPs, social workers, occupational therapists, community nurses and health visitors, or individual carers can initiate the contact themselves. Although the main aim of the service is to allow time off for carers, occasionally care attendants can be provided for people with chronic illness who live alone. The Winged Fellowship Trust also provides a respite care scheme, as well as arranging holidays for which escorts can be organised. The charity Counsel and Care for the Elderly administers a number of trust funds from which single payments for arranging respite care can be obtained. 'Sitters' can also be arranged through Age Concern.

Residential Care

In the later stages of the illness, when the symptoms have become acute and are no longer controlled by medication, the patient may become severely disabled and incapacitated. The loss of independent functions will mean that constant care is required for all daily activities such as bathing, dressing and feeding. Although most carers and families try to postpone the need for residential care and want to look after the patient at home for as long as possible, a time will come when the demands of caring make residential care an option to be considered. Charities such as Counsel and Care for the Elderly and The Elderly Accommodation Council have a nationwide register of sheltered accommodation, residential care and nursing homes. Advice about residential care can also be obtained from the head office of the Parkinson's Disease Society and about private residential care from Grace Link.

Sheltered accommodation combines independent living with access to help when required. Whether operated by local authorities, by voluntary groups or privately, it consists of a number of independent residential units, either houses or flats, with communal facilities such as a laundry, a shop and a social activities lounge, and a warden who can be contacted when needed.

Residential and *nursing homes* may also be run either by local authorities or privately, and are set up to provide more intensive care for their residents. Nursing homes have a qualified nurse on duty. Both residential and nursing homes are registered with local authorities, which inspect them to ensure that they meet a particular standard of care. If the Parkinson's patient is admitted to a long-stay hospital or a home run by the Social Services, he or she may not be able to choose the particular place he or she goes to. There *is* choice, of course, with privately run residential units and nursing homes, and admission to these does not exclude people on low incomes, as arrangements can be made for the Department of Social Security to make a contribution towards the fees. When a person stays in a nursing or residential home run by a local authority for longer than eight weeks, the charges paid are means-tested.

When it comes to choosing a suitable home, visit as many as you can, assess the premises and ease of access by car or public transport, talk to the staff, try to judge the quality of care offered, the social and leisure activities, and the interaction between staff and residents.

HOLIDAY BREAKS

Like all of us—or perhaps more than most—the Parkinson's patient as well as his or her carer will undoubtedly benefit from holidays away from home. In the initial phases of the illness no additional arrangements may be required, other than ensuring that an adequate supply of medication is available while away. But when disability sets in, both patient and carer may desperately want a break but be unable or unwilling to do so—for several reasons:

- The unpredictability of the illness, the fact that it may be difficult to foresee the physical condition of the individual over longish periods or even from one day to the next, makes advance booking relatively risky.
- The many modifications that may have been introduced into the home to cope with disability, such as wheelchair ramps, wider doorways and handrails in the bathroom, would not be available in the standard holiday resort or hotel.
- The difficulties associated with mobility and transport may seem insurmountable at first sight.
- The additional financial demands made by the illness on limited resources may mean that a holiday is not easily affordable.
- Given current negative public attitudes to disability, there may be the fear and embarrassment of being in public places and exposed to strangers who are not too sympathetic or understanding.

But all of these are problems that can be resolved with some forward planning and effort. Most travel agents and holiday companies offer holiday insurance that reimburses clients if the arrangements have to be cancelled because of ill-health. Holiday insurance is also a sensible option for other eventualities, such as the cost of medical care that might become necessary while away, or loss or damage to special equipment. There are two charities that are concerned with the provision of information, help and advice about holidays for people with disability or special needs: the Holiday Care Service and the Winged Fellowship Trust. The Holiday Care Service gives free information on holidays for people with special needs, suggests hotels and guest-houses that may be suitable, and gives advice about sources of charitable funds that may contribute towards the cost of a holiday. Information about hotels, guest-houses and resorts with appropriate facilities can also be obtained from *Holidays for Disabled People*, published each year by the Royal Association for Disability and Rehabilitation. The Winged

Fellowship Trust arranges holidays at its own centres in the UK.

When you are selecting a hotel or other accommodation, it is important that access to and circulation around it should suit the level of abilities of the Parkinson's disease patient. For someone who is wheelchair-bound, wheelchair access to all public rooms, and large enough lifts, are essential. The attitude of the hotel staff and their willingness to help if problems arise is another consideration. Out-of-season holidays are not only cheaper, but may ensure a friendlier and more helpful service from staff who are not rushed off their feet. As already mentioned, charities such as Holiday Care Service and Winged Fellowship Trust can arrange an escort to accompany the individual and his or her carer on holiday. Every year, the Parkinson's Disease Society also organises a number of holidays for individuals and their carers in conjunction with the Winged Fellowship Trust (contact the head office of the PDS for details).

ALTERNATIVE MEDICINE

When a person is ill, it is a natural reaction to want to try any and all paths that may lead to a cure, or at least to the control or suppression of the symptoms. Yoga, meditation, hypnosis, acupuncture and the Alexander technique are some of the alternative, or complementary, therapies that are on offer and that have undoubtedly been tried by some people with Parkinson's disease. Meditation and yoga, techniques developed in the East to achieve relaxation, may be useful for the reduction of muscle stiffness, as may hypnosis. Acupuncture, which involves the insertion of special needles at specific points of the body, has been used for a variety of ills, and in Parkinson's disease it may be tried for the relief of pain. The Alexander technique is a method that teaches awareness of balance and posture in everyday activities, so that the individual learns to get rid of unnecessary muscle tension.

Although no systematic information about the value of these approaches to the treatment of Parkinson's disease exists, it is important not to be too dismissive of their possible value. In individual cases they may prove helpful, largely by reducing anxiety and inducing relaxation and a sense of self-control in the patient. However, caution is necessary when investigating these techniques:

- Obtain full information about the aims and procedures of each technique before embarking on a course, to ensure that at least no harm is done and that money is not wasted.
- Consult an accredited practitioner.

- Maintain an open mind and a balanced approach and know when to stop—being overzealous in a quest for a 'cure' or effective therapy can sometimes have dire emotional and financial consequences.
- Consult your GP before embarking on a course of alternative medicine—it may help you to keep a balanced attitude.

In his book, Ivan Vaughan gives an account of the various hypotheses that an individual can fall prey to, not only concerning the possible causes of the illness but also about what, other than the standard medical treatments, might help to control the symptoms. He describes his hypnosis trials in Hampstead, his investigations into meditation, his forays into yoga and shiatsu, his week on the Matham diet in Norfolk eliminating gluten and animal fat from his diet, and his fava bean period. None proved of much value in relieving his symptoms—and some left him with other problems:

> I had beans on their own, beans in stews—enough beans, I felt sure, to provide the same amount of L-dopa as I took in the tablets. I was full of beans but still not jumping! The lack of any noticeable effect left us with the problem of how to use up the huge sack of beans in the cupboard.

THE PARKINSON'S DISEASE SOCIETY

The Parkinson's Disease Society of the United Kingdom is a charity founded in 1969 by Miss Mali Jenkins (1904–89), whose sister had the illness. The Society has grown to become one of the largest medical charities in the UK. It is governed by a council of management which has the benefit of advice from a medical and a welfare advisory panel. The members of the medical panel, which gives advice on medical issues and directs the PDS research programme, are neurologists, neurosurgeons, scientists, a GP and a geriatrician. The welfare panel advises the council of management on welfare issues concerning patients and carers, and in addition to lay members includes a health visitor and speech therapist. The income of the Society, which has many local branches, comes from fund-raising, donations and bequests. The three main stated aims are:

- to help patients and their relatives with the problems arising from Parkinson's disease
- to collect and disseminate information on Parkinson's
- to encourage and provide funds for research into the illness.

The PDS tries to meet the needs of people with Parkinson's disease and their relatives in several ways:

- by providing information about the disorder and its treatment through its numerous booklets and quarterly newsletter
- by providing individuals and their relatives with practical advice— for example, there is a helpline operated by a welfare and benefits officer
- through its network of two hundred local branches that operate as support and self-help groups—for younger individuals, there is the Young Alert Parkinson's Partners and Relatives (YAPP&Rs) group (see p. 201).

At the PDS's 'brain bank' at the Institute of Neurology, post-mortem investigations are conducted to further clarify the brain abnormalities associated with the disorder, and to provide clues as to the cause. The medical research funded by the PDS includes the first nationwide epidemiological survey of Parkinson's disease in the UK. The Society also funds research projects aimed at improving service provision for people with the illness and establishing models of good practice. The Society holds many workshops and education programmes targeting professionals, and issues publicity aimed at improving public awareness of the disorder.

Many organisations similar to the PDS in the UK exist elsewhere in the world (see the 'A–Z of Useful Organisations', pp. 323–6).

We have worked very closely with the PDS, and our experience prompts us to advise all those diagnosed as having Parkinson's disease to join a branch of the Society as soon as possible. Membership provides access to a source of expert knowledge. Most branches offer very useful information packs or booklets containing clear information, written in simple language, about, for instance, the most up-to-date forms of treatment available and where it can be obtained. In addition, some branches employ a number of associated professionals, such as health visitors, social workers, welfare and benefits officers and specialist nurse practitioners, who can provide advice or help in crisis management. Margaret, the optician referred to in Chapter 8, expressed her appreciation of the health visitor of her local PDS branch:

> The welfare visitor from the local Parkinson's Disease Society is a trained health visitor. She came to see me within three days of diagnosis. She has always been there when I needed her. She is worth her weight in gold.

People differ in their willingness to meet others who have the illness, particularly immediately after the diagnosis. Some welcome the opportunity to talk about their symptoms and the associated problems with others in a similar situation, and to be forewarned about problems that may develop later for which they can start preparing in advance. Others shy away from meeting others with Parkinson's disease, because they would rather not see people in the more advanced stages. For this reason, many join the Parkinson's Disease Society but do not attend meetings. However, their fears may be largely unfounded, since at any average PDS meeting one is likely to encounter as many people with mild disability, who are still leading an active life despite having had the illness for twenty years, as wheelchair-bound people incapacitated by the illness early on. In his booklet *The Parkinson's Challenge: A Beginner's Guide to the Good Life in the Slow Lane*, Jan Peter Stern wrote:

> I was very reluctant to make that first, crucial visit to a Parkinson's support group, fearing that I'd be too depressed by what I would see; thinking I was not yet in so 'bad a way' as to need it. To my surprise, I was immediately relieved to see how well people are coping after 10, 20 and even 30 years.

THE CARERS' NATIONAL ASSOCIATION

In the UK, there are about seven million carers—in other words, one in every seven adults is a carer. According to the Family Policy Studies Centre, the value of informal unpaid care by family and friends is estimated to be about £25 billion a year. Of those seven million carers, 2.9 million are men and 3.9 million are women. The figure also incorporates 10,000 children under the age of 16 who act as carers for a parent or other close relative. In 1993, a survey of over 1,000 people in the workforce was conducted by the Crossroads Care Attendant Scheme to assess views on caring. The majority (78 per cent) of people in employment had no direct experience of caring; about 16 per cent who work were also carers. Of these, 18 per cent had taken time off from work in the previous month to attend to their caring duties. Two-thirds of the carers in the workforce were women. Only 12 per cent had had any help from health or Social Services. The general household survey conducted in 1990 revealed that 23 per cent of carers spent more than 20 hours a week looking after the sick relative, 11 per cent of them more than 50 hours a week. Research on the personal impact of caring has shown that carers can experience considerable physical strain and emotional stress, with a sense of isolation and loneliness.

Carers of people with Parkinson's disease are often spouses, who are also elderly and, in some cases, ill themselves. Alternatively, a middle-aged daughter or son with a family of her or his own may be looking after an ageing parent. In the case of people with young-onset Parkinson's, a young spouse or partner who may also be working, or a child of school-age, may be the primary carer. The specific needs of these various carers will be different, but they all need relief from the emotional and physical burden of caring—particularly from the constant looking-after that may be required in the more severe phases of the illness.

To meet the needs of carers and provide them with support, the Carers' National Association was formed in 1988. Their stated aims are:

1   to encourage carers to recognise their own needs
2   to develop appropriate support for them
3   to provide them with information and advice
4   to bring the needs of carers to the attention of government and other policy-makers.

Membership of the association is open to anyone who is a carer. There is a national network of carers' support groups, which have regular meetings—these can be a venue for meeting others in a similar situation and for airing some of the difficulties experienced, without the carers feeling that they are betraying their sick relatives. This sharing of experiences also allows an exchange of possible remedies to practical problems. The association produces a twice-monthly journal, with up-to-date information relevant to carers. They also operate a CarersLine, a telephone advice and information service open to any carer, whether a member of the association or not.

KEY FACTS 9

There are many sources of help available both to the individual and to his or her carer.

Table 5 Sources of help for people with Parkinson's disease

Source	Nature of help	How to get it
Physiotherapist	Exercises to improve posture, balance and walking, and to reduce rigidity and pain	Referral by GP or neurologist
Speech therapist	Exercises with feedback to improve monotonous and low-volume speech, reduce swallowing problems	Referral by GP or neurologist
Occupational therapist	Assessment and alteration of the home with a view to safety; provision of aids and advice to improve mobility and performance of daily activities	Referral by GP or neurologist
Social worker	Advice on available benefits and access to other services; discussion of personal and family problems	Referral by GP or neurologist; contact Social Services
Psychotherapist/ counsellor	Someone to talk to and get expert advice from when depressed or anxious	Referral by GP
Nurse practitioner	Information about PD and available sources of help; referral to other resources; advice about practical	Referral by GP or neurologist

	problems; someone to talk to	
Community/district nurse/health visitor	Home-based care: help with bathing, dressing, feeding, changing dressings; advice on lifting and incontinence	Referral by GP
Dietitian	Advice on diet to avoid constipation, weight gain or loss; and on protein redistribution to prevent interference with levodopa absorption	Referral by GP
Chiropodist	Care of feet and toenails	Referral by GP
Care attendant/sitter	Help with bathing, dressing, feeding, shopping and cooking, to give carer time off	Contact Social Services or Crossroads Care Attendant Scheme
Home help	Help with shopping, housework and laundry	Contact Social Services
Day care	Provision of leisure activities and a meal at a day centre or hospital; a break for the carer	Contact Social Services or district health authority; referral by social worker
Respite care	Temporary breaks to give carers a rest	Contact Social Services; referral by GP
Residential care	Possibly long-term accommodation for patients	Contact Social Services or district health authority; referral by GP
Parkinson's Disease Society	At local branches, opportunities to meet others with the illness; a helpline and many other services, e.g. provision of nurse practitioners, arranging holidays; information booklets and tapes about Parkinson's disease (and see p. 236)	Contact directly

| Carers' National Association | Carers' support groups for airing and sharing problems and for mutual support; a CareLine advice and information service; booklets about caring (and see p. 238) | Contact directly |

10

Self-help Strategies for the Person with the Illness: Minimising Disability and Preventing Handicap

Richard Brown

Your ultimate goal in facing the challenge of Parkinson's is to be able to continue to lead a full life, despite the illness. As in Chapter 5, I cover in this chapter five main spheres of daily living: self-care, mobility, work and leisure activities, financial independence and relationships with others. In particular, I discuss self-help strategies that can help reduce disability and prevent handicap, and promote better coping. But first, an important general principle that applies to all of these areas—scheduling your daily activities.

SCHEDULING YOUR ACTIVITIES

One of the most obvious ways of minimising the effects of the symptoms on your daily activities is simply to allow more time to get things done, rather than rushing to finish the task in the usual time. Many people with Parkinson's disease find that the pressure caused by trying to do things quickly makes the symptoms worse, and means that everything takes even longer to achieve. But deliberately taking things slowly and steadily may take some additional planning, if the extra slowness is not to interfere with other aspects of your life. This may mean starting the daily routine of washing and dressing slightly earlier than you used to, or scheduling subsequent activities for a later time. But while such a strategy may work well for you, problems may arise when the extra time you take to do things impinges on the lives of others—particularly if you haven't prepared them for it.

Another approach centres on picking the best time to get things done. Once the early phase of the illness has passed, there will almost certainly be some daily variation in your symptoms and an accompanying difficulty in performing routine tasks. As noted earlier, for many, the period in the morning immediately after waking is the best part of the day—the so-called *sleep benefit time*. Happily, this fits in well with the daily routine of washing and dressing, preparing and eating breakfast. In contrast, getting ready for bed at night can be a more leisurely process, and it rarely matters if it takes longer than it used to.

During the day, there may be patterns in your functioning that reflect definite 'good' and 'bad' ('on' and 'off') times. If possible, try to organise your day to take maximum advantage of your on periods, and reduce the demands that you make on yourself during the off times. Again, this may require some flexibility, both in your life and in those of the people around you. Do remember that someone who insists on sticking rigidly to the old routines may find that he or she has more problems than an individual with the same level of physical impairment who is willing to change his or her daily schedule.

In the middle and late phases, one of your doctor's primary tasks in managing your illness will be to maximise the amount of time that you are on and minimise the time that you are off. However, you may decide that the timing of the on periods is more important than their length. In discussing your drug regime with your doctor it's a good idea to have a firm idea of what you want to achieve in your average day, or when you need maximum benefit from the treatment, and of when you are willing to accept a decrease in speed, mobility, and so on.

SELF-CARE

Make Use of Physical Aids

In Chapter 9 we talked about the ways in which clothing and eating utensils can be altered to make it easier for the person with Parkinson's disease to get dressed or undressed and to eat; we also discussed practical aids relevant to many other aspects of daily life (see p. 215). Three imperatives were mentioned:

1   Obtain and use appropriate aids *at the right time*.
2   Have *regular assessments* by your OT, so that any aids you may have can be readapted to your particular needs at the time.
3   Be positive in your attitude to use of aids.

Point 3 calls for elaboration. Some individuals view physical aids in a negative way, and even refuse them. They may see them as outward signs that they are disabled or handicapped in the everyday, almost derogatory, sense of the terms. They may prefer to struggle on with buttons and shoe-laces rather than switch to zip-fasteners and Velcro. If they are eventually forced, by necessity, to accept such help they may see it as a defeat—a confirmation that they have in some way 'given in' to the disease. While one may sympathise with this attitude, or even admire such individuals for their determination, it is not necessarily in their best interest. Aids and special equipment are really extensions of the many things that we take for granted in making our lives easier or more convenient. Television remote-controls, electric toothbrushes and electric razors are all 'artificial aids' which we accept and use without a second thought, and they are no different from the special aids for the 'disabled'. They are all simply tools—a means to an end—that increase our independence or the amount of time that we have available to do other, more important, things.

The value of simple aids is illustrated by James, a man who had had Parkinson's disease since the age of 51:

> A collapsible stool/stick, bought in Boots, enabled me to go on holidays where I couldn't stand about listening to the tour guides. This has since enabled us to continue our hobbies (e.g. bird-watching), and we keep it in the car all the time. I also use it at check-out queues and at bus stops and in stations and while waiting for taxis.

Keep Your Actions Simple

In their informative book *Moving Ahead with Parkinson's Disease*, Meg Morris, Robert Iansek and Beth Kirkwood suggest a number of general principles that can make it easier to carry out self-care activities:

● Consciously think about and rehearse movements in your head before doing them, especially actions that you have particular problems with.
● Pay attention to each movement as you are doing it. Talking through

the actions as you perform them is a good way to focus attention on what you are doing.

● Try not to do two things at once. For example, don't walk around the bedroom while doing up the buttons of your shirt. Either your walking will suffer, or you will take longer to do up the buttons, or both. For someone with balance problems, even standing up can be a distraction, so try sitting down while getting dressed.

● As mentioned earlier, breaking down complex actions or movements into a number of steps will enable you to carry them out more quickly and more efficiently. Do one step at a time. For instance, with dressing:

1   Choose and set out your clothes in the order in which you are going to put them on.
2   Sit on a stable chair.
3   Pick up a garment and talk yourself through putting it on—for example, 'I'll first put my right hand into the right sleeve, then my left hand and arm through the left sleeve and then pull it over my head', and so on.

MOBILITY

Many of the suggestions above can be applied to problems of mobility as well. The following strategies for improving general mobility and aspects of *walking* have been mainly arrived at by trial and error by people in the early to middle stages of Parkinson's disease. Such tricks work well for some but not for others, but they are certainly worth trying. If they don't work, modify them, or think up your own.

● Transform your shuffling steps into a normal stride by imagining lines on the floor, such as patterns on a carpet or marks on the pavement, then high-stepping over them.

● If you have problems starting to walk, or if you suddenly freeze, try rocking gently forwards and backwards before taking the first step on a forward movement; or hum a song or whistle, then start to walk in time with the tune; or step over a real or imagined object.

● Remember to put your heel down first, rather than walking on the balls of your feet or your toes. Achieve this by thinking 'Heel first' to yourself. Also, try to walk with a long stride.

● To make turning safe, walk in a large circle and avoid sudden changes in direction. This way you reduce the risk of falls.

● While walking, avoid carrying things in your hands. Use a small rucksack, which will leave your arms free to steady yourself if you lose your balance, or to hold on to rails on buses or in the Underground or when you are going up or down stairs.

In his booklet *The Parkinson's Challenge*, Jan Peter Stern describes a number of other self-help ideas that have helped him to avoid *falls*, particularly in the home, and to minimise the damage if they do happen. This list of tricks and tips is adapted from his suggestions, with some extras of our own:

- If you feel unsteady, or when you are in a situation where you may fall, keep your feet about eight inches apart so as to give yourself a wider, more stable base.
- Walk without shoes when possible, so that you can better feel the contact of your feet with the ground. Avoid shoes with high-grip soles. 'Slippery' soles are safer if you tend to shuffle or suffer from freezing.
- If you feel light-headed or dizzy when you get up, sit down again and put your head between your knees for a short while before carrying on.
- Use automatic night-lights all over the house, so that you can see any obstacles.
- Remove loose rugs, and don't let people place objects in the main transit areas, even briefly.
- Get a phone with an answering machine, so that you don't have to rush to answer it.
- If you have glass doors, replace them with plastic ones or cover them with a safety laminate.
- Learn how to relax and roll the body in a fall, so as to reduce the impact and protect the head—Jan Stern learned to do this from a martial arts instructor.
- Learn how to get up if you do fall.
- When climbing stairs, focus on the steps one at a time by counting them. Always hold the handrail.
- When approaching an obstacle such as a kerb, deliberately lift your foot extra-high—it will probably then be just about right.
- When opening doors, try to stand to one side so that you don't have to take a backward step.

If fear of falling prevents you from venturing far, you will find Jan Stern's recommendations for learning *how* to fall and how to get up again especially helpful. Other practical aids, such as a walking-stick or frame, may provide as much psychological as physical support. The important thing is to keep walking for as long as possible.

Getting out of a chair, getting out of a car, turning in bed

As mentioned elsewhere, getting up from a chair often presents problems. So break the process down into simple steps:

1   Move towards the edge of the seat, so that your feet are well supported on the ground.
2   Move your heels right back.
3   Lean forwards.
4   Use your arms to push on the arms of the chair, or clasp your hands and with your arms held straight push your hands in front of you.
5   Stand up.

In any event, avoid those tempting low, soft chairs and sofas that you sink into. For more tips on the subject, see pp. 119, 212 and 219.

A similar sequence of movements to those outlined above can be used for getting out of the car which, in addition, requires turning your body around and putting your feet out of the car and on to the ground. To achieve this, some people find it helpful to sit on a plastic bag— because it's slippery, it's easy to turn the body in order to swing the legs out. Purpose-made transfer boards are available to help people transfer from a car to a wheelchair.

Turning over in bed is another automatic action that may be lost. We all toss and turn throughout the night, shifting position many times so as to keep comfortable. We don't usually need to wake to do this. The person with Parkinson's disease, however, may have to concentrate so hard on turning and use so much effort that he or she—and his or her partner—are wide awake at the end of it. Again, solving the problem can involve a series of strategies: for details, see p. 213. For getting out of bed, bend your legs, swing them over the side of the bed and then push yourself into a sitting position. Both turning over and getting out of bed are easier if you have a firm mattress rather than one that leaves you stranded in a valley in the middle. In her book *Living Well with Parkinson's Disease*, Glenna Wotton Atwood recommends a king-size water-bed with satin sheets! Finally, a device like a trapeze bar, or a rope, can be fitted, which will give you something to hold on to while turning.

Keeping Mobile Outside

Walking

If walking in and around the house presents problems, there will also be difficulty when you are outside. And while you may make your home 'user-friendly', you have far less control over the outside environment. This makes it all the more important, when walking, to take things slowly and carefully. When travelling alone, you may need to rely on strangers for occasional assistance. *Self-confidence*, as much as physical ability, is the critical factor. Many of the strategies mentioned previously can be used here.

- Time your journeys, where possible, to fit in with your periods of maximum mobility.
- Allow plenty of time so that you do not feel stressed. Stress and haste are the enemies of the person with Parkinson's—they make the symptoms worse and accidents more likely.
- Pay extra attention to possible obstacles and problems. Make your movements even bigger than you think you need to—it's better to look a little ungainly than to risk a fall.
- Use physical aids and supports whenever you can. You might consider using a walking-stick when you are outside, even if it's not necessary for most of the time. The extra support may be useful if you suddenly feel wobbly. Some people find that stepping over the handle of a turned-round walking-stick is useful to unstick feet that are 'frozen' to the ground. And of course, the walking-stick can serve as a useful sign to others, such as car drivers and bus conductors, that you may need a little extra time.
- Don't put off getting a wheelchair if you need one. Unlike, for instance, people paralysed after a stroke who use wheelchairs independently, you will almost certainly need someone to push it and to deal with steps, ramps and so forth.
- Accept help from others when it is needed and offered—don't be too proud to ask.

Driving

In both urban and rural areas, driving is an important means of transport and a prime feature of independent living. So don't give up driving without careful thought, but do take these precautions:

- As with any activity, think about the timing—allow more time for your journey and avoid rushing and other causes of stress.

- Take extra care. Think about your actions. Consider changing to an automatic car so that you can forget about gears. Power steering can also be a great help, particularly when parking.
- Regularly review your capabilities. There may be special courses in your area for 'older' drivers, for refreshing skills and testing ability.
- Above all, do you feel confident driving? If you don't, then it may be time to stop, or to start relying less on the car.
- If you do decide to give up, don't necessarily do it overnight. It may be better to phase out the car gradually while building up alternative means of transport, so that your life can continue with the minimum of disruption.
- Contact your insurance company as soon as you receive the diagnosis from your doctor. If you encounter problems, or if the new premium seems unreasonable, contact the Parkinson's Disease Society, which will suggest a number of informed insurance companies who are aware of the nature of the illness and the problems it may cause during driving.
- If you have particular difficulty with walking for any length of time, you can obtain a Disabled Parking Badge (see p. 230).
- Find out whether you are eligible for any benefits that are available for people whose mobility is affected by illness, such as the mobility component of the Disability Living Allowance (see p. 228). Under some circumstances, those who receive the mobility component may be exempt from payment of road tax.
- You can obtain information about mobility benefits and other aspects of disabled mobility from the charities Motability, the Royal Association for Disability and Rehabilitation and the Disabled Drivers' Association. Among other services, Motability has negotiated discounts with car and wheelchair manufacturers for disabled people.
- If you need specific adaptations to your car in order to continue to drive, you can obtain detailed information about specialist centres that carry out such adaptations from the Disabled Drivers' Association.

For more on cars and driving, see p. 119.

Using public transport

If you don't drive or have given up, public transport may be your main form of travel when you go anywhere further than walking distance of your home. Public transport can help you lead an active and independent life, and a few tricks and tips will make using it easier.

Buses   Getting on and off a bus, particularly in the rush hour, can be a trial for anyone. A walking-stick, as mentioned before, serves as a useful reminder to others to be a little more patient, and may help the individual with Parkinson's to feel less rushed. Don't be embarrassed to accept a seat if one is offered. The sudden stops, starts and turns of buses seriously test the balance of us all—let alone that of someone whose mobility is impaired. And do stay in your seat until the bus has stopped, before standing up to get off. Ask someone else to ring the bell, if necessary.

Dial-a-Ride and mobility buses   Even if you have no need of these most of the time, it is worth having their details to hand, if they are available in your area. If you use a wheelchair, they could be your main form of transport. Your local Social Services department, as well as local charities and church groups, may also offer transport to shops, hospital and social events.

Taxis and minicabs   The main form of transport for some people. While expensive, they offer the advantage of a door-to-door service. Some taxis are adapted for wheelchairs. It's a good idea to cultivate a relationship with a local taxi or minicab company. If you are a regular user, it may be possible to run an account and obtain a discount. You will often be able to ask for a particular driver who knows your needs— and the advantage of a driver who knows you is that he or she is more likely to help you in and out of the car, carry your shopping to the front door, and avoid throwing the car around bends like a competitor in the Grand Prix.

Trains and the Underground   When aiming to catch a particular train, don't forget to leave extra time for 'emergencies' or delays. If you are travelling to or from an unfamiliar station, try to check in advance on access to platforms—particularly if you are using a wheel-chair. There may be many stairs or escalators, and not all stations have lifts. During off-peak hours many stations are unattended, so there will be no one available to help at those times.

WORK AND LEISURE

Work

It is difficult to offer detailed advice, given the vast differences in the work people do. Also, Parkinson's disease affects people's ability to work in different ways. When problems with mobility develop, arrang-ing to work from home, if possible, will allow you to avoid the journey to work.

The same advice for increasing mobility about the home can be

applied to the workplace, although it will probably be more difficult
to make physical changes there. However, it may be possible to reorgan-
ise your workspace so that everything is closer to hand and requires
you to move around less. If you work at a desk, having a comfortable
chair is important. Wheels on the chair may help you move around
without having to get up all the time, but for someone troubled by leg
dyskinesia, having the chair firmly anchored to the spot would be more
useful. The Disability Service Division of the Employment Services
may be able to help if particular adaptations such as a wheelchair lift
are required at your workplace, to enable you to continue work. An
electric typewriter or word-processor is to be recommended—your
typing speed may not be great, but errors can be corrected and the final
product will always be legible. If you need to speak regularly—for
example, in meetings, to clients or to customers—and have problems
making yourself heard or understood, speech therapy could be useful;
and you might consider using some sort of portable mini-amplifier/
loudspeaker. Also, it might be worth consulting the disablement
resettlement officer at your local JobCentre.

From the booklets compiled by John Williams, *Parkinson's Disease
and Employment: The Experiences of Forty-three Patients* and *Parkinson's Disease: Doctors as Patients: Eleven Autobiographical Accounts*,
three factors emerge as important in determining the individual's ability
to continue working:

1 the need for a flexible approach to work
2 the central role of fatigue as a limiting factor and the need to
   accommodate it
3 the importance of other people at work, such as employers and
   colleagues.

Be flexible

When weighing up the pros and cons of a job in the light of Parkinson's
disease, there are four main options—to carry on as before, to modify
the existing job to fit in with your limitations, to change jobs, or to
stop work altogether.

If your illness is having little impact on your ability to perform the
job, then *carrying on as usual* is the obvious thing to do. This will
have several positive effects. It will maintain your self-esteem and
sense of achievement, the feeling that you are making a contribution;
it will permit continuing daily social contact with others; and it will
enable you to remain financially independent. But many people try
to work on as before *despite increasing difficulty*. While this is an

understandable response, such persistence may bring with it considerable costs, both to the individual and to others. John Williams' booklet *Parkinson's Disease and Employment* illustrates this. R.C., a British Telecom manager, recalls:

> During the last two years it has been difficult to remain fully committed to my work: it takes all my resolve just to keep going, and giving top priority to my work has had a direct effect on my social and family life.

And Dr I., a general practitioner:

> When I was first diagnosed I felt it was important to keep working for as long as possible, so, for the good of the practice, I kept the news to myself for two or three years. I worked for eight years after the diagnosis was made, and at first there was little difficulty and patients were unaware of my problems ... However, this being a small town, it eventually became common knowledge that I had PD. I was treated very sympathetically by my patients. Nevertheless, it became more and more embarrassing to examine patients with my tremor, which hardly inspired confidence. By 1987, being then 58, I realised the time had come to retire since I was also having difficulty with speech, driving and night calls.

The pressure of trying to carry on as usual may increase the physical symptoms, which may increase the pressure, which may make work more difficult, and so on in a vicious circle. To avoid such a situation, you might consider *modifying your job*. If you are lucky enough to be self-employed, or if you work in an organisation with a sympathetic management, it may be possible to decrease the number of hours you work each day. If your symptoms follow a reasonably regular pattern, you could try to negotiate working those hours when you are most able. An alternative, taken by many of the people who figure in John Williams' booklet, is to negotiate a less demanding job role, with less pressure—a *change of job*, in effect. Sometimes this will be a sideways move with no reduction in pay or status. More likely, though, the new job *will* involve a reduction in pay.

However, in many of the cases described in the booklet, it seemed that doing less work for less pay was considered preferable to retirement. Such a move may extend the period of effective employment by several years and may enhance your pension. But the time may come when you have to ask yourself *'Should I stop work?'* When to stop is very much a matter of personal choice. It may be that there will be only a short time before you reach normal retirement age anyway. If so, it may be worth 'battling on'. But if you have longer to go, it is sensible to continually evaluate the pros and cons of working or giving up. In particular, do the benefits of working, both financial and personal, outweigh the disadvantages? Is there more frustration and failure than job satisfaction?

When you do decide to give up work, you may be able to negotiate a period of time to 'wind down' the job, so as to avoid the abrupt jump from being fully employed to being 'retired', and to give yourself time to plan your retirement. Do treat retirement as a *positive step*, not as 'giving in' to the disease. Plan what you will do with your new-found time—don't leave it to chance or circumstances. Think of the things that you enjoy, see it as an opportunity to rediscover old lost hobbies and pastimes and to discover new ones. The account given by Dr G. portrays one approach to remaining active despite retirement:

It was not until I had retired that I appreciated how much the stress of trying to carry out my duties aggravated my symptoms. Once I had retired, my family and friends were very understanding in that they did not treat me as an invalid but were always ready to help me with any physical task I found difficult. Retirement does not mean that I have become a 'couch-potato', since I set myself small tasks every day: short walks, minor DIY jobs and helping more around the house. To keep my brain active I attempt crossword puzzles and play weekly bridge. Despite my forebodings I am enjoying my retirement more than I dared hope, and as I am not yet too severely affected I am fully independent.

Coping with fatigue

Neither physical nor mental fatigue is likely to be helped by medication. Appropriate scheduling and structuring of your activities will help you to minimise the effects of fatigue on your performance. Set yourself priorities each day, or each week. Do the most important, urgent or demanding parts of your work first thing every day before fatigue sets in, or allocate them to the times of the day when you are at your best. Regular short breaks may help you to work more efficiently and prevent fatigue from building up: just sit quietly and rest with your eyes closed, or, alternatively, have a cup of tea or a chat with a colleague. In preventing fatigue, a shift of attitude is as important as any practical accommodations. Avoid overloading yourself—try not to take on too many responsibilities or tasks at the same time. Don't expect to be able to work as fast or as hard as before you became ill. Learn to make allowances for your illness, and don't drive yourself too hard to achieve deadlines or other goals.

Communicating with employers and colleagues

Although a few people work totally on their own, most of us work with others; these may be managers or bosses, or other colleagues with whom we share the workload. You may be in a managerial or supervisory role with staff of your own. Even if you work alone, there may be clients or customers whom you meet regularly. As far as the options mentioned above are concerned—carrying on your work just as before, modifying your present job, or changing jobs—clearly, much will depend on these other individuals.

To renegotiate your job or your working hours, or to plan early retirement, you will need the fullest co-operation and support of your employers. From the practical viewpoint, they may also help by modifying your working environment to accommodate any mobility problems, or provide you with the equipment to make your job easier. Colleagues may provide either a formal or an informal support service: while you may arrange to pass over some duties permanently, it may be enough for them to take over as the need arises, from day to day.

However, none of this will happen unless you tell them about your illness. The importance of honest communication was discussed in Chapter 5. But it can't be emphasised too strongly that you should not put off telling employers and colleagues that you have Parkinson's disease. And tell them which tasks you do need help with and which you can manage on your own. It can be as frustrating to have to contend with colleagues who want to take over as with unhelpful ones.

Leisure and Social Activities

In Chapter 5, we underlined the importance of avoiding the phenomenon of *premature social ageing*—that is, the gradual withdrawal from active participation in work, in personal responsibilities and in social interaction that can be associated with Parkinson's. There are ways of coping with each of the difficulties—financial constraints, mobility problems, increased fatigue, unpredictability of response to medication, social embarrassment—ways that can help to some extent to prevent premature social disengagement. What is important is to guard against the isolation setting in in the first place. It may be that the particular symptoms that make social situations difficult and embarrassing will improve at some point; new treatments or modifications in existing drug regimes may reduce on–off fluctuations or dyskinesia.

But do remember that it is difficult to regain the habit of going out, once it has been lost. Friends and relatives may stop inviting you, or even stop thinking of including you in social activities, if you have repeatedly declined previous invitations.

Perhaps social embarrassment is the single most important problem to overcome. The embarrassment associated with being stared at in public, with being considered as 'odd' or 'disabled', finally persuades many to avoid social situations completely. It's so much easier to say than to do, but it really is necessary to grow a thick skin. Be selfish and think about yourself, not what others may be thinking. Above all, force yourself to carry on as long as it is physically possible for you to be out and about. Sidney Dorros offers a wise word on the subject:

> I was so embarrassed I often closed my eyes, pretending I wasn't there. But as long as Debbie [his wife] and our friends were willing to drive me and to endure awkward situations, I decided to risk the discomfort we often experienced rather than withdraw into a private shell.

Describing their many trips to various locations in the USA and Canada, Dorros says:

> We saw and did more than many healthier travelers. How did we manage? Through very careful planning. This included dividing the trip into several side trips of a few days each with a return for rest and recuperation to our home base, our son's house, between trips.

Even when things are at their most difficult, you *can* make life easier, for yourself and for others. You may be able to 'juggle' your tablets, so that you have a good period when you need it. If you enjoy eating out, find a local restaurant and use it regularly. Get to know the staff, and explain Parkinson's disease to them. Order dishes that involve less cutting up, and that you can eat with a minimum of help. To prevent spilling, put only a little in your glass at a time. If you use special cutlery, bring it with you. You may be able to choose times when restaurants are less busy—mid-week, they are often practically empty in the early evenings. The same may apply to cinemas and theatres, where afternoon showings are less crowded and rushed.

Most of us tend to have a well defined circle of friends with whom we spend the larger part of our social lives. As these are people we have known for some time, we share with them varying degrees of intimacy, friendship and caring—which may well help to create enough understanding to make social situations, even in the later phases of the illness, less embarrassing and daunting. In John Williams' *Parkinson's Disease: Doctors as Patients*, Dr F. wrote:

> We continue to enjoy occasional lunch and dinner parties so long as we know our hosts and guests well.

Hobbies, too, play a key role in keeping us mentally and physically active. But your symptoms may make it necessary for you to modify them. The need to give up old pastimes is reflected by Dr H., a general practitioner with Parkinson's, who wrote:

> My fly fishing was inaccurate and I had a 'twitch' at the end of each cast. I used to play snooker once or twice a week and I found that using the cue was becoming more difficult. I used also to sing in a choir and found that my voice was higher and weaker.

But there is an endless list of alternatives: gardening, decorating; taking part in sports such as swimming, bowls, croquet; doing jigsaw or crossword puzzles, reading, knitting, building model planes; helping in charitable work, attending adult education classes. Whether your own particular bent is towards becoming an expert on eighteenth-century novelists, perfecting your appreciation of classical or folk music, learning a new language or games such as chess, backgammon, dominoes, draughts or bridge, or learning to paint or type—now is your chance. Replacing the daily habit of work with new ways of passing your time will make the transition easier. As long as you keep yourself motivated, and your curiosity and imagination alive, the range of leisure activities that you can still enjoy, despite Parkinson's, is infinite.

Above all, *keep yourself active*—mentally, physically and socially. Set yourself targets that are realistic and achievable, but still challenging. The aim is to keep a balance of activities, within the limitations of your illness but with you in control.

Set yourself targets

While it may be easy to say, 'I'll keep active' or 'I'll look for a new purpose in my life', it is sometimes difficult to know where to begin and not to be discouraged by what might appear to be failures. Here are a few ideas that can be applied to everyday tasks or to the grandest scheme:

- Try to set yourself concrete targets—something that can be achieved in a single session of work or recreation. It might be anything from polishing your shoes to getting yourself to the cinema and back. Avoid vague, open-ended goals, or ones that would take a long time to achieve. A 'session' may be ten minutes or ten hours, depending on what you can deal with at the time. The aim is to have achieved what you set out to do. If an activity is too long to be done in one go, think of ways in which you can break it up into manageable chunks.

- As part of your target-setting, build in a few rewards. Promise yourself something that you enjoy—even if it's only a chocolate biscuit with your coffee—but *only* if you achieve your goal. No cheating! The bigger the achievement, the bigger the reward—which might just be having a quiet time doing nothing in particular!

- Although your aim is to set *manageable* targets, there will be times when you will 'fail'. Indeed, if you were to achieve a goal 100 per cent of the time, you would probably be making it too easy, failing to push yourself. Setting your targets too low is little more use than setting them too high. And if you do fail, don't give up—try again another time. If you keep on failing, though, consider changing the target slightly.

FINANCIAL INDEPENDENCE

Careful financial planning is important—ideally, before the drop in your income. If you are working, it is advisable to start the ball rolling as soon as you learn that you have Parkinson's disease. You may be able to obtain advice through your employer, or through your bank or other financial adviser. If you are taking early retirement, it is essential to discuss carefully with an expert, or even two, any occupational or private pension scheme that you may have to consider the pros and cons of stopping contributions or continuing even after retirement, of freezing the scheme or taking some early payment. You may also consider other ways of generating capital, such as moving to a smaller house or flat or one better suited to your physical needs. Even if you rent rather than own, there may be savings to be made to the weekly bill. If you no longer need your car or plan to stop driving anyway, you can save money there. As well as whatever you get for the car, there will be savings in insurance and running costs—although these will have to be offset against the cost of alternative means of transport.

It is worth doing some careful calculations of the likely change to your weekly income. Calculate current income and outgoings, and what they will be after you finish work or reduce your hours. Don't forget to take into account savings that will be made through not working—travel costs, meals, special clothing and so on, together with any new income through pensions or extra benefits. Clearly, if there is a major shortfall in your estimated future income and current outgoings, some adjustment to your lifestyle is required. The most obvious choice for most people is to cut back on 'luxuries'. Unfortunately, for many people luxuries include going out, be it to the pub, to the cinema or to restaurants. Financial constraints, therefore, may precipitate the social withdrawal discussed earlier. So it's important, in drawing up a budget, to allow enough to continue some of your previous entertainments and social life, or look for cheaper alternatives. Also, don't be too proud to claim the benefits you are entitled to. Remember that while you or your spouse or partner were working, you made contributions towards these state benefits, and are therefore entitled to them.

RELATIONSHIPS

Most of us have relationships with other people, such as a spouse or partner, other family members, friends, colleagues and neighbours, all involving differing degrees of closeness and caring. Depending on the nature of our relationship with each of these various sources of *social support*, discussed in Chapter 4 (see p. 91), they will be more or less able to provide you with practical help, sympathy and understanding. But they can only be that buffer against the stress of chronic illness if you tell them about it. And not only must you decide *whom* to tell, but also *when* to tell them, *what* to tell them and *how* to tell them.

To Tell or Not to Tell?

The issue of telling people about the illness has cropped up several times in this book—hardly surprising, since it underpins all the relationships that the person with Parkinson's disease has.

What are the advantages of telling, and the disadvantages of not telling?

Inevitably, sooner or later your symptoms will begin to show, even if they don't yet interfere with your life. To put it at its most practical, there may come a time when you require help from the people around you. Clearly, if they are told about your illness in advance, they will be in a better position to offer you that help when it is needed. One consequence of keeping the Big Secret is that other people are unlikely to raise the subject themselves, even when it is obvious, and are therefore less likely to offer help. As mentioned earlier, there is also a risk that people may misunderstand some of the symptoms. The published writings of people with Parkinson's describe many instances of problems with walking and balance being taken for drunkenness, fatigue for laziness, tremor for nervousness, lack of facial and vocal expression for boredom or depression. Such misperceptions can seriously affect a relationship, whether at work or at home, with friends or with strangers.

What are the disadvantages of telling?

The main argument comes from the desire to keep everything the same—either from a wish to *deny* the disease and possible future problems, or from a desire to *fight against* it. Either way, some people reason that it will be difficult to carry on as before if everyone knows: people may treat you differently, label you as 'having Parkinson's disease' or 'being disabled'; offer help when it is not required; avoid you because of embarrassment, or assume that you are unable to do things that you are perfectly capable of doing. You may be afraid that you will lose your job or be passed over for promotion.

Even if you don't tell, people will still treat you differently as the symptoms start to become evident. But if their attitudes and behaviour are based on ignorance or misunderstanding, they will be very different from the attitudes they might have had if they had been able to base them on information about the true nature of the situation.

Sidney Dorros, in *Parkinson's Disease: A Patient's View*, comments:

Like many Parkinsonians, I was reluctant to tell people I had the ailment. However, when I thought that they were noticing and wondering about the symptoms, I did try to tell them the cause as matter-of-factly as possible. I learned that people often misinterpret some of the symptoms if they don't know their origin. When I told them about my illness and its effects, it eased some of their concerns.

I also wish that I had discussed my illness earlier and in more detail with some people. Somehow, I took for granted that they knew more than they did. In later years, I found that I had failed to talk about my Parkinsonism with some of the people most important to me. My children, my parents and brother, certain close friends and associates at work have all told me that they didn't learn what was wrong with me until long after they had started worrying about me.

When you have considered all the pros and cons of telling people about your Parkinson's disease, I believe that you will conclude that telling wins over not telling. Decisions about *when*, *what* and *how* to tell may be more variable—they depend on your circumstances and the nature of the individual relationship.

Your spouse or partner

As already noted, the pattern of a couple's relationship before the onset of Parkinson's disease is likely to continue afterwards. Relationships marked by communication, trust and warmth will continue as such. Couples who have tended not to talk about their personal needs and feelings may find it difficult to adjust to the extra demands on them both.

While the gradualness of the changes that happen in Parkinson's disease can allow a smooth transition, it may also allow the slow build-up of dissatisfaction. Small irritations can become major sources of resentment if they are bottled up. Although it may seem obvious that the best way to encourage smooth adaptation is through talking to each other, it is surprising how many couples fail to communicate the 'niggling' irritations, let alone any more important concerns. For some, it may be difficult to 'complain' without feeling guilty—how can they criticise someone who is having to cope with the problems of Parkinson's disease? Or the ill person may be afraid of offending his or her partner, who may have been working harder and taking on extra duties.

The most useful rule is probably this. Rather than criticising your partner's behaviour or the situation, say what it is that you would *like* to be happening. For example, rather than saying, 'It really gets on my nerves the way you sit around all day doing nothing', try 'I think we both need to make more effort to get out and about.' One very important aspect of such communication is that there should be *no blame*— remember that your annoyance or resentment comes as much from you as it is 'caused' by your partner or by the situation.

Even better, make some concrete suggestions for dealing with the current problem.

Unfortunately, it's not always easy to be so open, flexible and positive. Once problems build up, it may take the help of a third party (discussed in Chapter 9) to guide the couple through the situation. There are many ways of obtaining such help—through agencies such as Relate (previously the Marriage Guidance Council) or the clinical psychology department of your local general or psychiatric hospital, from private therapists or counsellors (see your *Yellow Pages*), through your GP, or from your church minister if he or she is trained in marital counselling.

How best to cope with problems in the *sexual relationship* was discussed in Chapter 8. And the advice for dealing with such problems is the same as for any other kind. Discussion and communication are essential. Avoid criticism and blame. The same sources that offer counselling on general relationship problems can help with specific sexual ones; and, more importantly, by facilitating discussion they can help to determine what both members of the relationship want from sex, then help to 'negotiate' an arrangement acceptable to both.

If, either with the help of a therapist or on their own, a couple decide to stop having sex, it is important that some substitute be found so as to maintain a level of physical intimacy in the relationship. It may be that they spend more time cuddling, or they start giving each other massage. It is often the case that when the pressure of having sex is removed by mutual agreement, a couple start to rediscover their sensuality. They are able to take pleasure in physical contact with their partner, and may even feel a rekindling of sexual desire.

Other Family Members, Friends and Colleagues

Close contact and intimate relationships with others are basic human needs. We feel part of the world when we care about others and receive care and love in return. As already mentioned, telling your family and friends about your illness is the first and most important step. Give them information gradually and at appropriate times, answering any questions they may have. Tell them what the disease means for you, about your medication and about your particular symptoms. Armed with information, they are going to feel more at ease and so, therefore, will you.

To make social situations easier and more enjoyable, think about when and where you meet. While, in the past, you may have met friends in the evening, it may be easier now to meet during the day if that fits in better with the times when you are most mobile. You may find crowded places physically difficult and stressful. Busy pubs and restaurants may present too many challenges, and stop you relaxing. Choose quieter places and less busy times. If your finances are strained, go to the cinema rather than the theatre, meet for a drink rather than for a meal. Even cheaper, go to their home or invite them to yours.

However willing you are to adapt your old patterns, though, there may be times when things get just too difficult. There is nothing wrong in saying you can't come to a party, for instance. But rather than just saying no or giving some tired excuse, keep them informed—say, 'Thanks, but I'm going through a bad patch at the moment with my Parkinson's—perhaps we could try to meet next week.' This way they know that you want to continue contact. Treating people like this is a sign of trust and respect—important aspects of friendship.

And don't forget that work colleagues need to be taken into your confidence, too.

What to Say to Strangers

Strangers' reactions to disability range from drawing attention to the symptoms in a mocking or derogatory fashion, to ignoring the disability completely in situations where acknowledging it would be the preliminary to providing some necessary help, to treating the disabled person as if he or she is mentally incapacitated. All these reactions to her Parkinson's disease figure in Helen Rose's book *An Old-age Pensioner at Eighteen: My Life with Parkinson's Disease*:

> While I was in the chemist's shop I started shaking all over, although it was more obvious in my hands. A woman customer approached me and with a hint of bitchiness in her voice enquired as to whether I had had my morning drink. If not, would I like her to get it for me? I was so stunned that I was left speechless and very upset, so much so that the tremor became worse.

Another extreme reaction, the implication that the disability may be feigned, was experienced when Helen and her husband joined the queue for a 'disabled persons'' check-out in a supermarket:

> Just because they cannot see callipers or walking-sticks and you are not in a wheelchair they simply don't stop to think that you may be disabled ... Then some kind person, not necessarily in the same queue, would point out that we were at the wrong check-out.

On another occasion, at the polling station for the local elections, Helen walked with difficulty and a very stooped posture.

> When we walked in, an official took our cards and handed them to another. This man looked at me, turned to Peter, and said: 'Can she write, is she able to put a mark on her own paper?' Nodding silently, we took our papers and proceeded to vote. We were both stunned. This was the first time I had been talked over like an idiot.

Such reactions are the product of ignorance—people feel uncomfortable with what they don't understand, and to hide this discomfort they resort to ridicule or denial, or draw absurd conclusions. Unfortunately, until such time that the public's understanding and acceptance of disability improve, the person with the disability and his or her companions will continue to bear the burden of such ignorance. And, as always, the best way to combat it is to inform.

Clearly, it is impractical and unnecessary to tell everyone that you meet about your illness. But for those times when it *is* necessary, it's useful to have a plan or a form of words that suits the situation. For example, you may be subject to freezing episodes, or to unpredictable 'off' periods. If you are alone at the time, passers-by may come to your help, or ask if you need an ambulance. So it's best to know what you need other people to do at such times, and ask them. It may be that you don't need any help, in which case, briefly explain that you will be all right in a minute. Alternatively, they might be able to 'unfreeze' you by gently rocking you from side to side—whatever you have found works. Having a prepared 'speech' and advice to offer will reduce the stress and embarrassment of such informal encounters, and make you better able to cope. Sidney Dorros dealt with off moments this way:

> No, I don't need an ambulance. It's a neurological disorder that isn't dangerous. My medication needs time to work.

Jan Peter Stern lists in his booklet *The Parkinson's Challenge* a series of common questions that he has learned to deal with from a usually well-wishing public.

Question	*Answer*
'Do you feel all right?'	'Yes, this is normal for me— thank you for asking.'
'Do you have a bad back?'	'Sometimes.'
'Are you in pain?'	'Fortunately not.'
'When will you get better?'	'Some days are better than others.'
'Is it contagious?'	'Definitely not.'
'Why are you so slow today?'	'My muscles are stiff.'
'Did you have a stroke since I last saw you?'	'No, actually I'm learning to live with Parkinson's.'

Don't forget that it may sometimes be helpful to prepare people in advance. Sidney Dorros describes how he prepared a tour guide before setting off on a walk:

> Don't be concerned if you see me having difficulty walking. I take medication for a neurological condition that works very erratically. Sometimes I move too freely and sometimes I get very stiff.

KEY FACTS 10

Make use of all *of the resources available to you*
Resources include your own personal strengths, the help and support of others close to you, and the expert help of professionals. In this way you will be able to minimise the impact of Parkinson's disease on your life.

Be flexible
There will almost always be something that you can do to reduce the impact of the disease on any particular aspect of your life. Be willing to adapt and change, to make adjustments, to try new ways of dealing with your limitations, to accept assistance and to look for new opportunities.

What self-help strategies are likely to be useful?
First, schedule activities that you find difficult for those times of day when you are at your best. Whatever you're doing, allow more time. Try breaking complex sequences of actions into manageable stages. Talk yourself through actions as you perform them. Try to avoid doing two things at once.

How can handicaps be minimised?
As well as the resources and support offered by others, make use of any available aids, and be ready to make physical changes to your home and working environment. Even apparently small changes can have a significant impact on a particular problem—for example, with eating or dressing. Take an active attitude to such changes—don't see them as 'giving in'. Changing the way you do things, or when you do them, or using some 'artificial aid', are all aimed at reducing handicap or removing it altogether.

Keep active, both physically and mentally
This is central to maintaining health, enjoyment in life and a sense of self-worth. Don't let your Parkinson's disease restrict your normal patterns of work, leisure and social activities any more than absolutely

necessary. Because things may be physically more difficult, too expensive, or embarrassing, individuals sometimes begin to turn in on themselves. Don't. Keep going with your existing activities, modify them as necessary, or find suitable alternatives.

Set yourself targets for your day
Targets should be neither so easy that you can achieve them without effort, nor so difficult that you continually fail. Keep each target concrete, rather than vague, and build in some reward for yourself when you've achieved it.

The more people know, the more they will understand
People are crucial in our lives—our families and friends, our colleagues, even strangers. Tell them what they need to know about your illness. As well as being better able to help, if and when help is needed, they will not misinterpret your symptoms or other problems.

11

Self-help Strategies for the Person with the Illness: Maintaining Emotional Well-being

In Chapter 4, we reviewed in detail the factors that affect a person's adaptation to stressful life events such as a chronic illness. So how can knowledge of these factors be translated into ways of coping better with Parkinson's disease? In a sense, what this chapter offers is a list of dos and don'ts for maintaining emotional well-being and preventing depression and anxiety. But, as we have said from the start, do bear in mind that each person's Parkinson's disease is different from the next person's. You will find no recommendations here that will be one hundred per cent effective in every case. But the suggested strategies have been found useful by other people in similar situations, and they may work for you. To find out whether they do, try them out for yourself.

ACCEPTING THAT YOU HAVE PARKINSON'S DISEASE

It would be somewhat unusual not to be upset by the news that you have Parkinson's disease, that you are no longer completely healthy. But following this initial phase of shock and disbelief, a gradual acceptance of the reality of the illness usually follows. This means that you are beginning to accept the physical limitations imposed by the illness and to let go of lost function without anger or regret. The process of *accommodation*—or acceptance and adjustment—has started.

This involves achieving a balance between finding ways of working around the illness so as to overcome the limitations imposed by the symptoms, and at the same time learning to make allowances for your illness and disability. Achieving such a balance is the best way of remaining socially active, for example. You need on the one hand *to push yourself* and motivate yourself to do and achieve despite the difficulties posed by Parkinson's disease, and on the other, *not to be hard on yourself.* It is only realistic *not* to expect yourself to meet your previous standards. Instead, set yourself new and more achievable ones. This kind of realism about your illness, and leniency with yourself, make it more likely that you will not give up, more likely that you will achieve your goals. For instance, to accommodate fatigue, you need to adjust your daily routine by doing the most important tasks before fatigue sets in, and alternating periods of activity with frequent short rests.

Active denial of the illness, pretending that nothing is wrong and carrying on as before, may work in the short term, but is likely to lead to poor long-term adjustment. The despair and depression that some people experience result from letting their imaginations run loose and magnifying the possible implications of the disease for their health, their daily functioning and their future prospects. Realistic acceptance of your illness means enjoying your mobility and physical abilities while they last, and *dealing with problems as they arise.* Your attitude to the illness and your outlook on the future are perhaps the most important determinants of how you choose to live and cope with Parkinson's disease.

Remember that every individual has his or her own challenge in life. Some, such as having a life-threatening illness such as cancer, or a handicapped child, are more demanding than others. As Alexander Burnfield, a doctor who has multiple sclerosis, writes in his book *Multiple Sclerosis: A Personal Exploration*, what is important is how one deals with such challenges:

> I no longer need to fight because I know that I have the power in me to respond to whatever has to be. Although I cannot change the cards that life has dealt me, I do have some choice about how I play my hand, about how I answer my fate.

Cecil Todes, a psychiatrist with Parkinson's disease who has figured several times in this book, commented:

> It has been said that we experience illness in the style that we live our lives.

It is up to you and your family to decide how to face the challenge, and what style you set yourself in coming to terms with and coping with Parkinson's disease. The importance of *choosing* how you react is succinctly put by Glenna Wotton Atwood in her book *Living Well with Parkinson's Disease*:

> After my diagnosis in 1981, I realized that I could not control the fact that I had Parkinson's disease, but I could control the amount of time I might waste sitting around and wishing I didn't have it. I am passing this thought on to you: let your Parkinson's make you a *better* person, not a *bitter* person.

She goes on:

> You did not choose to have Parkinson's, but you can choose how to live with it. Find the right doctor, join a support group, start the exercise program, eat to live, build your family relationships and friendships, pursue the activities that have meaning to you, and you will find that, yes, there is a life with Parkinson's. Only you can decide to make it happen.

INFORMATION PERMITS CHOICE

Obtain information about the illness and its medical treatment. People differ in how much they want to know—some try to find out as much as they can, others would rather know as little as possible. But, in general, information allows you to make informed decisions. It also prepares you for what to expect, and gives you a sense of control—both of which can help reduce anxiety and fear.

The information you need can be obtained from doctors, from reading books such as this one and any of the others listed in the Further Reading list on p. 327, or by contacting the Parkinson's Disease Society. Most books on the illness produced for patients and their carers can be obtained from major bookshops and local libraries; or, occasionally, copies can be borrowed from the PDS. If something is unclear, don't be afraid to ask your GP or neurologist for further explanation. You might, for instance, want to find out more about current thinking as regards causes—maybe just to be clear about what did *not* cause your illness—or about the medication and its side-effects, how the drug regime might change over the years, how much disability to expect in the future, whether there are other symptoms that might emerge over time. Most of this information can be found in Chapters 1, 2 and 3 of this book, but you may want to ask your doctor about how it applies to your particular case.

AVOIDING NEGATIVE THINKING STYLES

What we think, how we feel and the way we behave are very closely related to each other. Optimism breeds contentment and self-confidence, goal-directed and problem-orientated behaviour. On the other hand, negative ways of thinking ruin self-confidence, create sadness, sap motivation and paralyse the individual into inactivity. Some psychologists and psychiatrists refer to self-defeating negative thoughts and attitudes as *mind traps* that undermine self-esteem and successful coping behaviour. Such negative thoughts and attitudes immobilise the individual and prevent adaptive behaviour.

Our thoughts reflect the way we see the world and how we interpret events. When people are depressed they tend to think negatively about themselves, their future and the world. Similarly, feelings of anxiety can be triggered by negative thoughts and unrealistic anticipation of danger. Such biased interpretations of reality occur because of distorted ways of thinking. See whether any of the following figure in your own streams of thought.

Overgeneralising
You expand on a single experience or event to conclude that something unpleasant will always happen to you or that you will never have a pleasant experience. For example, after a fall you may think, 'I will *always* fall if I go out.' This overgeneralising will stop you from going out.

Personalising
You consider yourself personally and solely responsible for unpleasant events, overlooking the part played by others or by external factors beyond your control. This unrealistic sense of personal responsibility gives rise to self-blame and guilt. For example, if you wrongly blame yourself for your Parkinson's disease, thinking that failure to look after your body has brought it on, then you are personalising an event that was completely out of your control.

Black-and-white thinking
A tendency to evaluate yourself, your circumstances, other people and situations in extreme terms either as good or as bad, with no room for in-between states. An example of this is the person who labels him- or herself as *totally* helpless, *completely* unable to cope, if he or she fails to cope with *all* situations *all* of the time. With this style of thinking you will get caught in a 'no-win' situation, because neither you

nor anyone else will ever be able to meet the stringent and perfectionist standards you have set.

Driving yourself by 'should' statements

You drive yourself and those around you by ideas of what you 'should do' or 'ought to be able to do'. Similar to black-and-white thinking, this results in rigid and inflexible codes of behaviour that will probably not usually be met by you or by anyone else. This failure may in turn lead to frustration, anger and guilt, or be interpreted as yet another example of personal inadequacy and so reinforce low self-esteem. Believing that you 'should' be able to do everything as quickly and efficiently as before the onset of your illness is an instance of this kind of thing.

Jumping to conclusions

Arriving at conclusions on the basis of little or scanty evidence can prevent you from dealing with situations in a positive manner. On occasion, this type of distorted thinking can result in your drawing conclusions, usually negative, about the future, as if you were able to look through a crystal ball and predict it. The bleak picture that you paint for yourself will only make you feel helpless, and drain your motivation to meet the challenges of living with Parkinson's disease.

Catastrophising

You are catastrophising when you fail to see the positive aspects of your life or your personal qualities because you blow up the negative aspects out of proportion—thinking that your life is totally ruined by Parkinson's disease, that your situation is dreadful and unbearable, is typical of this frame of mind.

Disqualifying the positive

Similar to catastrophising, but entailing even more distortion. It involves not only ignoring the positive, but also changing the positive into negative. For example, a stranger may take the trouble to be helpful and sympathetic when seeing you in trouble. But rather than seeing the helpful gesture in a positive light, you turn it around and see it as a sign that you are useless and dependent on the charity of strangers. This virtual reversal of reality and facts can lead to unhappiness, because you are seeing yourself, your life, your experiences and the world around you through perpetually dark glasses.

The first step towards dealing with such negative thoughts is to become aware of them and to perceive their role in creating your moods and determining your behaviour. Over time, they may have become habitual and automatic. First, you need to catch yourself thinking these thoughts. Write each one down, together with the situation in which it occurred and the feeling that it triggered. See how such thoughts have made you feel sad or anxious, or undermined your confidence. Identify the particular error of thinking that each negative thought involves. Then question yourself—examine the evidence for each thought and whether alternative interpretations of events or situations may be possible. Try to challenge these negative thoughts and replace each with an alternative positive statement to yourself. This is the basis of the method called *positive self-talk*, which challenges and, hopefully, changes your habitual negative thinking into positive thinking. But don't expect positive self-talk to work overnight. It's a skill that has to be developed over time. Practise it consistently, and it won't be too long before you are rid of your negative thinking pattern and able to regain your sense of well-being and your confidence.

LEARNING TO DEAL WITH YOUR EMOTIONS

Anger

Like loss of any sort, the loss of mobility and independence in Parkinson's disease is associated with a spectrum of emotions. Anger and the thought, 'Why me?', may be your first reactions after diagnosis. Later on, frustration and anger may be triggered by changes in your level of disability or increasing physical dependence. In *Living Well with Parkinson's Disease*, Glenna Wotton Atwood describes how she deals with her feelings of anger:

> Anger, an emotion I have always tended to hide, reappears from time to time. I've never been good at expressing it . . . In coming to terms with my Parkinson's, I needed to give myself permission to be angry at times, because the disease had upset my life. I needed to learn to express a healthy amount of anger without feeling guilty about it. I decided to try to deal openly with my anger in positive ways. I could go outdoors and walk it off. I could tackle the housework and allow myself to slam the cupboard doors. I could go to the typewriter and write about my feelings. What worked for me won't necessarily work for you, but the important thing is for you to admit you have normal emotions, to take a look at how you deal with them, and to allow yourself not to feel guilty about having them.

Although some degree of anger can be useful if it relieves the pressure and helps you to feel better afterwards, with some people angry feelings can take over. If *you* experience anger, work out what thoughts or aspects of your situation trigger it. Examine the evidence for and against such thoughts, and try alternative and more positive ways of evaluating your situation. Since it is difficult to think straight in the middle of a fit of rage, this is best done after a 'cooling down' period. To contend with your anger, try distracting yourself, do something different, break off from whatever you were doing when the fit of rage took hold: take a walk, turn on the TV, read a book, ring a friend. Try the breathing exercises described on p. 274 to relax yourself. Above all, avoid venting your anger on innocent bystanders such as your spouse or partner or children.

Instead of cooling you down, angry outbursts can at times pump up your system to make you even more furious. Even if it is someone else's behaviour that has provoked you, it's best to talk to him or her about it *after* you have cooled off, when you can put your point of view across in an assertive and constructive, rather than an aggressive, manner.

Anxiety

In contrast to the way that anger builds up to a peak, anxiety may be present throughout the individual's waking day and even at night, interfering with sleep. Anxiety may be to do with worrying about your inability to cope in an emergency, fear of rapid progression of the illness, anticipation of helplessness and dependence and of the need for assistance in performing most of your personal functions, the fear of becoming a burden on your family. Glenna Wotton Atwood describes her particular feelings about it:

> Over the years, one of the hardest things to control has been worry. Worry, of course, uses a lot of energy. It is unproductive. It is useless. Despite these disincentives, I have to admit that I still do some worrying. Fortunately, in my set of mixed feelings there is a balance more positive than negative . . . I resent all the limitations, but at the same time, I'm so thankful for all the things I can still do.

When it is intense and persistent, anxiety may be treated with medication. In severe cases, though, anti-anxiety drugs, or tranquillisers, are now seen as only a short-term measure. In Parkinson's disease such medication may make rigidity and slowness worse and should only be taken after consulting your GP.

It's better, if you can, to learn to combat anxiety with psychological techniques such as *changing your perception and outlook*, or *using relaxation methods*. Try to prevent anxiety from building up in the first place by making a conscious effort to maintain a positive outlook and adopting a pragmatic approach. Convince yourself that you can tackle each problem as it arises, instead of expecting the worst from the outset. After all, you have evidence from previous episodes that you *can* cope effectively. Don't dismiss this. Use your successes to boost your confidence. The technique of *positive self-talk* is of value again here. As before, identify the negative thoughts that trigger your anxiety, challenge them, and replace them with positive statements. When applied consistently, this can neutralise the 'poisonous' effect of such thoughts and change your outlook.

The best antidote for anxiety is relaxation, since neither the body nor the mind can be anxious and relaxed at the same time. The quickest way of achieving mental and physical relaxation is to engage in *deep, slow breathing* and to use *mental imagery*.

Sit in a comfortable position, where you will not be disturbed. Close your eyes. Focus your attention on your breathing—try to establish a regular rhythm, deep and slow. Count slowly in your head, to pace your breaths. Breathe in, pause, and then breathe out. Once you have established this rhythm, try to relax mentally. Think of a relaxing scene. Imagine yourself by the sea, listening to the sound of the waves and feeling the warmth of the sun on your skin. Alternatively, see yourself, in your mind's eye, in the countryside—listening to the birds, smelling wild flowers and feeling a gentle breeze.

Once you have practised these relaxation techniques and have become proficient in using them, they are at your disposal anywhere and at any time. There are many excellent audio-cassettes available to help you develop these skills. The Parkinson's Disease Society produces one, and others can be obtained at some healthfood shops.

Depression

In Chapter 5 we dealt in some detail with why and when depression may strike in Parkinson's disease, and the question of who may be vulnerable to it.

Apart from making you feel awful, and making you difficult to live with, depression can be just as disabling as Parkinson's disease itself. As we noted earlier, it is probably most helpful to see it as a reaction to the disability and handicap caused by the disease. Viewing it in this way, as a reaction to real or anticipated handicap, offers the individual and his or her family the possibility of actively preventing depression or of dealing with it if it occurs—the strategy is to *minimise that handicap.*

- Obviously, effective medical control of your symptoms is crucial, if your primary task is to reduce the level of your handicap. Handicap can also be decreased if you take steps to minimise the impact of those symptoms that remain. All of the strategies discussed in previous chapters—changing the times when you do things, taking things more slowly, avoiding stress, making use of aids, involving others—are aimed at reducing the impact of the disease on your life, at reducing your handicap. And in turn, reducing the impact of the disease will guard against depression.
- Try to identify the aspects of your life that you most fear losing or most regret having lost. These are the areas where you should make maximum effort to find ways of maintaining or regaining roles, or looking for alternatives.
- The various negative thinking patterns that we described above can play a key role in bringing on depression. The depressed person thinks negatively about him- or herself, about the world, and about the future. One of the most effective self-help strategies for combating depression is to *break the spiral of negative thinking* by learning to recognise the distortions that it involves. To do this, practise the little exercise described on p. 272. Catch yourself thinking such negative thoughts. Write them down. Identify the distortions that each thought contains. Then challenge them, and tell yourself more realistic and positive things, thereby building up a more constructive and balanced point of view. You'll be surprised how this disposal of your mental 'dirty laundry' will liberate you and empower you to feel more cheerful!
- Although self-help techniques may be effective, there may be times when depression is more severe and you need to seek professional help. Changing aspects of one's life or one's outlook is never easy— and even less so for someone who is already depressed. When depressed a person finds it difficult to see a way out of the current situation, and may be poorly motivated to try. If your depression persists and appears intractable, do seek professional help. Psychologists, psychiatrists, psychotherapists and counsellors can all help with 'talking therapy'. Your consultant or GP will be able to refer you to your local NHS services (typically, clinical psychologists and psychiatrists), or you can seek private help (typically, psychotherapists and counsellors). If your depression is so severe that it requires

medication, your doctor will prescribe a course of antidepressants to treat the main symptoms. Even then, it's likely that some additional 'psychological' support will be useful, to prevent further episodes. Friends and family can be invaluable in providing emotional support at such times.

- Be aware of possible *vulnerable times* for depression, when your handicap is increasing or there's a risk of it increasing. Discuss your fears or concerns with others—family, friends, colleagues. Even though, given your state of mind, you may find it hard to believe, they *may* be able to help alleviate the problem. Merely talking about your feelings with others at an early stage may prevent you from getting into the spiral of negative thinking.

As a general rule, never let your emotions build up to fever pitch. Learn to occasionally air your feelings with your nearest and dearest, with a friend or colleague, or with your doctor. Hearing their reactions and interpretations can also help you adopt a more balanced view. Above all, in dealing with your emotions, bear in mind President J. F. Kennedy's comment, 'We should not let our fears hold us back from pursuing our hopes', and remember that this is the only shot that you will have at living your life.

MAINTAINING YOUR SELF-ESTEEM

'Self-concept' is that familiar sense that each of us has of the 'I' or 'me' we refer to, the ways in which this me is unique and different from others. Our self-concept has many facets—our own evaluation of our personality and behaviour, of our achievements at school, at university or at work, of our performance as a spouse or parent, our interests in politics, arts or sports, our feeling towards our bodies and our perceptions of how others perceive us; and of course, of our weaknesses. In addition, we expect people to behave in set and familiar ways towards us. Our self-esteem, or the respect we have for ourselves as persons, partly comes from the constancy of others' behaviour in their dealings with us. Furthermore, we are creatures of habit. Chronic illness interrupts our habitual ways of living, and may alter the ways in which others interact with us. As a result, a profound threat to self-esteem may ensue, that may make us feel inadequate, unworthy, incapable.

With the progression of Parkinson's, maintaining self-esteem despite increasing disability and handicap may be difficult. To protect your self-esteem, the core of your personal identity, from the assault of the illness, remind yourself that despite the physical changes, the real you, the person inside the body, has not changed. Parkinson's disease cannot reverse your past achievements or take away past happiness. Neither can it prevent you from achieving new goals, provided they are realistic. You may never win an Olympic medal in the marathon, but Parkinson's wouldn't stop you from obtaining an Open University degree or winning first prize for your roses.

Loss of self-esteem, which is also a characteristic feature of depression, is to do with negative self-critical thinking, particularly extreme black-and-white thinking. So, the most effective strategy for preventing this is positive self-talk (see 'positive self-talk' on p. 272 again, and also pp. 274 and 275). Remember that you are more than your physical body. Perhaps, instead of merely trying to keep your inner core untouched, you could give it a chance to grow—by putting maximum effort into adapting to your new circumstances. To mould a more adaptive sense of your personal identity, your abilities and limitations, a degree of restructuring may be called for. We are often our own worst critics. We tend to reserve compassion, appreciation and encouragement for others. Why not indulge yourself, by *acknowledging your efforts* in the context of your new abilities and your new limitations?

In her book, Helen Rose describes periods of negative thoughts and feelings, and how these undermined her self-esteem. From therapy sessions with a psychologist, she gained insight into her thinking about herself as well as into her reactions to outside help.

> I was finding it hard to accept that I just wasn't as able as I used to be. This feeling not only applied to housework but to other things as well. He [the psychologist] said it was obvious that up to now I had always managed to fight the disease and that, now that it had finally got the better of me, I felt totally and utterly useless. And because of these feelings I rejected anybody who wanted to help me. Now that I knew what was happening to me, it seemed easier to handle. The situation is better now, although there are still the odd occasions when I find something difficult and these feelings return.

Although coping behaviours are generally similar, each new stress sets its own challenges and demands in unfamiliar ways. When challenging your self-critical thoughts, remember that it's not as if you have been on a training course on how to cope with Parkinson's disease and have failed. You may have had other difficulties in life to cope with, such as loss of a loved one, divorce, business or exam failure, but nothing in life could have prepared you for the onset of Parkinson's.

COMMUNICATION OPENS DOORS

We have already dealt with the paramount importance of communication in Chapters 5 and 10. Since your psychological and emotional well-being is intricately linked with your relationships with others, it might be a good idea to remind yourself of what we said earlier, especially in the sections beginning on pp. 129 and 259.

- Remember that communication with doctors is a two-way process. Neither your GP nor your neurologist will know that you are depressed, anxious or angry or that you need outside help, unless you tell them. Don't assume that, without any clues from you, they will automatically refer you to the available sources of help covered in Chapter 9. It is up to you to tell them how you feel and what your needs are.
- Honest and regular discussion within the family prevents frustration and conflict. Above all, remember that marriage and family life are about warmth, trust and mutual respect. Show your spouse or partner and your children that you appreciate their concern and help. Express warmth with hugs, and occasional treats and presents. After all, Parkinson's disease doesn't alter your ability to be kind or to give pleasure to others!
- Avoid secrecy with friends and colleagues. This undermines trust and leads to deterioration of your relationships. Honest communication can prevent misunderstanding. You can not expect your employer or your colleagues to make allowances for your problems if you are not honest with them.
- One of the major subjective traumas of a chronic illness is the sense of solitude, the sense of being alone in one's experiences. But your experiences *can* be shared—and sharing them may go some way towards overcoming the feeling of solitude.

POSITIVE ACTION CAN BRING RELIEF

Helen Rose came to this conclusion:

There are two choices: give up or fight. I chose the latter.

These are some of the positive steps that you can take in your fight against the disabling effects of the illness:

- As part of adaptive ways of coping, ask your GP or neurologist for referrals to the various sources of adjunct therapy, if you think you can benefit from them.

- Keep your social network alive. We have all heard the saying, 'A friend in need is a friend indeed.' Remember, if the situation were reversed, you would want to help any friend or relative who had Parkinson's disease. At times, merely knowing that there are friends and family who care can make a difference. But friendships have to be nurtured, so take Glenna Wotton Atwood's advice:

> Be very deliberate about keeping in touch with your old friends, and make time to see them each week, or as often as possible. At the same time, establish new contacts and make new friends through church activities, interest clubs, fraternal clubs, adult education classes, and volunteer work. You need to be stimulated by other people, to interact in meaningful ways with other people, to reach out and socialize with others. What you don't want or need is a life of sitting at home alone.

Janet, a district nurse, who had gradually developed symptoms since the age of 41 and was moderately disabled by Parkinson's, writes:

> I try to lead a full social life. I need to go out and meet people frequently. I often ask friends in or go to them in the evenings, as I am usually slow and stiff and unable to do activities, and being with others cheers me up. I continue to have dinner parties courtesy of Marks & Spencer's and a helpful husband. Guests help with serving (I have swallowed my pride) as I prefer this routine to not entertaining at all. When meeting new people, I ask friends to explain Parkinson's disease and especially dyskinesia to them beforehand, or I look for a suitable opportunity to explain the basics of Parkinson's disease. This makes it less embarrassing for everyone.

- Try to remain active. Over time, inactivity and lack of productivity may be taken by the ill person as evidence of his or her 'uselessness', and lead to depression. *Staying active* can keep depression away, and prevent the sedentary lifestyle and social isolation that can be associated with Parkinson's disease. Activity can distract you from negative thoughts, give you a sense of being in control, make you feel more motivated to do other things. It doesn't matter what the activity is, as long as you find it enjoyable and it gives you a sense of achievement. In *An Old Age Pensioner at Eighteen*, Helen Rose describes her decision to learn to use a computer and take up word-processing:

> I would probably never have achieved what I have with the

computer nor would I have been in the paper or on the television or nominated for an award if I hadn't been cursed with this thing inside me.

Janet writes:

I have got myself fully occupied with activities which give me great pleasure, mainly handicrafts, but also recording many minor as well as major emotional experiences in the form of poetry.

- Keep the fight against the illness, even the treatment, within reasonable perspectives. While many kinds of complementary therapy (discussed in Chapter 9) may prove of some help, irreversible treatments such as surgery should be undertaken only after serious consideration.
- Above all, be flexible. Don't resist change that may be to your advantage, such as role reversal within the household, or seeking help from others, or obtaining state benefits.

BE WILLING TO ADJUST CONTINUALLY

An unfortunate aspect of a progressive disorder such as Parkinson's is that the stresses and strains are not 'one-offs' but recurrent, reflecting the changes that take place during the course of the illness.

Let's take the example of someone whose Parkinson's disease has progressed very slowly over many years. Initially the symptoms may have been very mild, requiring no treatment; subsequently, they may have been well controlled by medication. Then this individual reaches the point when the disease becomes more severe, the medication loses some of its efficacy, and disability becomes more evident. This is a period that requires *readjustment*. Sometimes even a slight worsening of the symptoms may bring with it disproportionate increases in disability, so that the individual has to modify plans and ways of doing things. Periods when he or she and his or her carer and family feel that they are adjusting well to their altered circumstances may be interspersed with times when they feel overwhelmed by the demands of the illness. In other words, coming to terms with change and coping with the demands of Parkinson's disease is *an ongoing process*.

Not knowing the precise course of the illness, how quickly it will progress, how long the medication will remain effective, how the later daily on–off fluctuations will affect you, all contribute to the uncertainty that is characteristic of Parkinson's. Added to this is the fact that you don't know how long you can continue working, driving, enjoying your favourite hobbies. One way of coping with such uncertainty is to *live life one day at a time*. It may sound like a cliché, but if you really think about it, it makes sense. This was the conclusion that Dr E., in John Williams' *Parkinson's Disease: Doctors as Patients*, arrived at:

> Since my student days I have generally been on some committee or other, looking ahead and planning for the future. However, when I retired I determined to stop this and to 'live each day as if it were my last'. I do not worry about what the future may bring.

KEY FACTS 11

There are strategies that can help you to adjust to the illness, maintain emotional well-being and prevent depression and anxiety. Here is a list of dos and don'ts.

Accepting that you have Parkinson's disease and developing a positive outlook

Your attitude and your outlook are very important in shaping how you live and cope with Parkinson's. With time, you should come to accept the limitations imposed by the illness and find ways of working around them. Adjust your daily routine to accommodate slowness, fatigue and involuntary movements. You are more likely to remain motivated and active, if you set yourself realistic goals and standards.

Obtaining relevant information

At every stage, information about the illness and its treatment can be helpful in many ways. It shows you what is on offer and what choices you have available to you. It makes it easier to arrive at informed decisions. It prepares you for what to expect and gives you a sense of control that can help reduce anxiety and fear. Relevant information can be obtained from doctors, books and the PDS.

Combating negative thinking styles

Thoughts, feelings and actions are closely related to each other. This means that the way you think affects the way you feel and behave. While optimism brings about contentment and confidence, pessimism undermines confidence and motivation, creates sadness and inactivity. Distorted ways of thinking can result in biased interpretations of reality. To combat negative thoughts, first, become aware of them and the part they play in how you feel. Catch yourself thinking negatively. Write the negative thoughts down. Identify the errors of thinking involved and then challenge their accuracy. Think of alternative ways of interpreting events. Banish the negative thoughts and speak positive statements to yourself. With practice such positive self-talk can help you combat pessimism and make you feel better.

Learning to deal with your emotions

Anger, depression and anxiety may be experienced at different stages of the illness. Such feelings are counterproductive, because they sap your energy and undermine your confidence. The first step towards dealing with them is to ask yourself what situations, events or thoughts have brought them on. When feeling angry, give yourself time to cool off, then deal with the cause of your anger in a calm and assertive but not confrontational fashion. The best antidote for anxiety is physical and mental relaxation through deep, slow breathing and relaxing mental imagery. The technique of positive self-talk can help you to combat depression. Learn to air your feelings to your friends and family—this can help you to develop a more balanced view. If depression and anxiety persist, seek professional help.

Maintaining your self-esteem

To protect your sense of self-esteem, remind yourself that despite the physical changes brought about by Parkinson's disease, the real you, the person inside, hasn't changed. The illness cannot change your past successes or prevent you from achieving new ones. But set yourself more realistic standards. Don't be your own worst enemy through excessively self-critical thinking. Acknowledge your current achievements in the context of your present abilities and limitations, and reward yourself from time to time.

Communicating with friends and family

Talking openly and often with your spouse or partner and family about how Parkinson's affects your daily lives and how you can get around the problems can prevent frustration from building up. Also, if each person is clear about his or her roles and duties, your household will run more efficiently. Telling your friends and colleagues about the illness and how it affects you will prevent misunderstanding. Similarly, your doctor will not know how you are feeling if you don't tell him or her. Communication with those around you may also help to reduce the sense of solitude that can be associated with illness.

Taking positive action

There are many positive ways in which you can minimise the effects of Parkinson's disease on your everyday life and your emotions:

- Ask your GP for referral to the various sources of help available, if you think that you can benefit from any of them.
- Keep your social network alive. Knowing that there are people who care and who are willing to help can make you feel less alone in your fight against the illness.
- Try to remain active. Don't give up your professional or social roles prematurely. Take up new activities and hobbies. Not only is activity pleasurable in the short term—in the long term it gives you a sense of control and achievement.
- Be flexible. Don't resist change that can help you live and cope better.

Be willing to adjust continually

The stresses and demands of Parkinson's disease are not one-offs, but recur in different forms during the course of the illness. The periods when you experience difficulty coping with the symptoms will be interspersed with longer spells when they are well controlled by medication. These changing phases make different demands on your personal and emotional resources, so prepare yourself for a continuous and ongoing process of adjustment.

12

Self-help Strategies for the Carer

Brigid MacCarthy and Marjan Jahanshahi

It is a popular misconception that families have given up their caring roles. This is not borne out by the facts. As we noted earlier, in Britain 1 household in every 5 contains a carer, and 1 in 7 of the adult population care for a relative who is disabled or elderly. But increased geographical mobility and changes in family structure—fewer children, more women working, and so on—mean that care of the chronically ill person is less likely to be shared by an extended family network and more likely to become the responsibility of one or two family members. So in addition to his or her other duties such as going to work or looking after the household, each individual carer is more likely to have to cope with all the stresses and strains of looking after the ill relative rather than being able to share them with others.

In this chapter we describe the strategies that carers can use to optimise their coping with the new challenges and demands that Parkinson's disease imposes on their lives. Some of this information emerged in the course of our interviews and conversations with carers.

Remember that no single strategy is right for everyone. What is important is that both carer and patient feel comfortable, and satisfied that they are achieving the best possible for themselves in the circumstances. A strategy which works for one of you, but leaves the other feeling guilty, overloaded or exposed, will not help you to forge a smooth-running partnership.

STRATEGIES FOR COPING IN THE MILD-TO-MODERATE PHASE

During our interviews and conversations, carers demonstrated a truly striking resilience, and an ability to discover ways of coping that alleviated both practical problems and emotional distress. We were impressed by the courage and humour with which difficulties were faced, as well as by the highly individual solutions arrived at. These strategies for coping that others have devised may or may not work for you. To find out, try them.

Your Attitude to the Illness

Sorting out a coherent attitude to the illness is an important aid to well-being. We found that in the early stages, older individuals and their carers viewed the onset of the disease and its restrictions simply as one way of growing old. This kind of acceptance prompts people to review their past lives, recognising and valuing their achievements and satisfactions, and encourages them to move to this new stage with different expectations. Seeing the illness as an event appropriate to their stage in life helps people to feel less alone, less singled out by misfortune. Others, who were able to accept that developing the illness reflected random misfortune, also tended to accept the consequences of the disease fairly tranquilly. Some, however, chose more personal explanations for its onset, or continued to ask 'Why me?', 'Why us?', and these were the ones who usually had more difficulty in tolerating the consequences. This is where obtaining accurate information about Parkinson's disease and its possible causes is particularly significant: knowledge can facilitate the process of coming to terms with it.

Some carers stressed the importance of holding on to realistic hopes for a breakthrough in treatment. Many of the people with the illness, and their carers, volunteered to take part in scientific trials of new interventions, and took an interest in all sorts of ideas about how to maintain health and well-being. This enabled both parties to take an active role in minimising disability, which effectively combated any sense of helplessness. Yet another attitude, which seemed to be much less helpful, is that of a wife who expressed a kind of magical optimism:

> I just hope one day he will change. He might change one day and it will all go away.

This strategy *appears* to maintain hope. But, in fact, with each day that passed, with her husband's Parkinson's disease neither improving nor 'going away', she became more and more desperate. So, keeping a hold on realistic hopes and an active interest in developments in the treatment of the disease, but avoiding wishful thinking, appears to be the most effective approach.

In order to establish a mutually acceptable attitude to living with Parkinson's, talk about the disease and its implications together, as much as you need to, particularly early on. Carers who suspect the patient of not trying very hard, or who mistakenly perceive real disabilities as shamming, find it extra-hard to deal effectively with practical day-to-day tasks. Some couples reported that when one or other partner became very preoccupied with the disease and had difficulty accommodating it, it came to dominate their lives unduly. Respecting one partner's desire to minimise the impact of the condition is very helpful, as long as minimising doesn't involve denying its reality. As we noted elsewhere, the couples who felt that they had reached a mutually acceptable approach early on seemed to have found the initial adjustment least traumatic. Usually, they had arrived at that position by compromises built on plenty of discussion. Some carers we spoke to found particular solace in religion, which helped them to deal with feelings of anger and futility about the onset of the disease, and to keep faith in the future alive.

Choosing a Doctor

Those who had managed to find a doctor that they felt they could trust and relate to early on, felt better equipped to face the challenge of the illness. As soon as possible after the diagnosis, ensure that you choose a doctor whom both of you trust and feel comfortable with. Because Parkinson's is a chronic disorder, you can expect to have a long relationship with whichever physician is going to manage your ill relative's medical care. You have the option of going to the patient's GP or to a specialist hospital clinic. It is important that you feel the doctor is aware of your needs as a carer as well as those of the ill person, and is able to give you the information and support that you require.

Getting Relevant Information

As we have already mentioned, accurate information, sensitively given shortly after the diagnosis, is invaluable in helping families to manage the process of coming to terms with the disease. Fears that go unacknowledged can drive a wedge between people at a time when they specially need to depend on their close relationships. These fears often prove groundless or exaggerated. Insight gained from a range of serious illnesses shows that being fully informed about the symptoms of a disease and its treatment, and about what to expect in the future, helps people cope more effectively, both practically and emotionally. You don't have to become an expert on Parkinson's disease, but make sure that you feel you have enough information to make sensible decisions about your relative's treatment, and that you understand everything you have been told. Some people prefer to find out just the basics, and not to become too involved with the details. Decide what information you need to plan your present and your immediate future effectively.

Coping with Your Relative's Disability

Managing the disabling consequences of the disease effectively has a major part to play in minimising carers' stress. In the early stages, they rarely need to take over specific tasks. But the person with the illness often needs to be encouraged not to give up activities that he or she is functionally able to perform because, unjustifiably, he or she has lost confidence. Several carers spoke of the difficulty their relative experienced in making choices—for instance, about what to wear, how to unpack the groceries or choose the next job to do around the house.

Encourage the ill person to take responsibility for his or her general health. The emphasis should be on wellness, not on illness. Encourage him or her to remain in full-time employment for as long as possible. Don't let him or her withdraw from engagement in daily responsibilities and decision-making—this would only accelerate the process of 'premature social ageing'. The focus should be on what he or she can still do, rather than on what is no longer feasible. At all stages of the illness, the independence of the sick person needs to be respected. Allow him or her to do as much as possible—self-care, household duties within reason, and whatever else he or she can manage. Don't be frustrated by slowness, and don't nag or pressurise. Remember that the more he or she carries on doing, the less *you* have to do. Also, as mentioned earlier, once skills are lost or your relative gets out of the habit of performing particular tasks, regaining them will be difficult. Later, when moderate disability sets in, you may find the fluctuations in the symptoms frustrating—the ill person may be able to do certain things in the 'on' phase, but become totally incapacitated when he or she goes 'off'. Remind yourself that such fluctuations are a feature of the illness—the best you can do is accept them and adapt your schedule accordingly.

Of course, respecting the individual's independence has to be balanced against other practical demands on the carer's time. Carers spoke frequently about how difficult it was to achieve the right balance, stepping in at the right moment without taking over, and dealing with their own frustration too.

> His slowness sort of frustrates me and I think, 'Oh, if only he'd leave things alone and leave me to get on with it.' But I still let him continue.

Some preferred to take over discreetly, and finish jobs off when the individual had done as much as he or she could.

> I come to the rescue in a quiet sort of way, because I don't want to deflate him.

Others negotiated things much more openly, sharing out tasks to ensure that the individual was making a contribution to their joint lives. Sometimes this entailed him or her learning new skills or duties, and where this was possible it was experienced as highly rewarding all round. One woman spoke jokingly of having 'banned' her husband from a range of tasks that he could no longer finish reliably. She admitted that she now stopped him from doing some things that he could do at least some of the time, but she felt that having clear rules was the only way she could keep worry within manageable limits. In contrast, one man had prioritised delaying his wife's disabilities for as long as possible:

> I don't help a lot. It may sound mean, but I think in the long run it's in her interest to continue doing as much as she can do. Also, if you get people to do everything for you, you feel a damn sight worse.

Sometimes carers have discovered idiosyncratic tricks to help the individual overcome particular problems. One woman whose husband had had a military career found she could help him unfreeze by shouting, 'Left, right, left, right'. Another man who had been very outgoing and had played competitive sport professionally could be helped to speak more coherently if his wife spoke to him in the manner of a sports coach:

> Calm down. Speak slowly, speak clearly. Calm, slow, clear. Calm, slow, clear.

Each of these strategies illustrates how personal the process of adjusting to living with the illness is. Choosing the right approach is so important. For some, managing uncertainty and worry is clearly a priority, and sacrificing some competence may be a small price to pay. But other couples find the challenge of continuing to perform tasks despite increasing disabilities very rewarding, and are less troubled by the risks entailed by that strategy. This approach is easier to adopt if neither partner has other pressing duties, such as work or children to care for.

Another factor worth bearing in mind is that there is nothing unique about dealing with illness. Chronic illness has many features in common with other situations with inherent stress. It may turn out that the most efficient way to deal with it is via methods that the family has success-fully used to deal with other major difficulties. Falling back on old and tested ways also induces a sense of control and familiarity. If avoiding confrontation is important, introduce changes more discreetly. But if open discussion or even a good argument is the preferred means to a solution, then use them—provided they don't cause long-term distress.

Nurturing Your Partnership

The quality of the carer's relationship with the person with the illness plays a major role in determining how stressful they each find the early to middle stages of the illness. Many carers we spoke to had found great strength in respecting the individual's efforts to cope. For some, coping together had improved their relationship; acknowledging that the illness was a joint life event increased mutual involvement in its management. Appreciation of the fact that lack of facial expression, a monotonous voice and apathy were features of the illness, rather than signs of the person's loss of interest in the carer, helped carers to accept and compensate for them. Some carers reported that the illness had made the person with Parkinson's gentler, more tolerant, more easy-going. Similar expectations about the right level of care, and some degree of reciprocity—the person with Parkinson's doing things for the carer, as well as vice versa—are valuable. Reminiscing about the past, sharing what can still be enjoyed together, learning to express affection, maintaining mutual respect and trust, talking about prob-lems—all these were strategies used in households that were coping well.

Couples who took care to safeguard their personal relationship against the stresses of the illness often did well. Despite the physical limitations imposed on the individual and the burden carried by the carer, such couples had managed to keep the core of their relationship alive by expressing warmth and appreciation. One husband expressed his appreciation in this way:

Every evening in bed, I give her a cuddle and a kiss. It's my way of saying thank you for everything she does for me during the day. After all, she has a lot to put up with—me and my Parkinson's disease are not a bed of roses.

A woman in her late fifties described how adopting a long-term perspective on her life with her husband of 35 years, who had had Parkinson's for eight, helped her:

When it all becomes too much, I remind myself of my wedding vows: for richer, for poorer, in sickness and in health, till death do us part. It helps me accept the disease as just another part of our lives. I sometimes look through our albums and try to remember him as handsome as he was when we first met, and review all the good times we've had together. Then I know that I can go on and do my best for him and for me.

As already emphasised, if conflict and resentment do build up, there is no substitute for direct and open discussion. Some of the people we interviewed told us they had arranged to put some special time aside to talk about the awkward issues in detail, making a commitment to be as open and honest as possible, sharing feelings and talking together about their needs and preferences. Others found it easier to have a third person present, perhaps a grown-up child or a close friend, to help sort out exactly what the problem was. These sessions work best when all parties stick to concrete issues such as who is going to feed the dog or manage the household bills. It is important that a plan of action be agreed before ending the session. If the relationship between the carer and the person with the illness has been under strain for some time, mere discussion may not suffice and outside help may be necessary. Organisations such as Relate, and others referred to in Chapter 9 or listed in the A–Z of Useful Organisations at the end of the book, can offer professional guidance in sorting out longer-standing relationship problems.

Maintaining Outside Contacts and Seeking Social Support

People with Parkinson's disease often find getting started on things or making major choices taxing. But if gently prompted to do things in their own time and at their own pace, they find old favourite occupations very rewarding. Developing a thick skin, and being familiar with local resources, can combat social embarrassment caused by the more noticeable symptoms. One couple had been active supporters of the local theatre for all their married lives. Seats at the ends of rows, near exits, were always available, and for them, seeing half a play was a lot better than giving up this major interest entirely.

Carers need persistence and flexibility if they are going to maintain a level of interest and engagement with the outside world that suits both partners. They can so easily become isolated and feel that they have no life of their own. Keeping their separate friends and interests is not a selfish preoccupation, but a vital lifeline to keep the carer–patient partnership in good shape. Maintaining an energetic involvement with their own independent interests was felt by some carers to be crucial for a variety of reasons—here are two:

I'm not a martyr—to be able to carry on I need to have a break.

I've started to go out more, which encourages him to try running things by himself, at least for a while. It seems to work.

Those who had built up close links with their extended family and friends in order to gain emotional support and practical help also fared well. One woman reported that her husband confided more in their daughter, which was a welcome sharing of burdens.

It's important for the carer, too, to avoid secrecy, since insisting on telling no one about the diagnosis imposes a severe strain. Also, openness allows you to seek support outside your relationship—from friends and family, or from your nearest branch of the Parkinson's Disease Society—if you want to. All these alternatives will help to ensure that you don't feel isolated with the problem. It's better to build or reinforce links early on, rather than allowing them to loosen while you cope alone—only to find later, when you need help, that you have lost your old network of contacts.

Looking After Yourself, Too

For the carer, chronic illness in a close relative means sleep disturbance, increased workload, change of future plans, the need for emotional and work-related adjustments, confinement, restriction of social activities, and financial strain. Unsurprisingly, research on a host of chronic physical illnesses has shown that the primary carer is also susceptible to major psychological stress and physical strain.

Unfortunately, carers often fail to look after themselves. One of the common worries of elderly carers is what would happen to their relative if they were to fall ill. Obviously, such worries can best be handled by carers putting time aside to look after themselves, so as to reduce the risk of ill-health. Making contingency plans such as arranging for close relatives to come and look after the sick person at home if the need arises, or temporary admission to a nursing home, can also help to allay such fears. The Carers' National Association has introduced an emergency identity card, which identifies the holder as a carer and gives the patient's name and address, as well as the names and telephone numbers of those who can be called on to help. The aim is to alert the emergency services, if the carer has an accident, that someone depends on him or her. To obtain copies of the emergency card, contact the Carers' National Association.

How is the task of looking after yourself as carer best achieved? The following strategies can help you maintain physical and psychological well-being.

- Have *regular daily breaks*, no matter how short, from the chores of caring. You may just want to sit quietly and have a cup of tea, look through a magazine, watch a favourite TV programme, or ring a friend up for a chat. Longer periods away from home can be a welcome break both for the person with Parkinson's disease and the carer. Accept invitations to stay with grown-up children, relatives or friends. Alternatively, use the methods for arranging holidays discussed in Chapter 9.
- Even though the task of caring for your relative may be physically exhausting, try to put aside some time every week for two or three sessions of *exercise*. Go for a swim with your ill relative, take the dog for a brisk walk. Take up ballroom or country dancing, which can be enjoyable as well as good exercise. Avoid pulling muscles or straining your back by learning proper ways of lifting from a physiotherapist or via the nursing services.
- Make sure you get a good night's sleep and enough rest during the day. If your spouse's or partner's illness disrupts your sleep, move to separate beds or bedrooms. Don't let sleepless nights build up—it becomes impossible to cope during the day when you are exhausted. Ensure that you and your partner are eating a healthy and balanced diet.

Remember, in addition, all those other ways of keeping yourself emotionally and physically healthy that we have mentioned elsewhere:

- Socialise, with or without your relative. Accept invitations.
- Give yourself a break from looking after your relative. Get someone

to fill in for you. Don't feel guilty about taking time off to recharge your batteries.

- Develop new interests—some of which you might share with your relative. Activities that take your mind off your duties as a carer are particularly worthwhile.
- Obtain all the benefits that you and your relative may be entitled to (see Chapter 9).
- Be flexible and adaptable. Don't hold on to old ways of doing things that no longer suit your altered circumstances.

Above all, don't try to be a martyr. Don't overdo your stoicism. Strike the right balance between caring and meeting your own needs.

Joining a Carers' Support Group

Amongst the carers we talked to, those who had joined a support group considered it to be a lifeline. They enjoyed the meetings and felt in consequence better equipped to cope with caring and combating stress. Such groups perform many functions for them. They are a place to exchange information about the illness and about the available services and benefits, as well as other practical advice. The social aspects of the support groups—the opportunity for conversation and for airing and sharing emotions and concerns, empathy and understanding; the exchange of ideas and opportunities for joint problem-solving, the development of friendships, the organised activities and outings—all these were considered equally important in reducing the carers' sense of isolation, served to relieve frustration, and helped them to develop a pragmatic approach to caring. One put it this way:

I have found that those in the support group I attend are the people I can relate to most. They all have been through similar experiences as me, and they seem to be the only ones who understand what I am going through.

Another carer highlighted why the support group provided such an important break from the duties of caring for her:

The only time that I really relax is when I go to the meetings of the carers' group. I feel I am among people who understand my situation. I have a chat with a couple of other people I have got to know well. We exchange news about the ups and downs, give each other tips about how to cope, but also manage to have a good laugh.

Contact the Parkinson's Disease Society or the Carers' National Association to find out whether there are any PD carers' support groups in your area. If there aren't any, and you know others in similar situations who may be interested in joining, why not start your own?

Living for the Present

Learning not to focus on the illness, mentally minimising rather than magnifying its consequences, making the most of daily pleasures, and focusing on the present rather than the future, are universally successful:

> I don't treat him as if there was anything major wrong with him. Maybe it's very selfish and maybe the day will come when it will be different, but right now this seems to be what we both want.

> I think everything is an attitude of mind. If you've got something and you can't get rid of it, then make the best of it. Be thankful you've got an arm—some people haven't got an arm—there's always someone worse off. When I wake up in the morning I say, 'Oh, thank God I'm here', and carry on. I don't think of the future as such.

Keeping Your Sense of Humour!

Some carers found humour a vital strategy in minimising and deflecting tension. They were not afraid of seeing the funny side of the predicaments the disease sometimes leaves them in. When humour is shared, Parkinson's patients are unlikely to experience it as belittling their difficulties.

> We laugh at it. You have to, otherwise there would be tears. We just have a laugh and start again.

> What's the good of keeping on bellowing? It only sets him shaking, then we're worse off than originally. We end up with a laugh, and so long as I can get a laugh from him, that's a reward.

STRATEGIES FOR COPING IN THE SEVERE PHASE

When disability has become severe, *the way* people cope makes an enormous difference to their sense of well-being and to their practical management of their individual circumstances. In our contacts with carers and patients, we were often moved and impressed by the courage and good humour with which they tackled overwhelmingly difficult situations.

Solving Practical Problems

Many of the strategies discussed earlier work equally well when it comes to severe disability, but the need to organise effective solutions to practical problems is more urgent at this stage. Evidence from other sources, as well as the experiences of the carers we talked to, indicates that no amount of effort expended in dealing with personal feelings, either with or without the help of others, can substitute for making good use of practical, problem-focused strategies. Only once the best possible practical solutions have been arrived at can working on personal feelings contribute to the carer's sense of well-being.

Those carers who put energy and enthusiasm into using any practical aid available seemed to gain something more than the simple mechanical advantage—it may be that a sense of increased control and mastery comes with the sense of efficiency:

Practical everyday things are just something to get around. At the moment I'm very much on top of it. I like to feel I will continue to be, but one never knows.

For example, one man with a severely disabled and totally dependent wife solved the problem of serving hot meals at times that fitted in with his wife's unpredictable on–off periods by learning to cook with a microwave oven. He reported feeling delighted at learning a new skill—something he had lacked the time or energy to do for several years—which also provided a solution to a major problem.

When the disease becomes incapacitating, it may be necessary to obtain appropriate eating utensils. Other self-care activities such as washing, bathing and dressing may no longer be possible to perform unaided, and may need the carer's help. The main priority here is to find ways of making these tasks easier (see Chapter 9, in particular p. 217, for available aids and equipment).

The sick person who is wheelchair- or bed-bound should be moved every few hours, to prevent pressure sores (see below) and pneumonia from developing. You will need to learn ways of lifting or moving him or her without damaging your own back or pulling any muscles—the community nurse can help here (see p. 222). Communication problems will increase as speech deteriorates—give the patient time to communicate, or develop alternative means of communication (see pp. 209,

220). Above all, be patient—frustration is not good for either party. In solving practical problems, you may often have to resort to the various sources of outside help discussed in Chapter 9.

Making Use of Outside Help

Besides the Carers' National Association, all the sources of outside help listed in Chapter 9—GP, neurologist, physiotherapist, occupational therapist, social worker, members of the various nursing services, psychotherapist or counsellor, the PDS and so on—are available to provide guidance and help for the carer as well as for the sick person. When Parkinson's disease becomes moderately to severely disabling, drawing on these various resources can provide major relief for the carer.

In our interviews with carers we discovered that the morale in households that were able to rely on paid help or on close and committed relatives for practical assistance was noticeably higher. When respite could be afforded by someone else providing the constant vigilance that many severely disabled people needed, carers felt more able to manage their daily routines and to snatch some time for their own interests. Not everyone can employ outside help privately, of course, but statutory help is available, and energy is well spent lobbying for entitlements. Local health and social services provide home helps and day care in a range of different contexts, from lunch clubs to full-time day centres, periods of respite care, and a range of sheltered accommodation (see Chapter 9). Individual needs are carefully assessed before offers of such services are made. Many statutory services employ advocacy workers to help people state their circumstances and needs clearly, and to help them fill in forms. Households that assemble for themselves a package of practical supports from a variety of sources, formal and informal, are in a strong position to tackle both daily stresses and sudden crises.

Balancing Your Partnership

With the progression of the illness and the sick person's increasing disability, the carer may begin to feel that he or she is constantly giving but receiving nothing in return. Although most people willingly undertake all the practical tasks dictated by their partner's illness, the main complaint is often lack of emotional support—particularly true if the ill partner becomes engulfed in the symptoms and the changes in disability, or totally wrapped up in his or her own emotions. The gradual dependence of the ill partner, if combined with a lack of communication and emotional give and take, may make the other partner feel that he or she is reduced to the role of nurse.

Many of the ways of coping used in earlier stages of the illness to protect and nurture the partnership seem to be just as useful at this later stage:

- Carers emphasise the importance of still being able to shout and argue occasionally without feeling guilty. One couple kept to a firm rule that they would not 'let the sun go down' on their bad temper, and it was agreed between them that they would argue but that no dispute should be allowed to last longer than the day it began. Bottling up anger or frustration can have serious consequences for both parties, particularly for the long-term security of their relationship.
- Acknowledging and promoting give and take, within the constraints imposed by severe disabilities, is also very important.

    I don't do anything with the bills, he deals with them. It's a responsibility that he cherishes. It makes him feel he is making a contribution to running our life.

- Many carers find that the courage and good humour of the ill person, in the face of all the problems, gives them the strength to continue.
- Not allowing the daily demands of Parkinson's to reduce life to a series of self-care routines is of paramount importance. Deliberately putting time aside, no matter how short, to gossip, to reminisce, to make decisions, to plan future activities, promotes interaction and involvement. At bedtime, expressions of warmth and appreciation through hugging, cuddling or kissing can make a demanding day more tolerable for both.
- Humour remains an invaluable resource, when there is little else to resort to.

Dealing with Your Emotions

Of course, Parkinson's disease evokes a range of emotions in the carer. The feelings that are perhaps most unjustified, as noted elsewhere, are *self-blame* and *guilt*. Sometimes, the healthy partner may feel guilty that he or she is not physically incapacitated and does not have to live through the ups and downs in mobility and dyskinesias that can characterise the late stages; another common source of guilt is simply taking time off. Carers may also blame themselves when things go wrong, even though there may have been nothing that they could have done to prevent accidents such as falls, or the distressing side-effects of medication. When one partner is ill, the other may feel guilty about becoming irritated or losing his or her temper.

These feelings are often rooted in a deep concern for the ill relative, but irrationality also contributes to them. Feelings of self-blame are misplaced in this context, because they are based on the assumption that you as carer should have control over situations which may in fact be uncontrollable. Also, they don't allow for the fact that we all make mistakes or judge situations wrongly. Furthermore, they are based on the assumption that the carer should somehow be selfless. Only angels are selfless, not human beings!

Whatever the nature of your emotions, don't lock them up. Don't feel guilty about talking about them with close friends or family. Don't think that you are betraying your partner. Airing your feelings will not only make you feel better, it may bring you a new perspective, or useful insight or advice. If you don't, you are more likely to feel strained by the demands imposed on you, and more likely to have outbursts when it all becomes too much for you to handle.

In learning to deal with your emotions as a carer, you will find that the techniques of mental and physical *relaxation* and *positive self-talk* described in the previous chapter (see pp. 274, 272) can work equally well for you. If you catch yourself thinking negative thoughts, identify your particular errors of thinking, challenge your negative thoughts and replace them with more positive statements—and with time you will feel better. Put aside time for doing the relaxation exercises. If you go through a particularly bad patch, when it all seems to have become too much for you, seeing a psychotherapist or counsellor may help you to develop new perspectives and coping strategies.

Keeping a Sense of Realism

Developing a realistic attitude about the future, without falling into pessimism, is a vital asset. Carers' individual efforts to deal with their feelings about their situation seem to focus on trying to achieve resignation while avoiding despair. The weariness brought on by coping with a very long-term problem can threaten to defeat people, unless ambitions and expectations are adjusted.

I've always got the hope that he won't get worse—or depressed.

The carers we spoke to identified some helpful strategies in trying to strike the right balance: recognising that major improvement is out of the question, being committed to maximising the use of functions that remain intact, leading a healthy lifestyle, hoping for plateaux to last as long as possible, and participating in trials of new treatments when opportunities come up.

Recognising the strengths of the ill person helps many carers to accept the daily difficulties they face. It is important to appreciate whatever abilities are preserved: for example, several carers emphasised the value to them of the intactness of their partners' mental capacities. Yet others stressed the patience or good humour of the ill person, preserved despite extensive physical deterioration.

Preparing for the Time When Your Caring Role May End

The time may come when your ill relative becomes so severely disabled that you can no longer look after his or her needs at home. This is the point at which you need to give careful consideration to some form of *residential care*. Discuss the pros and cons with your relative and with other members of your family. View potential homes and decide which is the most suitable for his or her particular needs (see Chapter 9).

When the time comes for the separation, you will need to have mentally prepared both yourself and your partner for the changes that are going to occur in your living circumstances and your daily routines. Discuss the likely changes together, so that you can both start accepting them. It's even more important to talk about your feelings, so that you don't end up feeling guilty because you think you are abandoning your relative. The reality will be that you have done your best in caring for him or her up to now, but with the current level of disability, his or her needs are going to be best met by an alternative arrangement. You are doing what is *best for both of you*.

The other feeling, commonly expressed, is a sense of uselessness, of no longer being needed, now that you have lost those caring duties that may well have dominated your life in the last few years. Feelings of loneliness may also prevail. One man in his mid-seventies put it this way:

> After living together for 50 years, the last 15 of them with her Parkinson's disease, my wife is now in a nursing home. Life is certainly less chaotic for me, but the house seems very empty, and at times I don't know what to do with myself now that she is no longer here to look after every day.

With time, you will learn to care for the person with Parkinson's disease in your new capacity. Frequent visits, taking with you news of friends and family and a supply of favourite foods and magazines, will be much appreciated. And now, if you have managed to keep up your contacts with friends and maintained your outside interests, you can pick up your own life again.

CAMPAIGNING FOR SERVICES THAT WILL MEET YOUR NEEDS

In their leaflet *Carers' Needs—a Ten-point Plan for Carers*, the Carers' National Association has set out the criteria for ensuring that carers and the people they care for can lead full and independent lives. According to this, carers' needs are:

1 Recognition of their contribution as carers and of their own needs as individuals in their own right.
2 Services tailored to their individual circumstances, needs and views, agreed upon through discussions at the time help is being planned.
3 Services equally accessible to carers of every race and ethnic origin, reflecting an awareness of differing racial, cultural and religious backgrounds and values.
4 Opportunities for a break, both for short spells (e.g. an afternoon) and for longer periods (a week or more), to relax and have time to themselves.
5 Practical help to lighten the tasks of caring, including domestic help, home adaptations, incontinence services and help with transport.
6 Someone to talk to about their own emotional needs—at the outset of caring, while they are caring and when the caring task is over.
7 Information about the available benefits and services, as well as about how to cope with the particular condition of the person cared for.
8 An income that covers the cost of caring and that does not preclude carers' taking employment or sharing the caring with others.
9 Opportunities to explore alternatives to family care, for both the immediate and the long-term future.
10 Services designed, at all levels of policy-planning, through consultation with carers.

Reflecting on your own experiences, you may feel that there is a large gap between this 'ideal' list and the actuality of being a carer. As a first step in bridging this gap, consider joining a pressure group,

302   PARKINSON'S DISEASE

to campaign for the provision of better services. Often, groups can voice their needs more effectively than individuals. Join a support group, if you haven't already. Also, as an individual carer, you may find this list useful as a guideline for obtaining the services that will help you to cope.

KEY FACTS 12

No single strategy works for everyone. Select and try out strategies that may work for you.

When the Illness Is Mildly to Moderately Disabling

Establishing a shared approach to living with Parkinson's

You and your ill relative need to arrive at a common approach to living with Parkinson's. Talk about the disease and its implications with your relative and with other members of the family. Accepting the reality of it while maintaining hope for new treatments will help you develop ways of accommodating it with minimal disruption and distress.

Choosing a doctor

Early on, you and your ill relative should choose a doctor—whether GP, hospital consultant or private neurologist—whom you both trust, feel comfortable with, can talk to easily, and consider able to appreciate your particular circumstances and needs. Continuity of care from such a doctor is likely to be beneficial for the medical management of the illness.

Getting relevant information

Knowing about the symptoms and about their impact on your ill relative's daily activities will help you to understand the limitations imposed on him or her and the fluctuations in ability. Accurate information about possible causes, likely course and available treatments will prepare you for what to expect and so prevent unnecessary anxiety and irrational fears. Information also allows both of you to make sensible decisions about treatments, about stopping work and about giving up driving or moving house.

Coping with your relative's disability

Knowing about the illness can prevent you from feeling frustrated, from pushing your partner too hard, and from nagging. For as long as the illness allows it, encourage him or her to continue work, to exercise, to take on new or different responsibilities, to do household tasks, to drive, to socialise as before. Even when disability sets in, let him or her continue to do as much as possible. Show appreciation for efforts made.

Nurturing your partnership

When the disease becomes moderately disabling, you and the ill person may be spending a considerable amount of time together. How you treat and interact with each other will be very important for the quality of your lives. Major setbacks and new pressures can be faced more effectively if you pool your resources, rather than fighting alone or in ways that would undermine your individual efforts. Respect each other's wishes and learn to compromise. Express affection and warmth and show your appreciation of your partner's efforts.

Maintaining your social contacts

When you are faced with the daily demands of the illness, keeping in touch with friends and family and pursuing your hobbies may seem your last consideration—but it should be precisely the opposite. It's now, perhaps more than ever, that you need to make social activities a priority. Don't deprive yourself of the practical help and emotional support that your friends and family can give you. Don't let social embarrassment turn you and your partner into hermits. Live for yourselves—don't be bothered by what other people—mostly strangers, anyway—may think. Explain to people in simple terms about Parkinson's disease and how it affects your relative.

Looking after yourself

- Have regular daily breaks from caring.
- Put aside some time every week for exercise.
- Make sure you get a good night's sleep and that you are eating healthily.
- Take time off.
- Be flexible and adaptable.
- Don't try to be a martyr.

Joining a carers' support group

Meeting other people who are in your situation will help reduce your sense of isolation, provide you with important sources of information about services and benefits and with practical advice; furnish opportunities for airing and sharing feelings and exchanging ideas; offer social support, organised activities and outings.

Living for the present

Enjoy life *now*. This doesn't mean that you shouldn't plan for the future. Simply, don't postpone what you can enjoy now until some indefinite later date.

Keeping your sense of humour

Having a good laugh can often help to relieve tension and lighten the burden for both of you.

When the Illness Becomes Severely Disabling

Solving practical problems

When Parkinson's disease becomes severely disabling, the ill person may need much more help with everyday activities. Making these tasks easier by obtaining appropriate equipment and by seeking help from available resources will be critical in lightening your workload. Remember that the various external resources—doctors, nurses, therapists and so on—are there to be used. So, instead of fighting alone, ask for whatever services you think you will both benefit from.

Achieving a balance in your partnership

Despite your partner's disability, building some form of reciprocity into your relationship will be most gratifying. Allow him or her to do things for you, no matter how small. Express appreciation of his or her patience and tolerance, and efforts to cope—this will in turn encourage him or her to show appreciation of your hard work.

Dealing with your emotions

Try the techniques of mental and physical relaxation and positive self-talk described in Chapter 11—they can work equally well for you. Catch yourself having negative thoughts, identify your errors of thinking, and replace your negative thoughts with more positive statements. Banish any feelings of guilt—you can't expect yourself to be completely selfless, or to be able to control situations that are beyond your control. Don't lock your emotions up—share them with friends and family. It may help you feel better and bring you a new perspective or useful insight or advice.

Maintaining a sense of realism

Developing a realistic attitude to increasing disability, and to the implications for you and the rest of the family, is difficult. But don't let pessimism and despair take over. The most adaptive coping strategies at this stage are realistic acceptance, a pragmatic attitude to problem-solving, living for the present, and not worrying about the future.

Preparing for the end of caring

A time may come when your partner's needs are best met in residential care. Accepting this as the best course of action may be difficult partly because you have unjustified feelings of guilt at 'abandoning' him or her. Discuss the practicalities as well as your feelings, so as to prepare both yourself and your partner for the changes in your daily routines. After his or her departure, you are likely to feel a void. It's easier to pick up your life again if you have kept in contact with friends and maintained outside interests.

Campaigning for Better Service Provision

Your needs should not be overshadowed by those of the ill person. Familiarise yourself with the Carers' National Association's list of priorities for meeting the needs of carers. Ensure that you obtain access to services that will allow you to fulfil these needs. Join others in campaigning for better service provision.

Tailpiece

13

Past Perspectives and Future Horizons

The history of Parkinson's disease is one of the best illustrations of the multitude of paths to scientific discovery and advancement. The gradual development of ideas combined with laborious observation and experimentation over many years, unusual insights leading to sudden leaps, natural experiments and accidental discovery, have all marked the history of the disorder and have played a role in our current knowledge. Since past achievements mould the shape of future advances, we outline here the major landmarks before moving on to consider what promise future research horizons hold.

THE HISTORY OF PARKINSON'S DISEASE

References to the symptoms of the illness in ancient texts suggest that Parkinson's disease has probably existed for centuries. However, it was not until 1817 that the various symptoms were described together as forming a single illness by James Parkinson.

The first of the six children of John and Mary Parkinson, James was born on 11 April 1755. His father was a pharmacist and surgeon who worked at 1 Hoxton Square in Shoreditch, then a village near London, where the family also lived. James studied medicine, then joined his father as a general practitioner, and he too both lived and worked at 1 Hoxton Square. He married Mary Daler, with whom he had six children, four of whom survived, and one qualified in medicine. Besides his essay on the 'shaking palsy', the name for Parkinson's disease at the time, he produced a number of other publications. He was also a political activist, and is described as a social reformer. He died on 21 December 1824.

An Essay on the Shaking Palsy, 66 pages long, was published in 1817.

In the first chapter, the history of the illness is outlined, a definition is given and six patients are described, not all of whom had been personally examined by Parkinson. The symptoms are described in more detail in Chapter II. Chapter III deals with distinguishing the 'shaking palsy' from other disorders, and chapters IV and V, respectively, cover possible causes and the methods of treatment.

Parkinson had the mark of a true scientist. In the preface, acknowledging the hypothetical nature of his statements about the illness, he wrote that 'mere conjecture takes the place of experiment'. Two major achievements of Parkinson's are evident from the essay. The first is that fact that, as already mentioned, although the disorder may have existed for many years it was not recognised as a separate disease until the publication of the essay, at the beginning of which he writes that the illness 'has not yet obtained a place in the classification of nosologists; some have regarded its characteristic symptoms as distinct and different diseases, and others have given its name to diseases differing essentially from it'. Second, Parkinson was an astute observer, and his descriptions of the age of onset, the slow mode of onset and the progressive and chronic nature of the disorder, as well as of the symptoms, are still valid today. This is remarkable because he had at his disposal none of the medical tools or tests that are now commonly used.

Parkinson mainly concentrated on describing tremor. The other main symptoms—bradykinesia, rigidity, balance and walking problems—were highlighted by Jean-Martin Charcot, the first professor of neurology at the Salpêtrière hospital in Paris. In the course of his famous Tuesday lectures, published in 1877, Charcot stated that the terms 'paralysis agitans', or 'shaking palsy', were inadequate, since the shaking or tremor was absent in some cases and there was no evidence of palsy or paralysis in any case. He proposed that, instead, since James Parkinson had provided the first detailed description of it as a separate illness, it should be known as the *maladie de Parkinson*, or Parkinson's disease.

Paralysis agitans was also considered in detail in William Gowers' *Manual of Diseases of the Nervous System*, published in 1886. Gowers, the prominent British neurologist working at the time at what is now the National Hospital for Neurology and Neurosurgery, included in his observations on the amplitude and frequency of tremor the fact that tremor could remain confined to one side of the body for many years but then spread to the other. Problems with balance and walking were also reviewed. However, Gowers placed more emphasis on rigidity, the monotonous speech and the expressionless face.

The epidemic of encephalitis lethargica in 1918, which lasted until 1926, gave rise to a large number of chronically disabled people with Parkinsonism. As described earlier, the illness started with flu-like symptoms, sleepiness, paralysis of the eye movements, rigidity, slowness of movement and behavioural change. About 40 per cent of sufferers died in the acute phase. Those who survived recovered to some extent, but after some years entered the chronic phase with all the predominant symptoms of Parkinsonism. These showed some similarities to, as well differences from, those of Parkinson's disease as described by Parkinson, Charcot and Gowers. This suffering on a vast scale served to demonstrate that Parkinsonian symptoms could have more than one cause, creating the concept of Parkinson*ism* and paving the way for the distinction between idiopathic Parkinson's disease and secondary Parkinsonism, and the subsequent refinement of diagnostic categories from the 1960s onwards.

Neither James Parkinson nor Charcot knew precisely which area of the brain was affected in Parkinson's disease and, as noted earlier, it was not until post-mortem examinations of the brain became possible that any progress was made. In 1893 in Paris, a patient with unilateral Parkinson's was found to have a small tumour pressing on the basal ganglia. So attention now focused on the basal ganglia as a possible site of damage in Parkinson's disease. A year later Édouard Brissaud, a French professor of neurology, suggested that damage to the substantia nigra in the brainstem, which has many close connections with the basal ganglia, might cause Parkinson's disease. The first major discovery confirming this was made by Tretiakoff as part of his doctoral thesis. On the basis of the post-mortem examination of nine cases of Parkinson's disease, Tretiakoff confirmed the loss of pigmented cells of the substantia nigra and the presence of the spherical bodies previously described by Frederick Lewy (Lewy bodies, p. 23) in those cells that remained.

In 1957, Montagu discovered the neurotransmitter dopamine in the brain. During 1957–9 the Swedish professor Arvid Carlsson demonstrated that dopamine was concentrated in the areas of the brain considered to be affected in Parkinson's disease. In experiments with rats, injections of the drug reserpine resulted in signs of Parkinsonism and the reduction of a number of neurotransmitters, including dopamine, in their brains. When the rats were injected with levodopa, the symptoms of Parkinsonism disappeared. In 1960, Ehringer and Hornykiewicz demonstrated the depletion of dopamine in the basal ganglia of the brains of people with Parkinson's. This was followed in 1961 by the administration of levodopa to patients by Birkmayer and Hornykiewicz, which started a new era in the medical treatment of the disorder. However, it was not until 1967 and the publication of George Cotzias' results of administering levodopa in larger doses that the therapeutic revolution started.

As described in Chapter 3, the first drawback of levodopa therapy was that many people developed nausea and vomiting, due to dopaminergic stimulation of the vomiting centres in the brain. The development and introduction of selective peripheral decarboxylase inhibitors such as carbidopa (Sinemet) and benserazide (Madopar) overcame this problem in most cases. The next therapeutic advance was the designing of synthetic directly acting dopamine agonists such as bromocriptine, pergolide and lisuride. This was followed by medication such as selegiline hydrochloride (Deprenyl), aiming to prolong the duration of dopamine action in the brain by inhibiting monoamine oxidase B, which causes the breakdown of dopamine.

The 1950s also saw another revolution: the development and use of neuroleptic medication for the treatment of the more severe mental disorders such as schizophrenia and manic-depressive psychosis. Although this class of medication effectively controlled the target mental illness, a frequent side-effect was the development of Parkinsonism, which could be reversed by withdrawing the medication. The report of such chemically induced and reversible Parkinsonism led to predictions that soon the cause of Parkinson's disease would be discovered.

In the late 1970s and 1980s, the 'MPTP story' unfolded (see p. 20), and from that 'natural experiment' a number of significant ideas have emerged:

- Using MPTP (1-methyl-4-phenyl-1,2,3,6-tetrahydropyridine) an 'animal model' of Parkinsonism has been developed: by inducing Parkinsonism in animals it is possible to conduct controlled experiments and trials of new medications before their use in clinical trials on patients.
- As described in Chapter 1, the MPTP story has opened up a whole new approach to the study of the possible causes of Parkinson's disease. It focused attention in impairment of mitochondrial mechanisms and the possible causal role of environmental or endogenous toxins.
- The protective effect of certain types of monoamine oxidase inhibitor medication against MPTP in laboratory animals led to the study of the possible neuroprotective effect of this class of medication in Parkinson's disease.

The MPTP story illustrates the fact that scientific advance does not necessarily occur at a steady pace, but may take the form of occasional hare-like leaps interspersed with periods of crawling.

THE WAY AHEAD

This short history of Parkinson's disease is convincing evidence that we have come a long way since 1817, when James Parkinson published his essay. In fact, Parkinson's disease is unique amongst neurological disorders, in that during the last 30 years research has revolutionised our understanding of the disorder and its treatment. The landmarks in this route of discovery were:

1960s   the discovery of the degeneration of dopamine-producing cells in the substantia nigra as the cause of the symptoms of Parkinson's disease
1970s   the discovery of dopamine replacement therapy with levodopa
1980s   the battle against the long-term complications of levodopa therapy

What will the 1990s be remembered for? We can spot important landmarks: brain implantation of foetal tissue, preventive therapy, important research into the causes of the disease, and the development of markers to detect the illness before the symptoms become manifest. What is particularly reassuring is that research into Parkinson's is at the top of the agenda in many fields of neuroscience. This is partly because progress in Parkinson's research also constitutes pioneering work in relation to our understanding of brain function. It is said that nothing succeeds like success! As a consequence of the relatively steady progress in unravelling the mysteries of the disorder that has occurred in the last 30 years, research into Parkinson's attracts a large number of first-rate scientists from a variety of disciplines. Research now and in the near future will take many different routes, and the journey along several of them is likely to prove fruitful.

The Search for the Cause

The foremost question in the mind of every person with Parkinson's disease is 'Will there be a cure in my lifetime?' To find a cure, we have to find the cause. In the search for the cause, the main question posed by scientists is 'What causes the degeneration process in Parkinson's disease?' Two sets of theories are currently dominant, and research effort centres on these. The first is the possibility that Parkinson's may be the result of a slow-acting viral infection; the second concerns the possible role of exposure to an environmental toxin.

If we knew what starts the degeneration process that results in dopamine deficiency in Parkinson's, it might be possible to halt it or even prevent it from occurring in the first place. Therefore, the research into the cause of the disease goes hand in hand with finding ways of detecting pre-symptomatic or early Parkinson's disease, and the development of neuroprotective therapy to halt its progression.

The elderly in the population exhibit in mild form some of the symptoms that are reminiscent of Parkinson's disease, such as slowness of movement, stooped posture and shorter strides, and a greater number of falls. Given that some of the pathological and chemical changes that occur in the brain in the process of ageing are similar to those found in Parkinson's disease, and since age is the most definite predisposing factor for the disorder, research to explore the hypothesis that Parkinson's is an accelerated ageing process may also be worthwhile.

The Search for Pre-symptomatic and Diagnostic Markers

From research findings, we know that symptoms of Parkinson's disease become evident only after striatal dopamine is depleted by about 80 per cent. This means that a number of years intervene between the start of the degenerative process and the first appearance of the symptoms. In light of this gradual process of dopamine depletion, scientists have been eager to develop tests that would allow them to identify the pre-symptomatic state. This has been coupled with efforts to develop tests that would allow reliable diagnosis of idiopathic Parkinson's disease, once the symptoms have become manifested.

The search for pre-symptomatic and diagnostic markers is important for several reasons:

- A diagnostic marker would permit a definite diagnosis of Parkinson's disease and the certainty of being able to differentiate it at an early stage from other, related, disorders.
- It would also serve as a measure of the underlying disease process— as a useful index of the severity of the illness and of the changes that occur as it progresses. In addition, it would provide a means of assessing the effectiveness of the various forms of treatment.
- With diagnostic markers, it might be possible to detect the disease before the symptoms become fully expressed, which in turn might make it possible to instigate preventive measures, such as neuroprotective therapy, that would halt the progression of the disease.

A number of tests have been explored as potential diagnostic markers, to do with reduced sense of smell, abnormalities in visual evoked potentials, and fluorodopa uptake patterns assessed with PET (see p. 49). However, none of these changes has proved to be specific to Parkinson's disease, and so none has proved particularly useful as a marker. But although no single useful diagnostic marker has yet emerged, a number of lines of enquiry hold particular promise. Research into mitochondrial abnormalities in Parkinson's disease is a most exciting area, and abnormalities in the metabolism of particular substances in the brain are also being pursued as potential biological markers. More sensitive PET scanning to detect subclinical levels of dopamine deficiency in the putamen, insufficient to produce overt symptoms, can also be useful in identifying the pre-symptomatic state. Other approaches to early diagnosis include the search for immunological markers of Lewy body degeneration in the cerebrospinal fluid, the assessment of extracerebral dopamine metabolism—changes induced by dopamine outside the cerebral cortices—as an index of what is happening in the brain, and the possible detection of Lewy bodies in extracerebral tissues.

The Search for Preventive Therapy

The focus of the search for preventive therapy is on two particular areas. First, the development and use of medication that will slow down, and others that may halt, the progression of the disease process altogether. The results of the DATATOP (see p. 77) and other studies have demonstrated that selegiline delays the need to start levodopa therapy. As selegiline produces a mild symptomatic benefit, it is unclear whether its effects are due to protective (slowing down progression of the illness) or symptomatic (simply improving symptoms) mechanisms. Research into the use of other monoamine oxidase B inhibitors to slow the progression of Parkinson's disease continues. The second focus of research in this area has been on the development of methods of protecting against the damage caused by free radicals (see p. 26) and other agents that increase 'oxidative stress', and that may be involved in the degeneration process. The use of growth factors that may promote sprouting in dopamine-producing neurones and anti-oxidant agents is also being explored.

The discovery of such neuroprotective therapy will, of course, have personal significance for those who have just developed the illness. Moreover, the search for preventive therapy is well justified in terms of health economics. It has been estimated that if a hypothetical drug slowed down the progression of Parkinson's disease by about 10 per cent, it would produce annual savings of £327 million for the US health care system. This figure is based on the prolongation of employment of people with Parkinson's disease and their continued payment of income tax, decreased disability payment, and the postponement of the need for hospitalisation and residential care.

The Search for Effective Treatments

The focus of the search for effective treatments is on finding medications that offer the benefits of levodopa but with longer-lasting effects and without levodopa's long-term complications. This could be achieved in several ways. First, by developing better means of delivering dopamine to the brain. Second, by using drugs that would prolong the effects of dopamine, such as monoamine oxidase inhibitors and catechol-O-methyltransferase. Third, by exploring neurotransmitter systems, other than the dopaminergic one, in treating the symptoms.

Many of the side-effects of levodopa arise from the fact that, in the course of its conversion to dopamine, levodopa indiscriminately stimulates all types of dopamine receptor. The future development of dopamine agonists that selectively stimulate subpopulations of dopamine receptors may reduce these side-effects. The development of new drug-delivery systems such as controlled-release pills, subcutaneous infusions and skin patches may also prove worthwhile, by maintaining steadier levels of dopamine. Some symptoms of Parkinson's disease which may be related to the impairment of other neurotransmitter systems in the brain, do not respond to dopaminergic medication, so classes of drugs other than dopaminergics may prove of value in treating them.

The further development of brain implantation techniques may improve the efficacy of this treatment. But many questions about the procedure remain to be addressed. With much more basic and applied research, brain implantation technology may advance to the point where it becomes possible to reverse the degeneration of neurones in the substantia nigra and the resulting dopamine deficiency by neural implants that take on the role of dopamine production. Further refinement of other surgical procedures such as pallidotomy, and pallidal, subthalamic nucleus and thalamic stimulation, will continue to provide better symptomatic relief in cases with severe rigidity or tremor.

The Search for Improved Service Provision

Medicine is a biological science, but healing is an art. The technological advances that have occurred in most fields of medicine during the last hundred years have somewhat distanced it from what should be its primary concern: ensuring people's health and well-being and preventing disease. In the course of present-day hi-tech medicine, technology sometimes takes precedence and the human approach is overshadowed or forgotten during medical consultations. Furthermore, as we noted in Chapter 4, the 'acute model' of illness—according to which the individual falls ill, seeks medical treatment and is then cured—prevails in much of medicine. This model is applicable to infectious diseases, but does not coincide with the reality of chronic illnesses such as Parkinson's, whose progressive nature must be a major concern in its medical management. Of prime consideration here must be a good 'quality of life', which depends not only on optimal symptomatic control, but also on the introduction of methods for promoting good coping, and emotional and practical adjustment to the illness.

A recent report by the Royal College of Physicians stated that in standard neurological practice, the psychosocial needs of patients with chronic neurological illness are rarely addressed. To overcome some of the shortcomings, the report recommended that 'districts should appoint and evaluate the effectiveness of "key-workers" assigned to individual patients'. Such key-workers, it was suggested, might be trained in nursing, social work or physiotherapy. As discussed in Chapter 9, we already have evidence that contact with key-workers such as a nurse practitioner is found to be very valuable by people with Parkinson's disease.

In the early 1990s the Patients' Charter was launched, the stated aim of which is to ensure a high-quality health service for everyone and to safeguard the rights of the individual patient. If the Patients' Charter is to be anything more than a public relations exercise, it is also necessary to introduce steps to address the needs of people with chronic illnesses such as Parkinson's. One way to do this would be through the nationwide development of key-worker services aimed at improving the quality of life of Parkinson's patients and their families. Unfortunately, with the restricted resources available, all services need to be justified in terms of cost. It is difficult to quantify improvements in 'quality of life' in financial terms. But although employing key-workers may in the short term be more costly, in the long term, if the need for hospitalisation or institutional care can be avoided or delayed, it is likely to lead to substantial savings for the NHS.

You could help

What we know about Parkinson's disease and its treatment is based on many years of research around the world on many thousands of people with the illness. The search for the cause, for pre-diagnostic and diagnostic markers, for effective treatments, for preventive therapy and for improved service provision will require many more years of dedicated and creative research by scientists and clinicians, as well as the willing participation of many thousands more patients in these studies. If you feel up to it, both patient and carer can contribute to this process of discovery in a number of ways:

- by giving up a few hours of your time every year to volunteer to participate in research studies
- by considering whether, after your death, you would be willing to donate your brain tissue to a brain bank—brain banks are at the forefront of the search for a cause of Parkinson's disease
- by spending time in fund-raising activities for the PDS and other associated charities—the money collected partly funds research studies.

In most research projects, including those involving the donation of tissue to a brain bank, the participation of the carer is equally appreciated, as it provides information on healthy individuals that can be compared with the information obtained from people with the disease. With such a comparison it is possible to assess the type and extent of change from normal.

What does all this mean for the person who has had Parkinson's disease for the last five, ten, twenty or thirty years, or for the person who has just been diagnosed as having it? Will a cure become available in time for them—a cure in the sense that a cough can be cured, with complete restoration to normal health? This is certainly a prospect for the future, if not on the immediate horizon. But effective treatments that may be as good as a cure *are* feasible, and within sight. More importantly, service provision can certainly be improved so as to ensure a high quality of life for everyone with Parkinson's disease and their carers and families.

We end on a note of optimism, by quoting the man whose powers of observation gave his name to the disease: 'There appears to be sufficient reason for hoping that some remedial process ere long be discovered.'

Appendix

AN A–Z OF USEFUL ORGANISATIONS

IN THE UK

Age Concern
Astral House
1268 London Road
London SW16 4ER
Tel: 0181 679 8000

Provides services for the elderly such as day centres, relatives' groups, shopping schemes and sitting services. They put out many useful publications relevant to the needs of the elderly, on topics such as making a will, heating requirements, sheltered accommodation and leisure activities.

Alzheimer's Disease Society
Gordon House
10 Greencoat Place
London SW1P 1PH
Tel: 0171 306 0606

Publishes many useful advice sheets about Alzheimer's disease. This charity has many local branches in the UK, some of which provide services to relieve the carer such as day care or sitters for the person with dementia.

Benefits Enquiry Line
Benefits Agency
Freephone 0800 882200

An executive agency of the Department of Social Security, it gives advice about available benefits and how to claim them.

British Association for Counselling
1 Regent Place
Rugby CV21 2PJ
Tel: 01788 578328

Supplies information about qualified and registered counsellors in particular areas of the country.

Carematch
286 Camden Road
London N7 0BJ
Tel: 0171 609 9966

A computerised service that finds residential care for people with disability or dementia.

Carers' National Association
20–25 Glasshouse Yard
London EC1A 4JS
Tel: 0171 490 8818
CarersLine 0171 490 8898

Provides information about caring for an ill person and advice on how best to cope with the task of caring. Others in a similar situation can be contacted through local groups. They operate a CarersLine, a telephone advice and information service. (See also p. 238.)

Citizens' Advice Bureau
115–123 Pentonville Road
London N1 9LZ
Tel: 0171 833 2181

Provides advice about any practical problem, whether legal, financial, employment- or housing-related, and about personal matters. Many local branches throughout the UK.

Counsel and Care for the Elderly
Twyman House
16 Bonny Street
London NW1 9LR
Tel: 0171 485 1566

Provides advice and information for older people and their families. This charity has a computerised database for nationwide information about nursing agencies and home care, and can provide advice on residential care and nursing homes. They administer a number of trust funds from which single payments can be made for home improvement or respite care.

Crossroads Care Attendant Scheme
10 Regent Place
Rugby CV21 2PN
Tel: 01788 573653
Fax: 01788 565498

Provides over 2 million hours of free respite care each year in the UK. Trained care attendants take over the caring role and provide time off for carers, to allow them to pursue social and leisure activities or to simply relax. This charity has regional offices throughout the UK.

Disability Scotland
Princes House
5 Shandwick Place
Edinburgh EH2 4RG
Tel: 0131 229 8632

Advises on public building design to ensure access to all, highlights problems with community care and campaigns for better service provision; deals with personal enquiries from disabled people and provides advice on equipment, employment, holidays, transport and clothing. Hosts the biennial Scottish Mobility Roadshow exhibiting the latest mobility aids and equipment.

Disability Services Division of the
Employment Service
Third Floor
Rockingham House
123 West Street
Sheffield S1 4ER
Tel: 0114 2595749
Fax: 0114 2596465

Helps people with a disability to find and keep jobs both by direct support and by working with employers to encourage a favourable attitude. Offers in-depth assessments, employment rehabilitation, subsidies for special equipment or adaptation of premises. Disability employment advisers work from Job Centres.

Disabled Drivers' Association
Ashwellthorpe
Norwich NR16 1EX
Tel: 01508 489449

Provides information and advice about all aspects of mobility including driving, benefits, and equipment for the disabled. It also gives advice on holidays, and some local groups have their own holiday facilities. Members are offered discounts on car ferries.

Disabled Living Foundation
380–384 Harrow Road
London W9 2HU
Tel: 0171 289 6111

Best source of up-to-date information on many aids and equipment, such as wheelchairs, walking-frames, and aids for bathing and eating. It also runs about 30 Disabled Living Centres around the UK, where a range of equipment is on display, with professional staff to demonstrate it and give advice.

Disablement Income Group
Unit 5, Archway Business Centre
19–23 Wedmore Street
London N19 4RZ
Tel: 0171 263 3981

Acts as a pressure group to secure and improve disability benefits. This organisation provides information and help in obtaining benefits and allowances for people with disability, as well as advice about financial problems.

Driver and Vehicle Licensing
Centre (DVLC)
Swansea SA6 7JL

See information on p. 120.

Elderly Accommodation Council
46A Chiswick High Road
London W4 1SZ
Tel: 0181 995 8320

Provides information and advice on suitable accommodation for the retired and the elderly. This charity has a nationwide register of residential care homes, sheltered housing, nursing homes and retirement housing for rent or sale, in both the public and the private sector.

Family Welfare Association
501–505 Kingsland Road
London E8 4AU
Tel: 0181 254 6251

Provides voluntary social work for families.

Grace Link
Upper Chambers
7 Derby Street
Leek ST13 6HN
Tel: 0345 023300

Helps with finding private residential care for those who are disabled or demented.

Healthline
College of Health
St Margaret's House
21 Old Fort Road
London E2 9PL
Freephone 0800 66 55 44

A health information service that provides information about NHS services in the London area and about 3,000 self-help groups, as well as taped information about 350 common diseases. Ring between 9 and 5, Monday to Friday, or write for information.

Holiday Care Service
2nd Floor
Imperial Building
Victoria Road
Horley RH6 7PZ
Tel: 01293 774535

Provides information and advice about holidays and travel facilities for people with special needs, and supplies volunteer escorts for those who may need extra care away from home.

MIND
(National Association for Mental
Health)
15–19 Broadway
London E15 4BD
Tel: 0181 519 2122

Campaigns for the rights of people with
mental illness. MIND publishes useful
books and advice leaflets about mental
disorders. The numerous local
associations engage in counselling, in
relatives' support groups, in meeting
employment and housing needs, and in
running workshops and day centres
(among other activities).

Motability
Gate House
West Gate
Harlow CM20 1HR
Tel: 01279 635666

This charity aims to help disabled people
use the higher-motability component of
the Disability Living Allowance to buy or
hire a car or wheelchair.

National Care Homes Association
5 Bloomsbury Place
London WC1A 2QA
Tel: 0171 436 1871

A federation of associations of private
residential homes that offers advice and
can provide information about private
residential care in your area.

Parkinson's Disease Society
215 Vauxhall Bridge Road
London SW1V 1EJ
Tel: 0171 931 8080

Provides information and advice for
people with Parkinson's disease and their
carers. A welfare and benefits officer
operates a helpline, and is available to
discuss practical and financial problems.
Over 200 local support groups exist. The
PDS produces many useful publications.
(See also p. 236.)

Relate
National Marriage Guidance
Herbert Gray College
Little Church Street
Rugby CV21 3AP
Tel: 01788 73241

Aims to enhance the quality of couple,
marital, parental and family relationships
generally and to prevent breakdown and
divorce. Marital, sexual and family
counselling is provided through 400
regional centres. Puts out publications on
family and marital relationships, divorce,
childhood and teenage years, emotional
well-being.

Royal Association for Disability
and Rehabilitation (RADAR)
12 City Forum
250 City Road
London EC1V 8AF
Tel: 0171 250 3222

Includes most of the major charities
concerned with disability; acts as a
pressure group promoting the rights and
meeting the needs of the disabled in
health, education, employment, housing,
mobility, benefits and holidays. Many
useful publications.

Samaritans
17 Uxbridge Road
Slough SL1 1SN
Tel: 01753 32713
(see local phone directory)

Volunteers are available by phone at any
hour of the day or night to help those
passing through personal crises and in
danger of taking their own lives.

Sexual and Personal Relationships
of the Disabled (SPOD)
286 Camden Road
London N7 1QH
Tel: 0171 607 8851

Provides information and telephone
counselling about personal and sexual
relationships for people with disability;
counsellors will reply to written
enquiries; referral to suitable local
counsellors can be arranged.

Tripscope
65 Esmond Road
London W4 1JE
Tel: 0181 994 9294

Provides advice on travel and transport
for people with disabilities.

Winged Fellowship Trust
Angel House
20–32 Pentonville Road
London N1 9XD
Tel: 0171 833 2594

Provides holidays and respite care for
handicapped people; escorts can also be
arranged.

Women's Royal Voluntary Service
Milton Hill House
Milton Hill
Abingdon
OX13 6AF
Tel: 01235 442900

A large voluntary organisation providing
local hospital, community and emergency
services. Best known for
meals-on-wheels; other services include
hospital visiting, 'books-on-wheels',
home support; they also run lunch clubs,
day centres, residential homes.

YAPP&Rs
(Young Alert Parkinson's Partners
and Relatives)
38 Wessex Drive, Harp Hill
Cheltenham GL52 5AU
Tel: 01242 236729

A special-interest group of the PDS, for
younger and more able people with the
disease; produce a magazine and have
regional meetings, a postal library service
and a computer link.

EUROPEAN PARKINSON'S DISEASE SOCIETIES

Austria
Austrian Parkinson's Patients' Association, Märzstraße 49 A–1150 Vienna. Tel:
(43) 1 9837383. Fax: (43) 1 9837393

Belgium
Belgische Parkinson Vereniging, J. Stobbaertslaan 43, B–1030 Brussels. Tel: (32)
2 2455945, (32) 10 430290. Fax: (32) 10 411972

Denmark
Dansk Parkinson Forening, Hornemansgade 36 St, 2100 Copenhagen 0. Tel: (45)
39 271555. Fax: (45) 31 182075

324 PARKINSON'S DISEASE

Estonia
Estonian Parkinson's Society, Sõle str 15–1, Tallinn EE0006. Tel: (3722) 49 15 03. Fax: (3722) 49 68 15

Finland
Findland Parkinson Forbound, Pitämäenk 4a, 20350 Turku. Tel: (358) 21 391233. Fax: (358) 21 391180

France
Association France Parkinson, 35 bis Rue la Fontaine, 75016 Paris. Tel: (33) 1 45202220. Fax: (33) 1 40501644

Association des Groupments de Parkinsoniens, 2 Rue des Gauvignets, 44600 St Nazaire. Tel: (33) 2 40709557

Germany
Deutsche Parkinson Vereinigung, Moselstrasse 31, 41464 Neuss. Tel: (49) 2131 41016/7. Fax: (49) 2131 45445

Iceland
Parkinsonsamtökin á Islandi, Laugaveg 26, PO Box 10182, 130 Ruik.

Italy
Associazione Italiana Parkinsoniani, via Zuretti 35, 20125 Milan. Tel: (39) 2 66713111. Fax: (39) 2 66713111

Azione Parkinson, Via Sesto Celere 6, 00152 Rome. Tel: (39) 6 58330678/5819183. Fax: (39) 6 5599200

Luxembourg
Association Luxembourgeoise de la Maladie de Parkinson, 12 Rue de la Resistance, L–2425 Howald. Tel: (352) 291998

The Netherlands
Parkinson Patienten Vereniging, Postbus 46, 3980 CA Bunnik. Tel: (31) 30 6561369. Fax: (31) 30 6571306.

Norway
Norges Parkinsonforbund, Schwigaardsgt. 34, Bygg F, Oppg. 1, 0191 Oslo. Tel: (47) 2 2175861. Fax: (47) 2 2175862

Portugal
Associação Portuguesa de Doentes de Parkinson, R. Duarte Galvão, 34–7° Dto, 1500 Lisbon.

Slovenia
Parkinson's Disease Society of Slovenia, University of Clinical Neurophysiology, 61105 Ljubljana.

Spain
Parkinson España, Calle de la Torre, 14 bajos, 08006 Barcelona. Tel: (34) 2 416 0320. Fax: (34) 3 416 1060

Sweden
Neurologiskt Handicappades Riksforbund, Box 3284, S–10365 Stockholm. Tel: (46) 8 6777010. Fax: (46) 8241315

The Swedish Parkinson's Disease Association, Box 121, S–428 22 Kallered. Tel: (46) 31 7953295

Switzerland
Schweizerische Parkinsonvereinigung, PO Box 123, CH–8132 Hinteregg. Tel: (41) 1 9840169. Fax: (41) 1 9840393

OTHER PARKINSON'S DISEASE SOCIETIES

Australia
Parkinson's Association of Western Australia Inc., 320 Rokeby Road, Subiaco, Western Australia 6008. Tel: (61) 9 381 8699

Parkinson's Disease Association (Victoria) Inc., 20 Kingston Road, Cheltenham, Victoria 3192. Tel: (61) 3 955 11122. Fax: (61) 3 955 11310

Parkinson's Syndrome Society of New South Wales Inc., Building 64, Concord Repatriation Hospital, Hospital Road, Concord, NSW 2139. Tel: (61) 2 736 7881

Brazil
Associação Brasil Parkinson, Rua Visconde de Indaiatuba 279, São Paulo–SP 05083.

Canada
The Parkinson Foundation of Canada (National), 710–390 Bay Street, Toronto, Ontario M5H 2Y2. Tel: (1) 416 366 0099. Fax: (1) 416 366 9190

Israel
Israel Parkinson Group, PO Box 635, Kiryat Bialik, 27100.

New Zealand
Parkinsonism Society (NZ) Inc., PO Box 11–900, Wellington.

Parkinson's Disease Society, c/o 148 England Street, Christchurch.

South Africa
Parkinson Association SA, Private Bag X36, Bryanston 2021. Tel/Fax: (27) 11 787 8792

USA
American Parkinson's Disease Association, 1250 Hylan Blvd., Suite 4b, Stuten Island, NY 10305. Freephone: 800 223 2732

National Parkinson Foundation, 1501 NW 9th Avenue, Miami, Florida 33136. Tel: (1) 305 547 6666. Freephone: 800 327 4545

Parkinson's Disease Foundation, William Black Medical Research Building, 640 West 168th Street, New York NY 10032–9982. Tel: (1) 212 923 4700. Freephone: 800 457 6676

Parkinson's Educational Program USA, 3900 Birch Street, No. 105, Newport Beach, California 92660. Tel: (1) 714 250 2975. Freephone: 800 344 7872

United Parkinson Foundation, 833 West Washington Boulevard, Chicago, Illinois 60607. Tel: (1) 312 733 1893.

FURTHER READING

Many of the books that appear in lists 1 and 2 below can be obtained from the Parkinson's Disease Society or YAPP&Rs.

1   FIRST-HAND ACCOUNTS OF LIVING WITH PARKINSON'S DISEASE

Atwood, G. W. (with L. Green Hunnewell), *Living Well with Parkinson's Disease*, John Wiley & Sons: New York, 1991.

Baynes, P., *Heading for Goal*, YAPP&Rs Publications: Scotland, 1989.

Dorros, D., and Dorros, S., *Path: The Route to Better Management of Parkinson's Disease: Coping Needs of the Parkinson Care Partner*, Sandoz, 1991.

Dorros, S., *Parkinson's Disease: A Patient's View*, Seven Locks Press: Santa Ana, CA, 1981.

Gordon, S., *Parkinson's: A Personal Story of Acceptance*, Branden Publishing: Brookline Village, MA, 1992.

Kennedy, R., and Lees, A. J., *Ray of Hope*, Pelham/Penguin Books: London, 1993.

McGoon, D. C., *The Parkinson's Handbook*, W. W. Norton: New York, 1990.

Monnot, M., *From Rage to Courage: The Road to Dignity Walk*, St Denis Press, 1988.

Pierce, J. R., *Living with Parkinson's Disease; or Don't Rush Me! I'm Coping as Fast as I Can*, Pectrum Communications, 1989.

Rose, H., *An Old-age Pensioner at Eighteen; or My Life with Parkinson's Disease*, PDS Publications: London, 1990.

Stern, J. P., *The Parkinson's Challenge: The Beginner's Guide to the Good Life in the Slow Lane*. Privately published, 1987.

Todes, C., *A Shadow over My Brain: My Struggle with Parkinson's Disease*, Windrush Press: Moreton-in-Marsh, 1990.

Vaughan, I., *Ivan: Living with Parkinson's Disease*, Macmillan: London, 1986.

Williams, J. (ed.), *Parkinson's Disease and Employment: The Experiences of Forty-three Patients*, PDS Publications: London, 1990.

Williams, J. (ed.), *Parkinson's Disease: Doctors as Patients: Eleven Autobiographical Accounts*, PDS Publications: London, 1992.

2   BOOKS BY PROFESSIONAL AUTHORS

Caird, F. I. (ed.), *Rehabilitation in Parkinson's Disease*, Chapman & Hall: London, 1991.
Duvoisin, R. C., *Parkinson's Disease: A Guide for Patient and Family*, 3rd ed, Raven Press, 1991.
Godwin-Austen, R. B., *The Parkinson's Disease Handbook*, Sheldon Press: London, 1984.
Hutton, J. T., and Dippel, R. L. (eds), *Caring for the Parkinson's Patient*, Prometheus Books: New York, 1989.
Kohner, N., *Caring at Home: A Handbook for People Looking after Someone at Home—Someone Young or Old, Handicapped or Disabled, Ill or Frail*, Health Education Authority and King's Fund: London.
Lieberman, A. N., and William, F., *Parkinson's Disease: The Complete Guide for Patients and Carers*, Simon & Schuster: New York, 1993.
Morris, M., Iansek, R., and Kirkwood, B., *Moving Ahead with Parkinson's Disease*, Kingston Centre, Warrigal Road, Cheltenham 3192, Australia, 1995.
Nutt, J. G., Hammerstad, J. P., and Gancher, S. T., *Parkinson's Disease: One Hundred Maxims*, Edward Arnold: London, 1992.
Oxtoby, M., and Williams, A., *Parkinson's at Your Fingertips*, Class Publishing: London, 1995.
Pearce, J. M. S., *Parkinson's Disease and Its Management*, Oxford University Press: Oxford, 1992.
Sacks, O. W., *Awakenings*, Pan Books: London, 1990.
Sagar, H., *Parkinson's Disease*, Optima, Positive Health Guides: London, 1991.
Stern, G., and Lees, A., *Parkinson's Disease: The Facts*, Oxford University Press: Oxford, 1982.
Wilcock, G., *Living with Alzheimer's Disease and Similar Conditions: The Complete Self-help Guide for Family and Professional Carers*, Penguin Books: London, 1990.
Woods, R. T., *Alzheimer's Disease: Coping with a Living Death*, Souvenir Press: London, 1989.

3   BOOKS AND BOOKLETS PRODUCED BY ORGANISATIONS

At Home in a Home   By Pat Young for Age Concern, 60 Pitcairn Road, Mitcham, Surrey CF4 3LL.

Caring at Home   4th ed, 1989. By Nancy Kohner for the King's Fund Informal Caring Support Unit, National Extension College, 18 Brooklands Avenue, Cambridge CB2 2HN.

Charities Digest   Family Welfare Association (address on p. 321): information about sources of charitable funding.

Coping with Dementia: A Handbook for Carers   Scottish Health Education Group, Woodburn House, Canaan Lane, Edinburgh EH10 4SG.

Coping with Disablement   Consumers Association, 14 Buckingham Street, London WC2N 6DS.

Directory of Grant-making Trusts   Charities Aid Foundation, Kings Hill Avenue, West Malling, Kent: information about sources of charitable funding.

Disability Rights Handbook   Disability Alliance Educational and Research Association, 25 Denmark Street, London WC2 8NJ.

Door to Door: A Guide to Transport for Disabled People   Department of Transport.

The Drug Treatment of Parkinson's Disease: Notes for Patients and Their Relatives   PDS Publications (address on p. 322).

Guide to Grants for Individuals in Need   Directory of Social Change, 24 Stephenson Way, London NW1: information about sources of charitable funding.

Help for Handicapped People   DSS; available from local DSS offices.

Holidays for Disabled People   Annual publication, Royal Association for Disability and Rehabilitation (address on p. 322).

How to Get Equipment for Disability   3rd edn, 1993. By M. Mandelstam for the Disabled Living Foundation (address on p. 321).

The Law and Vulnerable Elderly People   Age Concern, 60 Pitcairn Road, Mitcham, Surrey CR4 3LL.

Living with Parkinson's Disease   PDS Publications.

Parkinson's Disease: A Booklet for Patients and Their Families   By R. B. Godwin-Austen for PDS Publications.

Parkinson's Disease: Day to Day   PDS Publications.

Parkinson's Disease Patients and Their Social Needs   By M. Oxtoby, PDS Publications.

Someone-to-Talk-to Directory   Mental Health Foundation: names and addresses of about 10,000 self-help organisations in the UK.

Taking a Break: A Guide for People Caring at Home   King's Fund Informal Caring Programme, 1990. Free to carers from the Community Care Unit, King's Fund Centre, 126 Albert Street, London NW1.

Your Rights 1998–99: A Guide to Money Benefits for Older

330   PARKINSON'S DISEASE

People   By Sally West for Age Concern (annual publication), ACE
books (address on p. 319).

Your Taxes and Savings 1998–99: A Guide for Older People   By
Jennie Hawthorne and Sally West for Age Concern (annual publication), ACE books.

4   PARKINSON'S DISEASE ON THE INTERNET

It is now possible to obtain on the Internet information about the
symptoms and their medical and surgical treatment, and about living
and coping with Parkinson's disease. Addresses of some Internet sites
are given below. Many more websites are becoming available—you
may be able to access them from existing ones, or by searching the
Internet.

*The Parkinson's Web: Information on the Symptoms, Medical and
    Other Treatments*
http://neuro-chief-e.mgh.harvard.edu/Pweb
*The Parkinson's Web: List of Books on Parkinson's Disease and other
    Chronic Illness*
*http://neuro-chief-e.mgh.harvard.edu/parkinsonsweb/Main/Biblio/
    bibmenu.html*
The Parkinson's Web: The Caregiver's Handbook
http://neuro-chief-e.mgh.harvard.edu/parkinsonweb/Main/coping/
    caregiver.html
*Massachusetts General Hospital, Harvard Medical School: Information
    about Surgery*
http://neurosurgery.mgh.harvard.edu/fnctnlp.html
The Mulligan Foundation
http://www.frostbyte.com/mulligan/parkinsons

Index